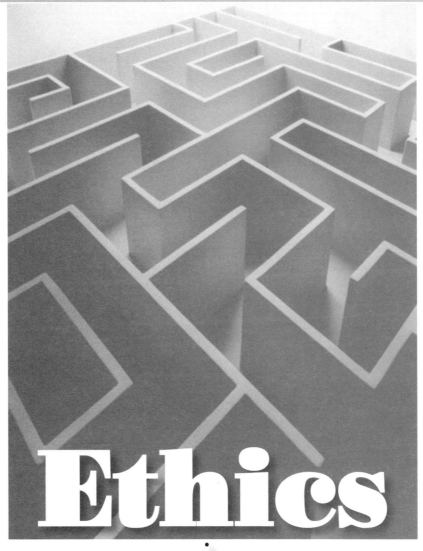

Ethics

in

Physical Therapy

Part 1: Overview of Ethical Issues in Physical Therapy

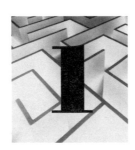

AMERICAN PHYSICAL THERAPY ASSOCIATION

This monograph is a compilation of official documents of the American Physical Therapy Association and articles originally published in *Physical Therapy* and *PT—Magazine of Physical Therapy*.

ISBN 1-931369-21-6

For more information about this and other APTA publications, contact the American Physical Therapy Association, 1111 North Fairfax Street, Alexandra, VA 22314-1488, 800/999-2782, ext 3395, www.apta.org. [Order No. P-152-05]

Table of Contents

Acknowledgements

We gratefully acknowledge Ruth Purtilo, PhD, PT, FAPTA, who contributed energy and vision to *PT Magazine* through the creation and fostering of "Habits of Thought" and related articles.

We also are grateful to the following individuals who reviewed the contents of the original edition as well as suggested additions for this second edition to ensure that the articles continue to be relevant, useful, and accurate. Thanks to Kathy Lewis, PT, MAPT, JD, Laura Lee (Dolly) Swisher, PT, PhD, Cathy Thut, PT, MBA, and Mary Ann Wharton, PT, MS.

And to the many authors of the articles that are included in this volume—thank you.

Introduction

> [The ancient philosophers] argued that a disciplined mind 'habitually' focuses attention on critical
> dimensions of a situation—the virtues inherent in it; the ethical principles involved; and the components
> governed by historical insight, law, economics, or other social norms. These habits of thought enable a per-
> son to move beyond merely private opinion to place a situation in its proper historical, ethical, and social
> context. ("To Move Beyond Private Opinion," *PT Magazine*, January 1993)

With this rich and thoughtful introduction, Ruth B Purtilo, PhD, PT, FAPTA, renowned ethicist and Fellow of the American Physical Therapy Association (APTA), launched a 3-year series in *PT—Magazine of Physical Therapy* that would challenge us to think beyond ourselves, beyond even our patients. "Habits of Thought," as the column was so aptly named, ranged from issues as broad as the theory of beneficence to those as focused as a patient's right to die. From "Habits of Thought" stemmed reader dialogue and debate, providing perspectives on ethical issues that might otherwise never have been shared in a public forum. "Judgment Call," for instance, a thought-provoking feature that appeared on numerous occasions in *PT Magazine*, took an ethical dilemma, usually suggested by a "Habits of Thought" reader—disclosure of information to patients, as an example—and presented commentary and feedback from other inspired readers on the topic.

Of course, *PT Magazine* was not the first APTA publication to approach the broad subject of ethics in physical therapy. For years, APTA's official peer-reviewed journal, *Physical Therapy*, has published manuscripts that have dealt with any number of ethical considerations. From these two publications came a wealth of discussion that in 1999 resulted in the first edition of the two-volume *Ethics in Physical Therapy*. This second edition is now part of APTA's *Risk Management in Physical Therapy* series, which also includes the two-volume *Law & Liability* and *Risk Management in Physical Therapy: A Quick Reference*. The second edition includes relevant articles published between 1999 and 2005, as well as the still-applicable articles from the first edition.

This volume, Part 1 of the two-part *Ethics in Physical Therapy,* is an entrée into the very wide world of health care ethics, and physical therapy ethics in particular. Here, in their entirety, are original articles dealing with ethical principles and considerations that have appeared in *PT Magazine* since its inception in 1993, along with several articles from *Physical Therapy* published during the last 20 years. Readers will notice that issues come up again and again, and that time not only adds insight but often brings us back to where we started. Additionally, we have provided relevant APTA core documents, such as the Association's *Code of Ethics* and *Guide for Professional Conduct*, and policy and position statements, such as the Association's Principles and Objectives for the United States Health Care System and the Delivery of Physical Therapy Services. These materials are essential to any student of physical therapy ethics.

Part 1: Overview of Ethical Issues in Physical Therapy begins with articles and other materials related to professional is-sues and considerations in ethics. From there, we move on to articles and positions on managed care and economics. *Part 2: The Patient and Society*, covers patient rights, welfare, and related issues; health issues, such as infectious/commu-nicable diseases and substance abuse; social issues, such as gender issues and cultural diversity; and the issues of sexual misconduct and nondiscrimination.

Purtilo reminded us regularly in "Habits of Thought," through her own reflections and those of her invited columnists, that physical therapists who are members of APTA are bound by a *Code of Ethics*. APTA spells out the following as among the key commitments of the Association:

> Promote physical therapy care and services through the establishment, maintenance, and promotion of ethical principles and quality standards for practice, education, and research ... [and] Facilitate a common understanding and appreciation for the diversity of the profession, the membership, and the communities we serve. (Mission Statement Fulfillment [HOD P06-93-06-07])

his collection of thought, opinion, study, and commentary is intended to generate ongoing dialogue on the subject of physical therapy and health care ethics—not only how ethical issues relate to the professional and the patient, but how they fit in the context of the world we live in, practice in, and experience today.

* Readers should note that APTA documents are current as of September 2005. They may change based on annual APTA House of Delegates actions. Visit APTA's Web site, www.apta.org, for the most current versions of all documents.

Professional Issues
and Considerations

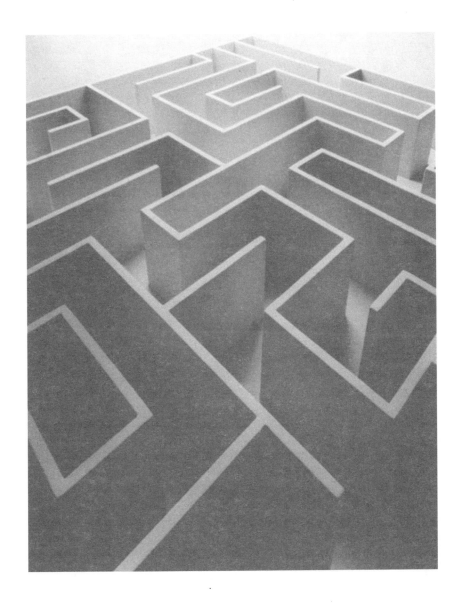

American Physical Therapy Association
Guide for Professional Conduct

✚APTA
American Physical Therapy Association
The Science of Healing. The Art of Caring.

Purpose

This *Guide for Professional Conduct* (Guide) is intended to serve physical therapists in interpreting the *Code of Ethics* (Code) of the American Physical Therapy Association (Association), in matters of professional conduct. The Guide provides guidelines by which physical therapists may determine the propriety of their conduct. It is also intended to guide the professional development of physical therapist students. The Code and the Guide apply to all physical therapists. These guidelines are subject to change as the dynamics of the profession change and as new patterns of health care delivery are developed and accepted by the professional community and the public. This Guide is subject to monitoring and timely revision by the Ethics and Judicial Committee of the Association.

Code of Ethics

Preamble

This *Code of Ethics* of the American Physical Therapy Association sets forth principles for the ethical practice of physical therapy. All physical therapists are responsible for maintaining and promoting ethical practice. To this end, the physical therapist shall act in the best interest of the patient/client. This Code of Ethics shall be binding on all physical therapists.

Principle 1

A physical therapist shall respect the rights and dignity of all individuals and shall provide compassionate care.

Principle 2

A physical therapist shall act in a trustworthy manner toward patients/clients and in all other aspects of physical therapy practice.

Principle 3

A physical therapist shall comply with laws and regulations governing physical therapy and shall strive to effect changes that benefit patients/clients.

Principle 4

A physical therapist shall exercise sound professional judgment.

Principle 5

A physical therapist shall achieve and maintain professional competence.

Principle 6

A physical therapist shall maintain and promote high standards for physical therapy practice, education, and research.

Principle 7

A physical therapist shall seek only such remuneration as is deserved and reasonable for physical therapy services.

Principle 8

A physical therapist shall provide and make available accurate and relevant information to patients/clients about their care and to the public about physical therapy services.

Principle 9

A physical therapist shall protect the public and the profession from unethical, incompetent, and illegal acts.

Principle 10

A physical therapist shall endeavor to address the health needs of society.

Principle 11

A physical therapist shall respect the rights, knowledge, and skills of colleagues and other health care professionals.

Adopted by the House of Delegates
June 1981
Last amended June 2000

Interpreting Ethical Principles

The interpretations expressed in this Guide reflect the opinions, decisions, and advice of the Ethics and Judicial Committee. These interpretations are intended to assist a physical therapist in applying general ethical principles to specific situations. They should not be considered inclusive of all situations that could evolve.

PRINCIPLE 1

A physical therapist shall respect the rights and dignity of all individuals and shall provide compassionate care.

1.1 Attitudes of a Physical Therapist

A. A physical therapist shall recognize, respect, and respond to individual and cultural differences with compassion and sensitivity.

B. A physical therapist shall be guided at all times by concern for the physical, psychological, and socioeconomic welfare of patients/clients.

C. A physical therapist shall not harass, abuse, or discriminate against others.

PRINCIPLE 2

A physical therapist shall act in a trustworthy manner toward patients/clients, and in all other aspects of physical therapy practice.

2.1 Patient/Physical Therapist Relationship

A. A physical therapist shall place the patient's/client's interest(s) above those of the physical therapist. Working in the patient/client's best interest requires knowledge of the patient's/client's needs from the patient's/client's perspective. Patients/clients often come to the physical therapist in a vulnerable state and normally will rely on the physical therapist's advice, which they perceive to be based on superior knowledge, skill, and experience. The trustworthy physical therapist acts to ameliorate the patient's/client's vulnerability, not to exploit it.

B. A physical therapist shall not exploit any aspect of the physical therapist/patient relationship.

C. A physical therapist shall not engage in any sexual relationship or activity, whether consensual or noncensensual, with any patient while a physical therapist/patient relationship exists. Termination of the physical therapist/patient relationship does not eliminate the possibility that a sexual or intimate relationship may exploit the vulnerability of the former patient/client.

D. A physical therapist shall encourage an open and collaborative dialogue with the patient/client.

E. In the event the physical therapist or patient terminates the physical therapist/patient relationship while the patient continues to need physical therapy services, the physical therapist should take steps to transfer the care of the patient to another provider.

2.2 Truthfulness

A physical therapist has an obligation to provide accurate and truthful information. A physical therapist shall not make statements that he/she knows or should know are false, deceptive, fraudulent, or misleading. See Section 8.2.C and D.

2.3 Confidential Information

A. Information relating to the physical therapist/patient relationship is confidential and may not be communicated to a third party not involved in that patient's care without the prior consent of the patient, subject to applicable law.

B. Information derived from peer review shall be held confidential by the reviewer unless the physical therapist who was reviewed consents to the release of the information.

C. A physical therapist may disclose information to appropriate authorities when it is necessary to protect the welfare of an individual or the community or when required by law. Such disclosure shall be in accordance with applicable law.

2.4 Patient Autonomy and Consent

A. A physical therapist shall respect the patient's/client's right to make decisions regarding the recommended plan of care, including consent, modification, or refusal.

B. A physical therapist shall communicate to the patient/client the findings of his/her examination, evaluation, diagnosis, and prognosis.

C. A physical therapist shall collaborate with the patient/client to establish the goals of treatment and the plan of care.

D. A physical therapist shall use sound professional judgment in informing the patient/client of any substantial risks of the recommended examination and intervention.

E. A physical therapist shall not restrict patients' freedom to select their provider of physical therapy.

PRINCIPLE 3

A physical therapist shall comply with laws and regulations governing physical therapy and shall strive to effect changes that benefit patients/clients.

3.1 Professional Practice

A physical therapist shall comply with laws governing the qualifications, functions, and duties of a physical therapist.

3.2 Just Laws and Regulations

A physical therapist shall advocate the adoption of laws, regulations, and policies by providers, employers, third-party payers, legislatures, and regulatory agencies to provide and improve access to necessary health care services for all individuals.

3.3 Unjust Laws and Regulations

A physical therapist shall endeavor to change unjust laws, regulations, and policies that govern the practice of physical therapy. See Section 10.2.

PRINCIPLE 4

A physical therapist shall exercise sound professional judgment.

4.1 Professional Responsibility

A. A physical therapist shall make professional judgments that are in the patient's/client's best interests.

B. Regardless of practice setting, a physical therapist has primary responsibility for the physical therapy care of a patient and shall make independent judgments regarding that care consistent with accepted professional standards. See Sections 2.4 and 6.1.

C. A physical therapist shall not provide physical therapy services to a patient/

client while his/her ability to do so safely is impaired.

D. A physical therapist shall exercise sound professional judgment based upon his/her knowledge, skill, education, training, and experience.

E. Upon accepting a patient/client for physical therapy services, a physical therapist shall be responsible for: the examination, evaluation, and diagnosis of that individual; the prognosis and intervention; re-examination and modification of the plan of care; and the maintenance of adequate records, including progress reports. A physical therapist shall establish the plan of care and shall provide and/or supervise and direct the appropriate interventions. See Section 2.4.

F. If the diagnostic process reveals findings that are outside the scope of the physical therapist's knowledge, experience, or expertise, the physical therapist shall so inform the patient/client and refer to an appropriate practitioner..

G. When the patient has been referred from another practitioner, the physical therapist shall communicate pertinent findings and/or information to the referring practitioner.

H. A physical therapist shall determine when a patient/client will no longer benefit from physical therapy services. See Section 7.1.D.

4.2 Direction and Supervision

A. The supervising physical therapist has primary responsibility for the physical therapy care rendered to a patient/client.

B. A physical therapist shall not delegate to a less qualified person any activity that requires the professional skill, knowledge, and judgment of the physical therapist.

4.3 Practice Arrangements

A. Participation in a business, partnership, corporation, or other entity does not exempt physical therapists, whether employers, partners, or stockholders, either individually or collectively, from the obligation to promote, maintain, and comply with the ethical principles of the Association.

B. A physical therapist shall advise his/her employer(s) of any employer practice that causes a physical therapist to be in conflict with the ethical principles of the Association. A physical therapist shall seek to eliminate aspects of his/her employment that are in conflict with the ethical principles of the Association.

4.4 Gifts and Other Consideration(s)

A. A physical therapist shall not invite, accept, or offer gifts, monetary incentives, or other considerations that affect or give an appearance of affecting his/her professional judgment.

B. A physical therapist shall not offer or accept kickbacks in exchange for patient referrals. See Sections 7.1.F and G and 9.1.D.

PRINCIPLE 5

A physical therapist shall achieve and maintain professional competence.

5.1 Scope of Competence

A physical therapist shall practice within the scope of his/her competence and commensurate with his/her level of education, training, and experience.

5.2 Self-Assessment

A physical therapist has a lifelong professional responsibility for maintaining competence through on-going self-assessment, education, and enhancement of knowledge and skills.

5.3 Professional Development

A physical therapist shall participate in educational activities that enhance his/her basic knowledge and skills. See Section 6.1.

PRINCIPLE 6

A physical therapist shall maintain and promote high standards for physical therapy practice, education and research.

6.1 Professional Standards

A physical therapist's practice shall be consistent with accepted professional standards. A physical therapist shall continuously engage in assessment activities to determine compliance with these standards.

6.2 Practice

A. A physical therapist shall achieve and maintain professional competence. See Section 5.

B. A physical therapist shall demonstrate his/her commitment to quality improvement by engaging in peer and utilization review and other self-assessment activities.

6.3 Professional Education

A. A physical therapist shall support high-quality education in academic and clinical settings.

B. A physical therapist participating in the educational process is responsible to the students, the academic institutions, and the clinical settings for promoting ethical conduct. A physical therapist shall model ethical behavior and provide the student with information about the *Code of Ethics*, opportunities to discuss ethical conflicts, and procedures for reporting unresolved ethical conflicts. See Section 9.

6.4 Continuing Education

A. A physical therapist providing continuing education must be competent in the content area.

B. When a physical therapist provides continuing education, he/she shall ensure that course content, objectives, faculty credentials, and responsibilities of the instructional staff are accurately stated in the promotional and instructional course materials.

C. A physical therapist shall evaluate the efficacy and effectiveness of information and techniques presented in continuing education programs before integrating them into his/her practice.

6.5 Research

A. A physical therapist participating in research shall abide by ethical standards governing protection of human subjects and dissemination of results.

B. A physical therapist shall support research activities that contribute knowledge for improved patient care.

C. A physical therapist shall report to appropriate authorities any acts in the conduct or presentation of research that appear unethical or illegal. See Section 9.

PRINCIPLE 7

A physical therapist shall seek only such remuneration as is deserved and reasonable for physical therapy services.

7.1 Business and Employment Practices

A. A physical therapist's business/employment practices shall be consistent with the ethical principles of the Association.

B. A physical therapist shall never place her/his own financial interest above the welfare of individuals under his/her care.

C. A physical therapist shall recognize that third-party payer contracts may limit, in one form or another, the provision of physical therapy services. Third-party limitations do not absolve the physical therapist from making sound professional judgments that are in the patient's best interest. A physical therapist shall avoid underutilization of physical therapy services.

D. When a physical therapist's judgment is that a patient will receive negligible benefit from physical therapy services, the physical therapist shall not provide or continue to provide such services if the primary reason for doing so is to further the financial self-interest of the physical therapist or his/her employer. A physical therapist shall avoid overutilization of physical therapy services. See Section 4.1.H.

E. Fees for physical therapy services should be reasonable for the service performed, considering the setting in which it is provided, practice costs in the geographic area, judgment of other organizations, and other relevant factors.

F. A physical therapist shall not directly or indirectly request, receive, or participate in the dividing, transferring, assigning, or rebating of an unearned fee. See Sections 4.4.A and B.

G. A physical therapist shall not profit by means of a credit or other valuable consideration, such as an unearned commission, discount, or gratuity, in connection with the furnishing of physical therapy services. See Sections 4.4.A and B.

H. Unless laws impose restrictions to the contrary, physical therapists who provide physical therapy services within a business entity may pool fees and monies received. Physical therapists may divide or apportion these fees and monies in accordance with the business agreement.

I. A physical therapist may enter into agreements with organizations to provide physical therapy services if such agreements do not violate the ethical principles of the Association or applicable laws.

7.2 Endorsement of Products or Services

A. A physical therapist shall not exert influence on individuals under his/her care or their families to use products or services based on the direct or indirect financial interest of the physical therapist in such products or services. Realizing that these individuals will normally rely on the physical therapist's advice, their best interest must always be maintained, as must their right of free choice relating to the use of any product or service. Although it cannot be considered unethical for physical therapists to own or have a financial interest in the production, sale, or distribution of products or services, they must act in accordance with law and make full disclosure of their interest whenever individuals under their care use such products or services.

B. A physical therapist may receive remuneration for endorsement or advertisement of products or services to the public, physical therapists, or other health professionals provided he/she discloses any financial interest in the production, sale, or distribution of said products or services.

C. When endorsing or advertising products or services, a physical therapist shall use sound professional judgment and shall not give the appearance of Association endorsement unless the Association has formally endorsed the products or services.

7.3 Disclosure

A physical therapist shall disclose to the patient if the referring practitioner derives compensation from the provision of physical therapy.

PRINCIPLE 8

A physical therapist shall provide and make available accurate and relevant information to patients/clients about their care and to the public about physical therapy services.

8.1 Accurate and Relevant Information to the Patient

A. A physical therapist shall provide the patient/client accurate and relevant information about his/her condition and plan of care. See Section 2.4.

B. Upon the request of the patient, the physical therapist shall provide, or make available, the medical record to the patient or a patient-designated third party.

C. A physical therapist shall inform patients of any known financial limitations that may affect their care.

D. A physical therapist shall inform the patient when, in his/her judgment, the patient will receive negligible benefit from further care. See Section 7.1.C.

8.2 Accurate and Relevant Information to the Public

A. A physical therapist shall inform the public about the societal benefits of the profession and who is qualified to provide physical therapy services.

B. Information given to the public shall emphasize that individual problems cannot be treated without individualized examination and plans/programs of care.

C. A physical therapist may advertise his/her services to the public. See Section 2.2.

D. A physical therapist shall not use, or participate in the use of, any form of communication containing a false, plagiarized, fraudulent, deceptive, unfair, or sensational statement or claim. See Section 2.2.

E. A physical therapist who places a paid advertisement shall identify it as such unless it is apparent from the context that it is a paid advertisement.

PRINCIPLE 9

A physical therapist shall protect the public and the profession from unethical, incompetent, and illegal acts.

9.1 Consumer Protection

A. A physical therapist shall provide care that is within the scope of practice as defined by the state practice act.

B. A physical therapist shall not engage in any conduct that is unethical, incompetent, or illegal.

C. A physical therapist shall report any conduct that appears to be unethical, incompetent, or illegal.

D. A physical therapist may not participate in any arrangements in which patients are exploited due to the referring sources' enhancing their personal incomes as a result of referring for, prescribing, or recommending physical therapy. See Sections 2.1.B, 4, and 7.

PRINCIPLE 10

A physical therapist shall endeavor to address the health needs of society.

10.1 Pro Bono Service

A physical therapist shall render pro bono publico (reduced or no fee) services to patients lacking the ability to pay for services, as each physical therapist's practice permits.

10.2 Individual and Community Health

A. A physical therapist shall be aware of the patient's health-related needs and act in a manner that facilitates meeting those needs.

B. A physical therapist shall endeavor to support activities that benefit the health status of the community. See Section 3.

PRINCIPLE 11

A physical therapist shall respect the rights, knowledge, and skills of colleagues and other health care professionals.

11.1 Consultation

A physical therapist shall seek consultation whenever the welfare of the patient will be safeguarded or advanced by consulting those who have special skills, knowledge, and experience.

11.2 Patient/Provider Relationships

A physical therapist shall not undermine the relationship(s) between his/her patient and other health care professionals.

11.3 Disparagement

Physical therapists shall not disparage colleagues and other health care professionals. See Section 9 and Section 2.4.A.

Issued by the Ethics and Judicial Committee
American Physical Therapy Association
October 1981, Last amended 2004   P-6

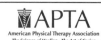

American Physical Therapy Association

Guide for Conduct of the Physical Therapist Assistant

APTA
American Physical Therapy Association
The Science of Healing. The Art of Caring.

Purpose

This *Guide for Conduct of the Physical Therapist Assistant* (Guide) is intended to serve physical therapist assistants in interpreting the *Standards of Ethical Conduct for the Physical Therapist Assistant* (Standards) of the American Physical Therapy Association (APTA). The Guide provides guidelines by which physical therapist assistants may determine the propriety of their conduct. It is also intended to guide the development of physical therapist assistant students. The Standards and Guide apply to all physical therapist assistants. These guidelines are subject to change as the dynamics of the profession change and as new patterns of health care delivery are developed and accepted by the professional community and the public. This Guide is subject to monitoring and timely revision by the Ethics and Judicial Committee of the Association.

Interpreting Standards

The interpretations expressed in this Guide reflect the opinions, decisions, and advice of the Ethics and Judicial Committee. These interpretations are intended to guide a physical therapist assistant in applying general ethical principles to specific situations. They

should not be considered inclusive of all situations that a physical therapist assistant may encounter.

STANDARD 1

A physical therapist assistant shall respect the rights and dignity of all individuals and shall provide compassionate care.

1.1 Attitude of a Physical Therapist Assistant

A. A physical therapist assistant shall recognize, respect, and respond to individual and cultural differences with compassion and sensitivity.

B. A physical therapist assistant shall be guided at all times by concern for the physical and psychological welfare of patients/clients.

C. A physical therapist assistant shall not harass, abuse, or discriminate against others.

STANDARD 2

A physical therapist assistant shall act in a trustworthy manner towards patients/clients.

2.1 Trustworthiness

A. The physical therapist assistant shall place the patient's/client's interest(s) above those of the physical therapist assistant. Working in the patient's/client's best interest requires sensitivity to the patient's/client's vulnerability and an effective working relationship between the physical therapist and the physical therapist assistant.

B. A physical therapist assistant shall not exploit any aspect of the physical therapist assistant–patient/client relationship.

C. A physical therapist assistant shall clearly identify him/herself as a physical therapist assistant to patients/clients.

D. A physical therapist assistant shall conduct him/herself in a manner that supports the physical therapist–patient/client relationship.

E. A physical therapist assistant shall not engage in any sexual relationship or activity, whether consensual or nonconsensual, with any patient entrusted to his/her care. Termination of patient/client care does not eliminate the possibility that a sexual or intimate relationship may exploit the vulnerability of the former patient/client.

F. A physical therapist assistant shall not invite, accept, or offer gifts, monetary incentives or other considerations that affect or give an appearance of affecting his/her provision of physical therapy interventions. See Section 6.3.

2.2 Exploitation of Patients

A physical therapist assistant shall not participate in any arrangements in which patients/clients are exploited. Such arrangements include situations where referring sources enhance their personal income by referring to or recommend-ding physical therapy services.

2.3 Truthfulness

A. A physical therapist assistant shall not make statements that he/she knows or should know are false, deceptive, fraudulent, or misleading.

B. Although it cannot be considered unethical for a physical therapist assistant to own or have a finan-cial interest in the production, sale, or distribution of products/services, he/she must act in accordance with law and make full disclosure of his/her interest to patients/clients.

2.4 Confidential Information

A. Information relating to the patient/client is confidential and shall not be communicated to a third party not involved in that patient's care without the prior

---

Standards of Ethical Conduct for the Physical Therapist Assistant

Adopted by the House of Delegates June 1981, Last amended June 2000

Preamble

This document of the American Physical Therapy Association sets forth standards for the ethical conduct of the physical therapist assistant. All physical therapist assistants are responsible for maintaining high standards of conduct while assisting physical therapists. The physical therapist assistant shall act in the best interest of the patient/client. These standards of conduct shall be binding on all physical therapist assistants.

consent of the patient, subject to applicable law.

B. A physical therapist assistant shall refer all requests for release of confidential information to the supervising physical therapist.

STANDARD 3

A physical therapist assistant shall provide selected physical therapy interventions only under the supervision and direction of a physical therapist.

3.1 Supervisory Relationship

A. A physical therapist assistant shall provide interventions only under the supervision and direction of a physical therapist.

B. A physical therapist assistant shall provide only those interventions that have been selected by the physical therapist.

C. A physical therapist assistant shall not provide any interventions that are outside his/her education, training, experience, or skill, and shall notify the responsible physical therapist of his/her inability to carry out the intervention. See Sections 5.1 and 6.1(B).

D. A physical therapist assistant may modify specific interventions within the plan of care established by the physical therapist in response to changes in the patient's/client's status.

E. A physical therapist assistant shall not perform examinations and evaluations, determine diagnoses and prognoses, or establish or change a plan of care.

F. Consistent with the physical therapist assistant's education, training, knowledge, and experience, he/she may respond to the patient's/client's inquiries regarding interventions that are within the established plan of care.

G. A physical therapist assistant shall have regular and ongoing communication with the physical therapist regarding the patient's/client's status.

STANDARD 4

A physical therapist assistant shall comply with laws and regulations governing physical therapy.

4.1 Supervision

A physical therapist assistant shall know and comply with applicable law. Regardless of the content of any law, a physical therapist assistant shall provide services only under the supervision and direction of a physical therapist.

4.2 Representation

A physical therapist assistant shall not hold him/herself out as a physical therapist.

STANDARD 5

A physical therapist assistant shall achieve and maintain competence in the provision of selected physical therapy interventions.

5.1 Competence

A physical therapist assistant shall provide interventions consistent with his/her level of education, training, experience, and skill. See Sections 3.1(C) and 6.1(B).

5.2 Self-assessment

A physical therapist assistant shall engage in self-assessment in order to maintain competence.

5.3 Development

A physical therapist assistant shall participate in educational activities that enhance his/her knowledge and skills.

STANDARD 6

A physical therapist assistant shall make judgments that are commensurate with his/her educational and legal qualifications as a physical therapist assistant.

6.1 Patient Safety

A. A physical therapist assistant shall discontinue immediately any intervention(s) that, in his/her judgment, may be harmful to the patient/client and shall discuss his/her concerns with the physical therapist.

B. A physical therapist assistant shall not provide any intervention(s) that are outside his/her education, training, experience, or skill, and shall notify the responsible physical therapist of his/her inability to carry out the intervention. See Section 3.1(C) and 5.1.

C. A physical therapist assistant shall not perform interventions while his/her ability to do so safely is impaired.

6.2 Judgments About Patient Status

If in the judgment of the physical therapist assistant there is a change in the patient/client status, he/she shall report this to the responsible physical therapist. See Section 3.1.

6.3 Gifts and Other Considerations

A physical therapist assistant shall not invite, accept, or offer gifts, monetary incentives or other considerations that affect or give an appearance of affecting his/her provision of physical therapy interventions. See Section 2.1(F).

STANDARD 7

A physical therapist assistant shall protect the public and the profession from unethical, incompetent, and illegal acts.

7.1 Consumer Protection

A physical therapist assistant shall report any conduct that appears to be unethical or illegal.

7.2 Organizational Employment

A. A physical therapist assistant shall inform his/her employer(s) and/or appropriate physical therapist of any employer practice that causes him or her to be in conflict with the *Standards of Ethical Conduct for the Physical Therapist Assistant*.

B. A physical therapist assistant shall not engage in any activity that puts him or her in conflict with the *Standards of Ethical Conduct for the Physical Therapist Assistant*, regardless of directives from a physical therapist or employer.

Issued by the Ethics and Judicial Committee
American Physical Therapy Association
October 1981, Last amended 2004   P-135

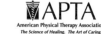

American Physical Therapy Association
Criteria for Standards of Practice For Physical Therapy

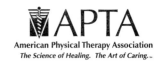

The *Standards of Practice for Physical Therapy* are promulgated by APTA's House of Delegates; Criteria for the Standards are promulgated by APTA's Board of Directors. Criteria are italicized beneath the Standards to which they apply.

Preamble

The physical therapy profession's commitment to society is to promote optimal health and function in individuals by pursuing excellence in practice. The American Physical Therapy Association attests to this commitment by adopting and promoting the following Standards of Practice for Physical Therapy. These Standards are the profession's statement of conditions and performances that are essential for provision of high quality professional service to society, and provide a foundation for assessment of physical therapist practice.

I. Ethical/Legal Considerations

A. Ethical Considerations

The physical therapist practices according to the *Code of Ethics* of the American Physical Therapy Association.

The physical therapist assistant complies with the *Standards of Ethical Conduct for the Physical Therapist Assistant* of the American Physical Therapy Association.

B. Legal Considerations

The physical therapist complies with all the legal requirements of jurisdictions regulating the practice of physical therapy.

The physical therapist assistant complies with all the legal requirements of jurisdictions regulating the work of the assistant.

II. Administration of the Physical Therapy Service

A. Statement of Mission, Purposes, and Goals

The physical therapy service has a statement of mission, purposes, and goals that reflects the needs and interests of the patients/clients served, the physical therapy personnel affiliated with the service, and the community.

The statement of mission, purposes, and goals:

- *Defines the scope and limitations of the physical therapy service.*
- *Identifies the goals and objectives of the service.*
- *Is reviewed annually.*

B. Organizational Plan

The physical therapy service has a written organizational plan.

The organizational plan:

- *Describes relationships among components within the physical therapy service and, where the service is part of a larger organization, between the service and the other components of that organization.*
- *Ensures that the service is directed by a physical therapist.*
- *Defines supervisory structures within the service.*
- *Reflects current personnel functions.*

C. Policies and Procedures

The physical therapy service has written policies and procedures that reflect the operation, mission, purposes, and goals of the service, and are consistent with the Association's standards, policies, positions, guidelines, and *Code of Ethics*.

The written policies and procedures:

- *Are reviewed regularly and revised as necessary.*
- *Meet the requirements of federal and state law and external agencies.*
- *Apply to, but are not limited to:*
  - *Care of patients/clients, including guidelines*
  - *Clinical education*
  - *Clinical research*
  - *Collaboration*

- *Competency assessment*
- *Criteria for access to care*
- *Criteria for initiation and continuation of care*
- *Criteria for referral to other appropriate health care providers*
- *Criteria for termination of care*
- *Documentation*
- *Environmental safety*
- *Equipment maintenance*
- *Fiscal management*
- *Improvement of quality of care and performance of services*
- *Infection control*
- *Job/position descriptions*
- *Medical emergencies*
- *Personnel-related policies*
- *Rights of patients/clients*
- *Staff orientation*

D. Administration

A physical therapist is responsible for the direction of the physical therapy service.

The physical therapist responsible for the direction of the physical therapy service:

- *Ensures compliance with local, state, and federal requirements.*
- *Ensures compliance with current APTA documents, including Standards of Practice for Physical Therapy and the Criteria, Guide to Physical Therapist Practice, Code of Ethics, Guide for Professional Conduct, Standards of Ethical Conduct for the Physical Therapist Assistant, and Guide for Conduct of the Affiliate Member.*
- *Ensures that services are consistent with the mission, purposes, and goals of the physical therapy service.*
- *Ensures that services are provided in accordance with established policies and procedures.*
- *Ensures that the process for assignment and reassignment of physical therapist staff supports individual physical therapist*

responsibility to their patients and meets the needs of the patients/clients.

- Reviews and updates policies and procedures.
- Provides for training of physical therapy support personnel that ensures continued competence for their job description.
- Provides for continuous in-service training on safety issues and for periodic safety inspection of equipment by qualified individuals.

E. Fiscal Management

The director of the physical therapy service, in consultation with physical therapy staff and appropriate administrative personnel, participates in planning for, and allocation of, resources. Fiscal planning and management of the service is based on sound accounting principles.

The fiscal management plan:

- Includes a budget that provides for optimal use of resources.
- Ensures accurate recording and reporting of financial information.
- Ensures compliance with legal requirements.
- Allows for cost-effective utilization of resources.
- Uses a fee schedule that is consistent with the cost of physical therapy services and that is within customary norms of fairness and reasonableness.
- Considers option of providing pro bono services.

F. Improvement of Quality of Care and Performance

The physical therapy service has a written plan for continuous improvement of quality of care and performance of services.

The improvement plan:

- Provides evidence of ongoing review and evaluation of the physical therapy service.
- Provides a mechanism for documenting improvement in quality of care and performance.
- Is consistent with requirements of external agencies, as applicable.

G. Staffing

The physical therapy personnel affiliated with the physical therapy service have demonstrated competence and

are sufficient to achieve the mission, purposes, and goals of the service.

The physical therapy service:

- Meets all legal requirements regarding licensure and certification of appropriate personnel.
- Ensures that the level of expertise within the service is appropriate to the needs of the patients/clients served.
- Provides appropriate professional and support personnel to meet the needs of the patient/client population.

H. Staff Development

The physical therapy service has a written plan that provides for appropriate and ongoing staff development.

The staff development plan:

- Includes self-assessment, individual goal setting, and organizational needs in directing continuing education and learning activities.
- Includes strategies for lifelong learning and professional and career development.
- Includes mechanisms to foster mentorship activities.

I. Physical Setting

The physical setting is designed to provide a safe and accessible environment that facilitates fulfillment of the mission, purposes, and goals of the physical therapy service. The equipment is safe and sufficient to achieve the purposes and goals of physical therapy.

The physical setting:

- Meets all applicable legal requirements for health and safety.
- Meets space needs appropriate for the number and type of patients/clients served.

The equipment:

- Meets all applicable legal requirements for health and safety.
- Is inspected routinely.

J. Collaboration

The physical therapy service collaborates with all disciplines as appropriate.

The collaboration when appropriate:

- Uses a team approach to the care of patients/clients.
- Provides instruction of patients/clients and families.

- Ensures professional development and continuing education.

III. Patient/Client Management

A. Patient/Client Collaboration

Within the patient/client management process, the physical therapist and the patient/client establish and maintain an ongoing collaborative process of decision making that exists throughout the provision of services.

B. Initial Examination/Evaluation/ Diagnosis/Prognosis

The physical therapist performs an initial examination and evaluation to establish a diagnosis and prognosis prior to intervention.

The physical therapist examination:

- Is documented, dated, and appropriately authenticated by the physical therapist who performed it.
- Identifies the physical therapy needs of the patient/client.
- Incorporates appropriate tests and measures to facilitate outcome measurement.
- Produces data that are sufficient to allow evaluation, diagnosis, prognosis, and the establishment of a plan of care.
- May result in recommendations for additional services to meet the needs of the patient/client.

C. Plan of Care

The physical therapist establishes a plan of care and manages the needs of the patient/client based on the examination, evaluation, diagnosis, prognosis, goals, and outcomes of the planned interventions for identified impairments, functional limitations, and disabilities.

The physical therapist involves the patient/client and appropriate others in the planning, implementation, and assessment of the plan of care.

The physical therapist, in consultation with appropriate disciplines, plans for discharge of the patient/client taking into consideration achievement of anticipated goals and expected outcomes, and provides for appropriate follow-up or referral.

The plan of care:

- *Is based on the examination, evaluation, diagnosis, and prognosis.*
- *Identifies goals and outcomes.*
- *Describes the proposed intervention, including frequency and duration.*
- *Includes documentation that is dated and appropriately authenticated by the physical therapist who established the plan of care.*

D. Intervention

The physical therapist provides, or directs and supervises, the physical therapy intervention consistent with the results of the examination, evaluation, diagnosis, prognosis, and plan of care.

The intervention:

- *Is based on the examination, evaluation, diagnosis, prognosis, and plan of care.*
- *Is provided under the ongoing direction and supervision of the physical therapist.*
- *Is provided in such a way that directed and supervised responsibilities are commensurate with the qualifications and the legal limitations of the physical therapist assistant.*
- *Is altered in accordance with changes in response or status.*
- *Is provided at a level that is consistent with current physical therapy practice.*
- *Is interdisciplinary when necessary to meet the needs of the patient/client.*
- *Documentation of the intervention is consistent with the Guidelines: Physical Therapy Documentation of Patient/Client Management (BOD G03-05-16-41).*
- *Is dated and appropriately authenticated by the physical therapist or, when permissible by law, by the physical therapist assistant.*

E. Reexamination

The physical therapist reexamines the patient/client as necessary during an episode of care to evaluate progress or change in patient/client status and modifies the plan of care accordingly or discontinues physical therapy services.

The physical therapist reexamination:

- *Is documented, dated, and appropriately authenticated by the physical therapist who performs it.*
- *Includes modifications to the plan of care.*

Glossary Standards and Criteria

Client. Individuals who engage the services of a physical therapist and who can benefit from the physical therapist's consultation, interventions, professional advice, health promotion, fitness, wellness, or prevention services. Clients also are businesses, school systems, and others to whom physical therapists provide services.

Diagnosis. Diagnosis is both a process and a label. The diagnostic process includes integrating and evaluating the data that are obtained during the examination to describe the patient/client condition in terms that will guide the prognosis, the plan of care, and intervention strategies. Physical therapists use diagnostic labels that identify the impact of a condition on function at the level of the system (especially the movement system) and at the level of the whole person.

Evaluation. A dynamic process in which the physical therapist makes clinical judgments based on data gathered during the examination.

Examination. A comprehensive screening and specific testing process leading to diagnostic classification or, as appropriate, to a referral to another practitioner. The examination has three components: the patient/client history, the systems review, and tests and measures.

Intervention. The purposeful interaction of the physical therapist with the patient/client and, when appropriate, with other individuals involved in patient/client care, using various physical therapy procedures and techniques to produce changes in the condition.

Patient. Individuals who are the recipients of physical therapy examination, evaluation, diagnosis, prognosis, and intervention and who have a disease, disorder, condition, impairment, functional limitation, or disability.

Physical therapist patient/client management model. The model on which physical therapists base management of the patient or client throughout the episode of care, including the following elements: examination, evaluation and reexamination, diagnosis, prognosis, and intervention leading to the outcome.

Plan of care. Statements that specify the goals and the outcomes, predicted level of optimal improvement, specific interventions to be used, and proposed duration and frequency of the interventions that are required to reach the goals and outcomes. The plan of care includes the anticipated discharge plans.

Prognosis. The determination of the predicted optimal level of improvement in function and the amount of time needed to reach that level.

Treatment. The sum of all interventions provided by the physical therapist to a patient/client during an episode of care.

F. Discharge/Discontinuation of Intervention

The physical therapist discharges the patient/client from physical therapy services when the anticipated goals or expected outcomes for the patient/client have been achieved.

The physical therapist discontinues intervention when the patient/client is unable to continue to progress toward goals or when the physical therapist determines that the patient/client will no longer benefit from physical therapy.

Discharge documentation:

- *Includes the status of the patient/client at discharge and the goals and outcomes attained.*
- *Is dated and appropriately authenticated by the physical therapist who performed the discharge.*
- *Includes, when a patient/client is discharged prior to attainment of goals and outcomes, the status of the patient/client and the rationale for discontinuation.*

G. Communication/Coordination/Documentation

The physical therapist communicates, coordinates, and documents all aspects of patient/client management including the results of the initial examination and evaluation, diagnosis, prognosis, plan of care, interventions, response to interventions, changes in patient/client status relative to the interventions, reexamination, and discharge/discontinuation of intervention and other patient/client management activities.

Physical therapist documentation:

- *Is dated and appropriately authenticated by the physical therapist who performed the examination and established the plan of care.*

- *Is dated and appropriately authenticated by the physical therapist who performed the intervention or, when allowable by law or regulations, by the physical therapist assistant who performed specific components of the intervention as selected by the supervising physical therapist.*

- *Is dated and appropriately authenticated by the physical therapist who performed the reexamination, and includes modifications to the plan of care.*

- *Is dated and appropriately authenticated by the physical therapist who performed the discharge, and includes the status of the patient/client and the goals and outcomes achieved.*

- *Includes, when a patient/client is discharged prior to achievement of goals and outcomes, the status of the patient/client and the rationale for discontinuation.*

IV. Education

The physical therapist is responsible for individual professional development. The physical therapist assistant is responsible for individual career development.

The physical therapist, and the physical therapist assistant under the direction and supervision of the physical therapist, participate in the education of students.

The physical therapist educates and provides consultation to consumers and the general public regarding the purposes and benefits of physical therapy.

The physical therapist educates and provides consultation to consumers and the general public regarding the roles of the physical therapist and the physical therapist assistant.

The physical therapist:

- *Educates and provides consultation to consumers and the general public regarding the roles of the physical therapist, the physical therapist assistant, and other support personnel.*

V. Research

The physical therapist applies research findings to practice and encourages, participates in, and promotes activities that establish the outcomes of patient/client management provided by the physical therapist.

The physical therapist:

- *Ensures that their knowledge of research literature related to practice is current.*

- *Ensures that the rights of research subjects are protected, and the integrity of research is maintained.*

- *Participates in the research process as appropriate to individual education, experience, and expertise.*

- *Educates physical therapists, physical therapist assistants, students, other health professionals, and the general public about the outcomes of physical therapist practice.*

VI. Community Responsibility

The physical therapist demonstrates community responsibility by participating in community and community agency activities, educating the public, formulating public policy, or providing pro bono physical therapy services.

The physical therapist:

- *Participates in community and community agency activities.*

- *Educates the public, including prevention, education, and health promotion.*

- *Helps formulate public policy.*

- *Provides pro bono physical therapy services.*

HOD S06-03-09-10
Adopted by the House of Delegates
June 1980
Last amended June 2003

BOD S03-05-14-38
Adopted by the Board of Directors
November 1985
Last amended March 2005   A-3

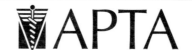

American Physical Therapy Association
The Science of Healing. The Art of Caring.℠

American Physical Therapy Association
Disciplinary Action Procedural Document

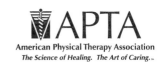

The American Physical Therapy Association (Association or APTA) has developed this *Procedural Document on Disciplinary Action* (Procedural Document) to establish a procedure to process claims that a member of the Association has violated the Association's *Code of Ethics* (Code) or *Standards of Ethical Conduct for the Physical Therapist Assistant* (Standards). This document encompasses the procedures for the investigation and hearing of such claims.

This Procedural Document will be followed when a Chapter President receives a signed complaint relating to a member of the Association or otherwise becomes aware of information indicating that a member has violated the Code or the Standards. The Appendix accompanying this Procedural Document is for informational purposes only. All time periods provided herein may be varied only for good cause consistent with fundamental fairness. Wherever this Procedural Document calls for the use of certified mail, return request requested, an alternative form of delivery may be used, provided that it generates a reliable record of receipt.

The Ethics and Judicial Committee of the American Physical Therapy Association will review all complaints, records, and recommendations that are initiated or generated at the Chapter level. At any time in the course of the disciplinary process the Ethics and Judicial Committee has the authority to assume responsibility for management of the ethics proceeding at the Chapter level. Questions of a legal nature may be addressed to Association headquarters.

1. INITIATION OF ETHICS PROCEEDING BY CHAPTER PRESIDENT

A Chapter President may initiate an ethics proceeding in response to a complaint or on the basis of reliable information that comes to his/her attention.

(a) Complaint.

(1) **Receipt, Forwarding, and Acknowledgment.** Any person who believes that a member has acted in violation of the ethical principles or standards of the Association may submit a signed written complaint to the President of the Chapter to which the member is assigned. The President may proceed on the basis of a signed complaint submitted by fax but not on the basis of any email complaint. A complaint must describe the conduct which the complainant believes constitutes an ethical violation, but it need not cite specific sections of the Code or Standards. Within three (3) days of receiving a complaint, the President must forward a copy to the attention of the Ethics and Judicial Committee at Association headquarters (1111 North Fairfax Street, Alexandria, Virginia 22314). Upon receipt of a copy of a complaint Association staff shall assign a case number for use on all documents in the proceeding and shall communicate the case number to the Chapter President. The Chapter President and the Chapter Ethics

Committee (CEC) must use this case number on all documents he/she or it issues in the proceeding. <u>The Chapter President and the CEC may not send any communication to a complainant or respondent unless its heading includes the case number assigned by Association staff.</u> Within fifteen (15) days after being advised of the case number, the President shall give the complainant written acknowledgment of receipt of the complaint, which acknowledgment shall enclose a copy of the Procedural Document and shall advise the complainant of the respondent's right to learn the identity of the complainant.

(2) **Alternative Recipient of Complaint.** In any case in which a person has a complaint against a Chapter President, a member closely associated with the Chapter President, or an elected or appointed leader of the Association or of any APTA chapter or section (or in which other circumstances exist which give rise to the appearance that the Chapter President may be unable to act impartially), the complainant may address the complaint to the Association's Ethics and Judicial Committee at the Association's headquarters. The Ethics and Judicial Committee, upon determining that the complaint falls within the foregoing sentence, shall proceed to carry out the functions hereunder of the Chapter President with respect to the complaint; in such a case, references in this Procedural Document to the Chapter President shall be deemed to be to the alternative recipient. The Ethics and Judicial Committee, upon determining that this paragraph does not apply, shall so notify the complainant (who will remain free to resubmit the complaint to the Chapter President).

(b) Chapter President's Action With Respect to a Complaint.
The responsibility of a Chapter President with respect to a signed complaint is to decide whether to initiate an APTA ethics proceeding by issuing a notice of charges as described in subsection (b)(2)(C) below. The Chapter President shall consult with the Chair of the CEC in making this decision.

The Chapter President first shall determine whether the complaint, fairly construed, alleges conduct by the Association member that would constitute a violation of the Code or Standards. For purposes of this analysis, the President shall assume that the specific facts alleged are true, unless the allegations are plainly baseless.

(1) **No Allegation of Ethical Violation.** If the Chapter President determines that the conduct alleged would not constitute an ethical violation, he/she must send the Ethics and Judicial Committee written notice advising that he/she is declining to issue a notice of charges and briefly explaining his/her rationale. The Chapter President shall send the complainant a copy of such notice of decision not to initiate an ethics proceeding.

(2) Allegation of Ethical Violation. If the Chapter President determines that the conduct alleged would constitute an ethical violation, he/she still must exercise his/her best judgment as to whether to refer the case to the CEC, taking into account the nature of the alleged conduct, the ability of the CEC to investigate and dispose of the case, and other relevant considerations. The Chapter President may decline to issue a notice of charges on the ground that:

(i) the conduct alleged would constitute only a de minimis violation such that referral to the CEC is not warranted;

(ii) the conduct alleged occurred sufficiently long ago that referral to the CEC is not warranted; or

(iii) the ultimate determination whether the conduct violates the Code or Standards would require resolution of legal or other issues beyond the competence of the CEC and/or the Ethics and Judicial Committee, so that referral to the CEC is not warranted.

(A) Decision Not To Initiate an Ethics Proceeding. If the Chapter President makes a discretionary decision not to refer the case to the CEC, he/she must send the Ethics and Judicial Committee written notice advising that he/she is declining to issue a notice of charges and briefly explaining his/her rationale. At the same time the Chapter President shall forward the complete file to the Ethics and Judicial Committee and shall send the complainant a copy of the notice of decision not to initiate an ethics proceeding.

(B) Decision To Initiate an Ethics Proceeding; Notice of Charges. If the Chapter President decides that a complaint's allegations of ethical misconduct should be referred to the CEC, he/she shall initiate an ethics proceeding against the member (respondent) by promptly sending a notice of charges to the respondent, with copies to the Ethics and Judicial Committee and the CEC. The President shall send the notice of charges to the respondent by certified mail, return receipt requested.

(C) Notice of Charges. The notice of charges shall describe, in the President's words, the conduct which, if proven, would constitute a violation of the Code or the Standards. The notice must describe the conduct in sufficient detail to apprise a reader unfamiliar with the case of the behavior in which the respondent allegedly engaged. The notice must specify which provision(s) of the Code or Standards the conduct, if proven, would violate. The notice of charges may, but need not, specify any provision(s) of the *Guide for Professional Conduct* or the *Guide for Conduct of the Physical Therapist Assistant* which the Chapter President believes is (are) relevant to the conduct in question. The notice of charges shall state that the President is referring the matter to the CEC and shall identify the Chair of the CEC (name, address, and telephone number). The President shall enclose a copy of the complaint with the notice of charges, and the notice shall advise the respondent that a copy of the complaint is enclosed. The President shall refer the matter to the CEC by sending it a copy of the notice of charges and shall transmit also the underlying complaint, and any other documents in the President's possession that may be relevant to the proceeding.

(c) Chapter President's Action Based on Reliable Information. A Chapter President may initiate an ethics proceeding without having received a signed complaint, but only in accordance with this subsection. A proceeding may be initiated on the basis of written information that is available publicly, obtained from authorized agencies, or otherwise properly obtained, if such information reliably indicates that an APTA member engaged in conduct that would constitute a violation of the Code or Standards. Such information may include evidence that a member has violated a state or federal criminal law or that a state licensing agency has taken disciplinary action against a member.

(1) Receipt of Information. Association staff may forward to a Chapter President reliable information that might be the basis for initiation of an ethics proceeding, in which case staff shall assign a case number to the matter and communicate that case number to the Chapter President.

A Chapter President who obtains reliable information that might be the basis for initiation of an ethics proceeding from a source other than Association staff must forward a copy of the information to the attention of the Ethics and Judicial Committee at Association headquarters within three (3) days of obtaining such information. Upon receipt of a copy of such information, Association staff shall assign a case number for use on all documents in the proceeding and shall communicate the case number to the Chapter President. The Chapter President and the Chapter Ethics Committee (CEC) must use the case number assigned by Association staff on all documents he/she or it issues in the proceeding. The Chapter President and the CEC may not send any communication to a respondent unless its heading includes the case number assigned by Association staff.

(2) Chapter President's Action With Respect to Information Reliably Indicating Misconduct. The responsibility of a Chapter President with respect to information reliably indicating that a member engaged in unethical conduct is to decide whether to initiate an APTA ethics proceeding issuing a notice of charges as described in subsection (b)(2)(C) above. The Chapter President shall consult with the Chair of the CEC in making this decision.

The Chapter President first shall determine the facts that have been reliably established (e.g., by a guilty plea or verdict in a criminal proceeding or by a consent decree in a licensing action). Because such determinations often involve the interpretation of legal documents, the Chapter President shall consult with the Association's legal counsel as needed.

(A) No Evidence of Ethical Violation. If the Chapter President determines that the conduct reliably established would not constitute an ethical violation, he/she must send the Ethics and Judicial Committee written notice advising that he/she is declining to issue a notice of charges and briefly explaining his/her rationale.

(B) Evidence of Ethical Violation. If the Chapter President determines that the conduct reliably established would constitute an ethical violation, he/she still must exercise his/her best judgment as to whether to refer the case to the CEC, taking into account the nature of the conduct, the ability of the CEC to investigate and dispose of the case, and other relevant considerations. The Chapter President may decline to issue a notice of charges on any ground specified in subsection (b)(2) above.

(i) Decision Not To Initiate an Ethics Proceeding. If the Chapter President makes a discretionary decision not to refer the case to the CEC, he/she must send the Ethics and Judicial Committee written notice advising that he/she is declining to issue a notice of charges and briefly explaining his/her rationale.

(ii) Decision To Initiate an Ethics Proceeding. If the Chapter President decides that an ethics proceeding based on reliable information should be initiated, he/she shall do so by promptly sending a notice of charges to the member (respondent), with copies to the Ethics and Judicial Committee and the CEC, in accordance with the requirements specified in subsection (b)(2)(C) above.

2. PROCEEDING BASED ON SERIOUS CRIME OR REVOCATION OF LICENSURE

(a) Serious Crimes. A member's commission of a crime which (i) is substantially related to the qualifications, functions, or duties of a physical therapist or physical therapist assistant and (ii) is classified as a felony by the applicable federal, state, or territorial law, or is punishable by imprisonment for six months or more, is *prima facie* evidence of a violation of the ethical principles or standards of the Association. The procedures in this section shall apply in the event of (a) a member's plea of guilty or nolo contendere to a charge involving such a serious crime, (b) a finding of guilt after trial, or (c) a member's conviction of such a serious crime. Such a plea (if not withdrawn), finding, or conviction shall be deemed presumptive evidence that the member has engaged in the activity alleged in the criminal charges to which he/she pleaded, as to which there was a finding of guilt, or of which he/she was convicted.

(b) Revocation of Licensure. A member's engaging in conduct which would justify revocation of professional licensure is *prima facie* evidence of a violation of the ethical principles or standards of the Association. The procedures in this section shall apply in the event a state licensing agency revokes a member's license (except that this section shall not apply if the revocation of the member's license is stayed). Such a revocation shall be deemed presumptive evidence that the member has engaged in the conduct on which the revocation was based.

(c) Chapter Responsibilities. If a Chapter President, through receipt of a complaint or other information, becomes aware that a member has committed a crime such as described in subsection (a) above or has had his/her license revoked as described in subsection (b) above, the President shall forward the complaint or other information to the Ethics and Judicial Committee. If a CEC becomes aware of information such as described in subsection (a) or (b) above concerning a member who is a respondent in a case before the CEC that relates to the crime or the basis for the license revocation, the CEC shall forward the information and the complete record of the case to the Ethics and Judicial Committee.

(d) Ethics and Judicial Committee Responsibilities. If the Ethics and Judicial Committee receives reliable information (from a Chapter President or any other source) indicating that a member has made a plea (which has not been withdrawn), been found guilty, or been the subject of a criminal conviction such as described in subsection (a) or that a state licensing agency has taken action such as described in subsection (b), the Ethics and Judicial Committee shall initiate (or continue) an ethics proceeding by preparing and sending a notice of suspension and charges to the member (respondent) by certified mail, return receipt requested.

(e) Notice of Suspension and Charges. The notice of suspension and charges shall advise the respondent that the Ethics and Judicial Committee has preliminarily suspended the respondent (ie, temporarily removed his/her membership rights as provided in Section 4), effective thirty (30) days after the date of the notice and continuing until the Ethics and Judicial Committee's decision. The notice shall describe the conduct which appears to constitute a violation of the Code or the Standards and shall specify which provision(s) of the Code or Standards the conduct appears to have violated. The notice of charges may, but need not, specify any provision(s) of the *Guide for Professional Conduct* or the *Guide for Conduct of the Affiliate Member* which the Ethics and Judicial Committee believes is (are) relevant to the conduct in question. The notice shall advise the respondent that the Ethics and Judicial Committee will consider the case at its next regularly scheduled meeting (or, if the date of the notice is sixty (60) or fewer days before the start of that meeting, at the first regularly scheduled meeting thereafter) and that the respondent may choose to appear before the Committee or to submit a written statement.

(f) Ethics and Judicial Committee Action. At the appropriate regularly scheduled meeting the Ethics and Judicial Committee shall consider the respondent's case. If the respondent exercises his/her right to appear before the Ethics and Judicial Committee, the hearing shall be limited to one hour.

(1) **Serious Crime.** With respect to any proceeding based on commission of a serious crime, the Ethics and Judicial Committee shall consider: whether the respondent in fact entered a plea of guilty or nolo contendere, was found guilty, or was convicted; the nature of the conduct underlying the criminal charges to which the respondent pleaded or was found guilty or convicted; the relationship of the criminal conduct to the qualifications, functions, or duties of a physical therapist or physical therapist assistant; the relationship of the criminal conduct to the provision(s) of the Code or Standards specified in the notice of suspension and charges; and any other matters which the Committee in its discretion deems relevant.

(2) **Licensure Revocation.** With respect to any proceeding based on revocation of licensure, the Ethics and Judicial Committee shall consider: whether the respondent in fact was the subject of administrative action resulting in revocation of licensure; the nature of the conduct upon which the licensing authority based its adverse action; the relationship of such conduct to the qualifications, functions, or duties of a physical therapist or physical therapist assistant; the relationship of such conduct to the provision(s) of the Code or Standards specified in the notice of suspension and charges; and any other matters which the Committee in its discretion deems relevant.

(3) **Ethics and Judicial Committee Decision.** The Ethics and Judicial Committee shall make a decision, based on the information available to it, to dismiss the charges or to impose any form of disciplinary action described in Section 4. The Ethics and Judicial Committee shall mail notice of its decision to the respondent, by certified mail, return receipt requested, within fifteen (15) days following the decision. If the Ethics and Judicial Committee decides to continue the suspension the notice of decision shall specify the length of the continuation (which shall be deemed the specified time of initial suspension for purposes of any future termination of suspension).

3. CHAPTER ETHICS COMMITTEE PROCEEDINGS

The CEC shall be responsible for processing any proceeding the Chapter President refers to it under Section 1. All CEC decisions shall be determined by a majority vote of members present and voting. The Chapter President, after referring a matter to the CEC, shall not participate any further in the proceeding.

(a) **Appointment of Investigator.** Within 30 days after receipt of the notice of charges, the CEC by letter (with a copy to the Ethics and Judicial Committee) shall appoint an investigator (who may be a member of the CEC and who need not be an Association member) to conduct and investigation of the charges set forth in the President's notice of charges. The CEC shall provide the investigator with the complaint (if any), the documentation underlying any proceeding initiated by the President under Section 1(e), the President's notice of charges, and any other documents or information the CEC determines to be relevant to the investigation.

(b) **Investigation.** The investigation shall be an appropriately comprehensive and unbiased review of the circumstances of the alleged unethical activity. As a part of the investigation, the complainant and the respondent will be offered an opportunity to submit a statement of position or other evidence with respect to the allegations against the respondent. The investigator shall advise the respondent of all adverse evidence developed in the course of the investigation and shall give the respondent the opportunity to respond to all adverse evidence.

(c) **Investigative File; Date of Receipt.** The investigator shall prepare an investigative file which includes the complaint (if any), any documentation on which the President relied in initiating a proceeding under Section 1(e), the President's notice of charges, and other information and documents acquired or created during the investigation. The investigative file shall not include a recommendation concerning the CEC's action on the case. The investigator, within ninety (90) days of his/her appointment, shall submit to the CEC a cover letter enclosing the investigative file. The investigator shall be available to be called at the hearing (if any) to clarify the contents of the investigative file. The CEC shall make a record of the date of its receipt of the investigative file (e.g., by memorandum to file).

(d) **Confidentiality.** In order to protect the legitimate interests of the respondent, complainant, witnesses, and others, the confidential nature of a proceeding under this Procedural Document shall be preserved (except as explicitly provided herein). The Chapter President, the members of the CEC, and the investigator shall take due precautions to assure the confidential nature of the proceeding; they shall endeavor to restrict knowledge of the existence and substance of any proceeding to those individuals having a need to know (e.g., witnesses, legal counsel, expert advisors or witnesses, stenographers, Chapter or Association staff with support responsibilities, etc.). The Chapter President, the CEC, and the investigator may seek information and documentation from state licensing agencies (and courts) relating to disciplinary (or criminal) proceedings involving the respondent, but they shall not reveal to state licensing agencies (or other parties) information or documentation developed in the course of the proceeding under this Procedural Document. Upon the respondent's request, the investigator shall disclose to the respondent any publicly available documents or information upon which the Chapter President relied in initiating a proceeding under Section 1(e). Except when the CEC dismisses the charges summarily without a hearing, the respondent shall have the right to obtain a copy of the complete investigative file, which shall contain a copy of the underlying complaint (if any). The Association's Chief Executive Officer or President may take appropriate steps (including cessation of the processing of ethics complaints and charges in a state) to protect the interests of individual participants in the ethics process (including respondents and witnesses), the Chapter, and the Association itself upon determining (i) that the law or practice of any state requires (or could require) the disclosure of the existence of a complaint or proceeding under this Procedural Document or the reporting or disclosure of information or documentation developed hereunder and (ii) that such requirement would be unfair to affected parties or could expose any participant, the Chapter, or the Association itself to an undue risk of civil or criminal liability.

(e) **Summary Dismissal Without a Hearing.** If the CEC determines, based upon its preliminary review of the investigative file, that the evidence does not substantiate the violation(s) specified in the notice of charges, the CEC may dismiss the charges summarily. In such a case the CEC shall prepare a notice of summary dismissal, which shall state the CEC's rationale. The CEC shall send the notice of summary dismissal to the respondent by certified mail, return receipt requested, with copies to the Ethics and Judicial Committee, the Chapter President, and the complainant (if any).

(f) **Notice of Right to Copy of Investigative File and Hearing.** If the CEC does not dismiss the charges against the respondent summarily under subsection (e) above, the respondent shall have the right (i) to obtain a copy of the investigative file, and (ii) if the respondent still is an APTA member, to have a hearing before the CEC.

In such a case, the CEC, after receiving the investigative file, shall send the respondent a notice of his/her rights, in substantially the following form:

> This Committee has conducted a preliminary review of the investigative file and determined that it contains evidence that could substantiate the charges against you specified in the [date] notice of charges that the Chapter President sent to you. Under the APTA's *Procedural Document on Disciplinary Action*, you have the right (i) to obtain a copy of the investigative file, and (ii) if you still are an APTA member, to have a hearing before the CEC. If you wish to exercise any such right, you must submit a written request for a copy of the investigative file or for a hearing within fifteen (15) days of your receipt of this notice.

The CEC shall send this notice by certified mail, return receipt requested, with a copy to the Ethics and Judicial Committee. The respondent shall have fifteen (15) days from receipt of the notice in which to request in writing a copy of the investigative file and/or a hearing.

(1) **Respondent's Election of Hearing.** If the respondent makes a timely election to have a hearing, then the CEC shall notify the respondent in writing of the date, time, and place of hearing at least thirty (30) days in advance. The hearing shall be scheduled within sixty (60) days of the CEC's receipt of the investigative file.

(2) **CEC's Calling of Hearing.** If the respondent declines the opportunity to have a hearing or fails to make a timely response, the CEC has the prerogative to call and convene a hearing (eg, if the CEC wishes to hear the respondent testify) to be held no later than sixty (60) days after the CEC's receipt of the investigative file. In such an event the CEC shall notify the respondent in writing of the date, time, and place of hearing at least thirty (30) days in advance.

(3) **No Hearing.** If no hearing is held the CEC shall proceed as described in Section 4 of this Procedural Document.

(g) **Hearing.** The CEC shall conduct the hearing to review the pertinent facts, including the calling of witnesses and the production of pertinent documents. Except for the purpose of offering testimony, attendance at the hearing is limited to members of the CEC, the respondent, the respondent's legal counsel (if any), the Chapter's legal counsel (if any), and a transcriber (if any). Additional persons may be allowed to attend with the mutual agreement of the CEC and the respondent. The respondent may call a witness(es) to the hearing. Witnesses, including the complainant, shall not be allowed to attend any part of the hearing in which they are not directly involved. The respondent shall have the right to appear at the hearing in person to present and question witnesses and examine evidence. If legal counsel for the respondent or the CEC is present at the hearing (or at any stage of the ethics proceeding including proceedings before the Ethics and Judicial Committee or Board of Directors of the Association) the scope of involvement of such counsel shall be to provide consultation and advice to the respective parties. Rules of evidence shall not be applied strictly, but the CEC shall exclude irrelevant or unduly repetitious evidence. An oral affirmation of truthfulness will be requested from each witness. All documents accepted by the CEC, including the investigative file, shall be made a part of the record of the hearing.

(h) **Failure of Complainant To Participate.** If a proceeding was based on a complaint and the situation arises where the complainant no longer participates, the CEC may continue the ethics proceeding.

(i) **Termination of Respondent's Membership During Proceeding.** If during an ethics proceeding the CEC learns that a respondent's membership in the Association has ended, the CEC shall still complete the collection of all available information to facilitate a later reopening of the case if the respondent at any time rejoins the Association. In such a case the CEC shall review the investigative file. The CEC may dismiss the charges summarily on the basis of the investigative file, in which case it shall send notice of such summary dismissal in accordance with subsection (e). Otherwise, the CEC shall notify the respondent in accordance with subsection (f) and shall conduct a hearing (if any) in accordance with subsection (g). If a hearing is held the CEC may dismiss the charges, in which case it shall so notify the respondent by certified mail, return receipt requested, with a copy of the notice to the Ethics and Judicial Committee. If the CEC does not determine to dismiss the charges against the respondent, the CEC shall forward the complete record of the case (including the investigative file and the record of any hearing) to the Ethics and Judicial Committee. In any such case the CEC may (but need not) make a recommendation to the Ethics and Judicial Committee concerning the disciplinary action that it deems would have been appropriate if the respondent had been a member throughout the time the proceeding was before the CEC. In any such case the Ethics and Judicial Committee shall proceed pursuant to Section 5(e).

(j) **Stay of Proceeding.** The CEC may (but need not) vote to stay any proceeding before it if the conduct in question is the subject of investigation or action by federal, state, or local governmental authorities. If the CEC stays any such proceeding it shall review its decision to stay at intervals of no more than six (6) months.

(k) **Communications With Ethics and Judicial Committee.** The Ethics and Judicial Committee may prescribe a form of Disciplinary Action Worksheet to be used to track the progress of any proceeding. The Chair of the CEC shall advise the Ethics and Judicial Committee periodically (and upon request) of the status of any matter pending before the CEC.

4. CHAPTER ETHICS COMMITTEE CONCLUSIONS AND RECOMMENDATIONS

(a) **Dismissal or Recommendations of Disciplinary Action.** The CEC shall take action based on the evidence contained in the investigative file and obtained at a hearing (if any). The CEC shall take one of the following actions:

(1) dismiss the charges; or

(2) recommend that the Ethics and Judicial Committee impose one of the following disciplinary actions:

(A) **Reprimand**—a statement of recognition that the respondent's behavior was contrary to the Code or Standards. A reprimand is issued with the understanding that the respondent will correct the violation immediately (if he/she has not done so already). Ongoing conditions may not be added to a reprimand.

(B) **Probation**—a stronger reprimand with conditions for corrective action that the respondent shall complete within a given time period, not less than six (6) months nor more than two (2) years. The CEC shall monitor compliance with the conditions of probation. Failure to comply with the conditions of probation shall result in review by the Ethics and Judicial Committee as described in Section 7(a).

(C) **Suspension**—a temporary removal for not less than one (1) year of the rights and privileges of membership as identified in Article IV, Section 2 of the Association's *Bylaws*, "Rights and Privileges of Members," with the exception of B.(11). The affected rights and privileges shall be restored after the termination of the specified time of initial suspension, in accordance with Section 7(b), provided that there has been compliance with Article IV, Section 5 of the *Bylaws*, "Good Standing," during the suspension;

(D) **Expulsion**—a removal of membership which is subject to reinstatement only as stipulated in Article IV, Section 7 of the Bylaws, "Reinstatement."

If the CEC recommends the imposition of disciplinary action, the recommendation must specify (i) the evidence that the CEC believes supports its recommendation and (ii) the Principle of the *Code of Ethics* or the Standard of the *Standards of Ethical Conduct for the Physical Therapist Assistant* that the CEC believes is implicated. The CEC shall not make any finding that the respondent has violated an ethical principle or any law or regulation.

(b) **Notice to Respondent.** The CEC shall mail a copy of its dismissal of the charges or its recommendation for disciplinary action to the respondent by certified mail, return receipt requested, within thirty (30) days of the hearing, or if no hearing is held, within seventy (70) days of the CEC's receipt of the investigative file. In either case the CEC shall send a copy to the Ethics and Judicial Committee. If the CEC recommends that the Ethics and Judicial Committee impose disciplinary action, the CEC must include notice of the respondent's right to have a hearing before the Ethics and Judicial Committee and to make a written submission. The notice shall be in terms substantially similar to the following:

Under the APTA's *Procedural Document on Disciplinary Action*, this Committee has authority to recommend but not to impose disciplinary action. The APTA's Ethics and Judicial Committee has authority to impose the disciplinary action recommended by this Committee, to impose less severe disciplinary action, or to dismiss the charges against you. You have thirty (30) days after your receipt of this letter in which (i) to request in writing a hearing before the Ethics and Judicial Committee and/or (ii) to make a written submission to the Ethics and Judicial Committee for its consideration.

(c) **Transmission of the Record.** The CEC, within the same time frame as above, shall mail to the Ethics and Judicial Committee the entire original of the record, including an updated Disciplinary Action Worksheet, the investigative file, the record of hearing (if any), and evidence of the receipt of all items required to be sent by certified mail, return receipt requested. The CEC shall retain a duplicate copy of the entire record until and unless directed by Association staff in writing to destroy such copy.

5. DECISION OF THE ETHICS AND JUDICIAL COMMITTEE

(a) **Time of Ethics and Judicial Committee Action.** The respondent, within thirty (30) days after receipt of the CEC's recommendation of disciplinary action, by written notice to the Ethics and Judicial Committee may request a hearing before the Ethics and Judicial Committee. Within the same period the respondent may make a written submission to the Ethics and Judicial Committee for its consideration. The Ethics and Judicial Committee shall consider the case at its first regularly scheduled meeting after the respondent's receipt of the CEC's recommendation of disciplinary action if: (i) the Ethics and Judicial Committee receives a timely written request for hearing, a timely written submission, or a written waiver of the unexercised right(s) forty (40) or more days before such meeting; or (ii) the period for the respondent to request a hearing and/or make a written submission expires forty (40) or more days before such meeting. Otherwise, the Ethics and Judicial Committee shall consider the case at the immediately succeeding regularly scheduled meeting.

(b) Notice of Hearing; Hearing. If the respondent elects to have a hearing then the Ethics and Judicial Committee shall mail the respondent notice of the date, time, and place of the hearing at least thirty (30) days before the hearing. If a hearing is held, the hearing shall be limited to one hour. The respondent's presentation shall be limited to matters relevant to the charges.

(c) Decision of Ethics and Judicial Committee. The decision of the Ethics and Judicial Committee shall be based on only the record of the CEC, any oral or written testimony presented by the respondent, and any other information that fairness requires to be heard. The Ethics and Judicial Committee shall not set aside the CEC's dismissal of charges unless it is not supported by substantial evidence, it resulted from a misinterpretation of procedures or of the Association's ethical principles or standards, or there is evidence of actual or apparent impropriety in the dismissal of the charges.

The decision of the Ethics and Judicial Committee with respect to a CEC's recommendation of disciplinary action shall be to:

- impose the disciplinary action recommended by the CEC and specify the effective dates thereof;
- impose less severe disciplinary action than recommended by the CEC or dismiss the charges; or
- remand to the CEC with appropriate directives.

If the Ethics and Judicial Committee decides to impose disciplinary action, its decision shall specify (i) its findings as to the conduct in which the respondent engaged and (ii) the Principle of the *Code of Ethics* or the Standard of the *Standards of Ethical Conduct for the Physical Therapist Assistant* that it believes was violated. Within thirty (30) days after the Ethics and Judicial Committee has considered the CEC's recommendations and any oral or written testimony, the Ethics and Judicial Committee shall prepare its decision and mail it to the respondent by certified mail, return receipt requested, with a copy to the CEC (and to the Chapter President who initiated the proceeding, if the decision is to approve a dismissal of charges). The Ethics and Judicial Committee shall include an explanation of the appeals procedure. All records of the proceeding shall be kept by the Ethics and Judicial Committee for at least the longer of three (3) years from the date of the decision or one (1) year after the termination of any probation or suspension, except that the records of any proceeding resulting in expulsion shall be kept for at least ten (10) years from the date of the decision.

(d) Publication of Disciplinary Action. If an Ethics and Judicial Committee decision that becomes final under Section 6 imposes suspension or expulsion, the Ethics and Judicial Committee shall publish the name of the respondent, the disciplinary action taken, and the effective date(s) of such action in *PT Magazine* and *Physical Therapy* and make appropriate communications regarding the matter wherever the public welfare requires.

(e) Non-Member Respondent. In a case where the respondent's membership has ended the Ethics and Judicial Committee may dismiss the charges if the evidence does not substantiate the violation(s) specified in the notice of charges, but it may not impose any disciplinary action upon a nonmember. If the Ethics and Judicial Committee does not dismiss the charges, it shall stay the proceeding until the respondent rejoins the Association. In such a case the Ethics and Judicial Committee shall maintain the record of the proceeding for at least ten (10) years from the date of the lapse and shall request the Association's staff to notify the Ethics and Judicial Committee upon the respondent's rejoining the Association so that the stay may be lifted and the proceeding brought to a conclusion.

6. APPEAL TO BOARD OF DIRECTORS

(a) Time for Taking Appeal; Notification of Finality If No Appeal. Within thirty (30) days after receiving the final decision of the Ethics and Judicial Committee, the respondent may appeal the decision by delivering a notice of appeal to (i) the Association's Board of Directors and (ii) the Ethics and Judicial Committee. If the Ethics and Judicial Committee does not receive a notice of appeal within thirty (30) days the decision shall become final and unappealable, and the Ethics and Judicial Committee shall forward a copy of its decision and a notice that the decision is final to the Chapter President, the CEC, the complainant (if any), and the Board of Directors.

(b) Time of Board Consideration. If the Ethics and Judicial Committee receives a timely notice of appeal, then the Committee shall assemble the record of the proceeding and forward it to the Association's Board of Directors. The Board of Directors shall hear the appeal at its next regularly scheduled meeting which is not scheduled concurrently with the Annual Conference, provided that meeting begins thirty-five (35) or more days after the date of delivery of the notice of appeal to the Board of Directors. Otherwise, the Board of Directors shall hear the appeal at the immediately succeeding regularly scheduled meeting which is not scheduled concurrently with the Annual Conference.

(c) Notice of Board Consideration. The Board of Directors, at least thirty (30) days prior to the date of its consideration of the appeal, shall mail the respondent a notice, by certified mail, return receipt requested, stating the date, time, and place of the consideration of the appeal. The Board's notice shall advise the respondent that he/she may elect to have a hearing before the Board of Directors and/or to make a written submission. The respondent must exercise any such election in such manner and within such time as the Board's notice prescribes. If the respondent timely elects to have a hearing he/she may appear and present testimony. The hearing shall be limited to one hour.

(d) Decision on Appeal. The Board shall base its decision on appeal upon the record before the Ethics and Judicial Committee and any newly available information which the Board may decide to consider. The Board of Directors shall restrict its consideration of the appeal to the question whether the decision of the Ethics and Judicial Committee is appropriate.

The decision of the Board of Directors on initial appeal shall be to:

- affirm the Ethics and Judicial Committee's decision;
- modify the decision by dismissing the charges or by imposing less severe disciplinary action than imposed by the Ethics and Judicial Committee; or
- remand to the Ethics and Judicial Committee with appropriate directives.

If the Board of Directors does not remand the case to the Ethics and Judicial Committee, then its decision to affirm or modify the Ethics and Judicial Committee's decision shall be final.

(e) Remand to Ethics and Judicial Committee. If the Board of Directors remands the case the Ethics and Judicial Committee shall follow the procedures (if any) prescribed by the Board in its remand. In the absence of any such prescription of procedures, the Ethics and Judicial Committee on remand shall afford the respondent the opportunity to elect to have a hearing before the Committee and/or to make a written submission. If the respondent elects to have a hearing, the hearing shall be limited to one hour. The Ethics and Judicial Committee shall make its decision on remand and give notice thereof to the respondent as in Section 5(c).

(f) Appeal From a Decision on Remand. The respondent shall have thirty (30) days after the receipt of the Ethics and Judicial Committee's decision on remand in which to appeal to the Board of Directors, in the same manner as in subsection (a).

(1) No Appeal From Decision on Remand. If the Ethics and Judicial Committee does not receive a copy of a notice of appeal within thirty (30) days, its decision on remand shall become final and unappealable, and it shall forward copies of its decision on remand to the Chapter President, the CEC, the complainant (if any), and the Board of Directors.

(2) Board Action on Appeal From Decision on Remand. If the Ethics and Judicial Committee receives a timely notice of appeal from its decision on remand it shall forward the record to the Board of Directors. On an appeal following a remand the Board of Directors shall either (i) affirm the Ethics and Judicial Committee's decision on remand or (ii) modify the decision on remand by dismissing the charges or by imposing less severe disciplinary action than imposed by the Ethics

and Judicial Committee. No further remand shall be ordered, and the Board of Directors' decision shall be final.

(g) Notice of Board's Final Decision. The Board of Directors shall notify the respondent of its decision, on initial appeal and upon appeal after remand, by certified mail, return receipt requested. The Board shall forward copies of a final decision (ie, one to affirm or modify the Ethics and Judicial Committee's initial decision or its decision on remand) to the Chapter President, the CEC, the complainant (if any), and the Ethics and Judicial Committee.

7. POST-DECISIONAL MATTERS

(a) Probation. In any case involving probation, responsibility for monitoring the respondent's compliance with the conditions of the probation shall lie with the CEC, which shall report to the Ethics and Judicial Committee as requested. If the Ethics and Judicial Committee determines that the period of probation has expired and that the respondent has complied with the conditions of probation, it shall send notice of the termination of the probation to the respondent by certified mail, return receipt requested, with a copy to the CEC (and appropriate notice to the staff of the Association responsible for maintaining membership records). If the CEC determines at any time that the respondent has violated the conditions of probation it shall promptly notify the Ethics and Judicial Committee in writing, with a copy to the respondent. Immediately upon receiving notification that a respondent has violated the terms of probation, the Ethics and Judicial Committee shall notify the respondent by certified mail, return receipt requested, that it will review the respondent's case.

(1) Notice of Review; Hearing or Written Submission; Time of Review. The notice of review shall advise the respondent that he/she may elect to appear before the Ethics and Judicial Committee (unless the Committee meets by conference call, in which case the respondent may participate in the call) and/or to make a written submission. The respondent must exercise any such election in such manner and within such time as the notice of review prescribes. If the respondent timely elects to appear before the Ethics and Judicial Committee (or participate in a conference call meeting), the hearing (or call) shall be limited to one hour. If the Ethics and Judicial Committee receives notification from the CEC forty (40) or more days before its next regularly scheduled meeting it shall review the case at that meeting. Otherwise, the Ethics and Judicial Committee shall review the case at the immediately succeeding regularly scheduled meeting or any special meeting. The Ethics and Judicial Committee shall notify the respondent of the date, time, and place of its review, by certified mail, return receipt requested.

(2) Ethics and Judicial Committee Action Upon Review. The Ethics and Judicial Committee, on the basis of the information available to it, shall have authority to impose more severe disciplinary action, including suspension or expulsion, as the circumstances warrant. The Ethics and Judicial Committee shall prepare its decision and mail it to the respondent by certified mail, return receipt requested, with a copy to the CEC, within fifteen (15) days after the decision. The respondent may appeal the Ethics and Judicial Committee's decision to the Board of Directors in accordance with Section 6, but only if the decision imposes more severe disciplinary action than the probation previously imposed.

(3) **Transfer of Responsibility for Monitoring Compliance.** If the respondent moves or changes his chapter assignment during the period of probation, the CEC or the respondent may seek to transfer the responsibility for monitoring compliance to another CEC by mailing a request to the Ethics and Judicial Committee with a copy to the other party. The Ethics and Judicial Committee in its discretion shall grant or deny the request.

(b) **Termination of Suspension.** A member suspended under Section 2(f) or Section 5 may seek restoration of the affected membership rights by submitting to the Ethics and Judicial Committee, at any time after the expiration of the specified time of initial suspension, a request for termination of the suspension. If the Ethics and Judicial Committee receives the request forty (40) or more days before the start of its next regularly scheduled meeting, then it shall consider the request at that meeting. Otherwise, it shall consider the request at the succeeding regularly scheduled meeting. The Ethics and Judicial Committee shall notify the respondent of the date, time, and place of its consideration of the request to terminate suspension.

(1) **Membership in Good Standing Determination.** The Ethics and Judicial Committee shall terminate the suspension of a member who complied with the conditions of Article IV, Section 5 of the *Bylaws*, "Good Standing," throughout the period of initial suspension. Accordingly, a request for termination shall include an answer to each of the following questions:

(i) Did the respondent remain a member of the Association throughout the period of initial suspension?

(ii) Did the respondent comply with the ethical principles or standards applicable to his/her membership class throughout the period of initial suspension?

(iii) Did the respondent make timely payment of all Association and chapter dues throughout the period of initial suspension?

(iv) Was the respondent under suspension or revocation of a license or certificate of registration to practice physical therapy or to act as a physical therapist assistant in any jurisdiction at any time during the period of initial suspension?

The request for termination may contain such other information as may be relevant to the Ethics and Judicial Committee's decision whether to extend the suspension in the event of a negative compliance determination. The Ethics and Judicial Committee, in determining whether the respondent was in compliance with the "Good Standing" conditions throughout the period of initial suspension, may rely upon the information contained in the request for termination of suspension and may make such further inquiry or investigation as it deems appropriate. If the Ethics and Judicial Committee proposes to make a negative determination based on information extrinsic to the request for termination, the Ethics and Judicial Committee first shall so notify the respondent and afford him/her reasonable opportunity to respond.

(2) **Termination Upon Affirmative Compliance Determination.** If the Ethics and Judicial Committee makes an affirmative compliance determination it shall terminate the suspension immediately, effective as of the expiration of the period of initial suspension. The Ethics and Judicial Committee shall send notice of the termination of suspension to the respondent by certified mail, return receipt requested, with a copy to the CEC (and appropriate notice to the staff of the Association responsible for maintaining membership records).

(3) **Action Upon Negative Compliance Determination.** If the Ethics and Judicial Committee makes a negative compliance determination it shall decide whether to terminate or extend the suspension. The Ethics and Judicial Committee in its discretion may terminate the suspension or extend it for any length of time (including an extension of less than one year). The Ethics and Judicial Committee shall mail its decision to terminate or extend the suspension to the respondent by certified mail, return receipt requested, with a copy to the CEC (and appropriate notice to the staff of the Association responsible for maintaining membership records).

(4) **Extended Suspension.** If the Ethics and Judicial Committee extends the suspension its decision shall specify the period of the extended suspension. Restoration of the affected membership rights shall be dependent upon compliance with the "Good Standing" conditions during the time of the extended suspension. A member under extended suspension may seek restoration of the affected membership rights by submitting to the Ethics and Judicial Committee, at any time after the expiration of the specified time of extended suspension, a request for termination of the suspension. Any such request shall be processed in the same manner as set forth above (substituting extended suspension for the initial suspension, as appropriate).

Appendix

Complainant's Responsibilities and Rights

1. Make written complaint to Chapter President (or Ethics and Judicial Committee) that a member has violated the ethical principles or standards of the Association. (Section 1(a))

2. Receive acknowledgment of receipt of complaint. (Sections 1(a))

3. Have the opportunity to submit to investigator a statement of position or other evidence with respect to the allegations. (Section 3(b))

4. May act as witness if hearing takes place. (Section 3(g))

5. Receive notice of final action of the Ethics and Judicial Committee or the Board of Directors. (Section 6(a) or 6(g))

Chapter President's Responsibilities

1. Obtain legal consultation from Association headquarters, as appropriate. (Introduction)

2. Receive written complaint. (Section 1(a))

3. Immediately forward copy of complaint to Ethics and Judicial Committee. (Section 1(a)(1))

4. Obtain a case number from APTA staff (Section 1(a)(1))

5. Send complainant acknowledgment of receipt of complaint. (Section 1(a)(1))

6. Decide whether to initiate an APTA ethics proceeding, in consultation with Chair of Chapter Ethics Committee (CEC). (Section 1(b))

7. Notify the Ethics and Judicial Committee if the President declines to issue a notice of charges based on complaint (Section 1(b)(1), Section 1(b)(2)(A))

8. Notify complainant of decision not to initiate an ethics proceeding. (Section 1(b)(1))

9. Forward to Ethics and Judicial Committee copy of any reliable information that might be the basis for an ethics proceeding (Section 1(c)(1))

10. Determine whether to initiate a proceeding based on reliable information indicating an ethical violation. (Section 1(c)(2))

11. Notify the Ethics and Judicial Committee if the President declines to issue a notice of charges based on reliable information (Section 1(c)(2)(a), Section 1(c)(2)(B)(i))

12. Prepare notice of charges describing conduct at issue, citing ethical Principle(s)/Standard(s), and referring case to CEC. (Section 1(b)(2)(C))

13. Send respondent notice of charges, with copy of complaint (if any), copy to CEC and Ethics and Judicial Committee. (Section 1(b)(2)(C))

14. Receive notice of final action of the Ethics and Judicial Committee or the Board of Directors. (Section 6(a) or 6(g))

Chair of Chapter Ethics Committee's Responsibilities

1. Consult with Chapter President as to whether to initiate an APTA ethics proceeding. (Section 1(b), Section 1(c)(2))

Chapter Ethics Committee's Responsibilities

1. Obtain legal consultation from Association headquarters, when appropriate. (Introduction)

2. Accept referral of case from Chapter President. (Section 1(b)(2)(C) or 1(c))

3. Appoint investigator. (Section 3(a))

4. Receive the investigative file and make record of date of receipt. (Section 3(c))

5. Determine whether investigative file has evidence tending to substantiate the charges in the President's notice. (Section 3(e))

6. Notify respondent, Ethics and Judicial Committee, Chapter President, and complainant (if any) of summary dismissal of charges. (Section 3(e))

7. Notify respondent of rights to obtain copy of investigative file and (if respondent is still a member) to have a hearing before the CEC. (Section 3(f))

8. Provide respondent copy of investigative file, if requested. (Section 3(f))

9. Notify respondent of date, time, and place of hearing (if any). (Section 3(f)(1))

10. Conduct hearing (if demanded by respondent or chosen by CEC). (Section 3(g))

11. If respondent ceases to be a member complete collection of available information to facilitate later reopening, and forward record to Ethics and Judicial Committee. (Section 3(i))

12. Report status of case to Ethics and Judicial Committee. (Section 3(k))

13. Issue a decision dismissing the charges or recommending disciplinary action. (Section 4(a))

14. Mail to respondent CEC's decision, including notice of right to request a hearing before Ethics and Judicial Committee and to make written submission, with copy to Ethics and Judicial Committee. (Section 4(b))

15. Mail entire original record to Ethics and Judicial Committee. (Section 4(c))

16. Retain duplicate copy of entire record until and unless directed by APTA staff in writing to destroy such copy. (Section 4(c))

17. Receive notice of Ethics and Judicial Committee's action with respect to CEC's recommendation of disciplinary action. (Section 5(c))

18. Receive notice of final action of the Ethics and Judicial Committee or the Board of Directors. (Section 6(a) or 6(g))

19. Monitor probation and report noncompliance to Ethics and Judicial Committee. (Sections 7(a))

Ethics and Judicial Committee's Responsibilities

1. Receive copy of complaint filed with Chapter President. (Section 1(a)(1))

2. Serve as alternative recipient of complaint -- for responsibilities, see Chapter President's responsibilities. (Section 1(a)(2))

3. Assign case number to proceeding. (Section 1(a)(1) and 1(c))

4. Receive copy of Chapter President's decision not to initiate an ethics proceeding. (Section 1(b)(1), 1(b)(2)(A))

5. Receive copy of notice of charges prepared by Chapter President. (Section 1(b)(2)(C) or 1(c)(2)(b)(ii))

6. Forward to Chapter President reliable information indicating an ethical violation. (Section 1(c))

7. Receive from Chapter President or CEC complaint (or other documentation) indicating commission of serious crime or revocation of licensure. (Section 2(c))

8. Prepare and send notice of suspension and charges in case of serious crime or revocation of licensure. (Section 2(d) and 2(e))

9. Dismiss charges based on serious crime or revocation of licensure or impose disciplinary action or impose disciplinary action. (Section 2(f)(3))

10. Receive copy of CEC notice of summary dismissal. (Section 3(e))

11. Receive copy of CEC notice of respondent's right to hearing and to obtain copy of investigative file. (Section 3(f))

12. Receive copy of CEC decision to dismiss or to recommend disciplinary action. (Section 4(b))

13. Receive entire original record together with CEC's dismissal of charges or recommendation for disciplinary action (if any). (Section 3(i) and 4(c))

14. Receive from respondent request for hearing or written submission. (Section 5(a))

15. Notify respondent notice of date, time, and place of hearing. (Section 5(b))

16. Make decision on CEC's recommendation and notify respondent and CEC. (Section 5(c))

17. Retain record of the proceeding for time required. (Section 5(c))

18. Publish fact of suspension or expulsion in PT Magazine and Physical Therapy after decision becomes final. (Section 5(d))

19. Alert staff as to respondent whose membership lapsed and maintain record of case for reactivation. (Section 5(e))

20. Forward copies of unappealed decision to Chapter President, CEC, complainant, and Board of Directors. (Section 6(a) and 6(f)(1))

21. Receive copy of notice of appeal and forward record to Board of Directors. (Section 6(b) and 6(f)(2))

22. Make decision on remand in accordance with directions from Board of Directors and Procedural Document. (Section 6(e))

23. Receive CEC notice of noncompliance with conditions of probation; send notice of review to respondent; review case; notify respondent and CEC of decision. (Section 7(a)(1) and 7(a)(2))

24. Receive respondent's request for termination of suspension; determine compliance with "Good Standing" conditions of Bylaws; give respondent opportunity to respond to proposal to make negative compliance determination. (Section 7(b)(1))

25. Terminate suspension and notify respondent, CEC, and staff if compliance determination is affirmative. (Section 7(b)(2))

26. Decide whether to terminate or extend suspension if compliance determination is negative; notify respondent. (Section 7(b)(3))

Respondent's Responsibilities and Rights

1. Right to receive from Chapter President notice of charges describing conduct at issue and citing ethical Principle(s)/Standard(s) allegedly violated. (Section 1(b)(2)(C) or 1(c))

2. Receive notice of suspension and charges from Ethics and Judicial Committee in case involving commission of serious crime or revocation of licensure. (Section 2(d))

3. Right to have hearing before or make written submission to Ethics and Judicial Committee concerning serious crime or revocation of licensure. (Section 2(e))

4. Receive notice of Ethics and Judicial Committee's decision concerning serious crime or revocation of licensure. (Section 2(f)(3))

5. Right to submit statement of position or other evidence with respect to charges against respondent. (Section 3(b))

6. Right to be advised by investigator of adverse evidence and to respond. (Section 3(b))

7. Right to confidentiality as provided in Procedural Document. (Section 3(d))

8. Receive notice of CEC's summary dismissal of charges. (Section 3(e))

9. Receive notice of right to obtain copy of investigative file and (if still an APTA member) to have a hearing before CEC. (Section 3(f))

10. Receive CEC's notice of date, time, and place of hearing. (Section 3(f)(1) or 3(f)(2))

11. Attend the CEC hearing; right to examine and cross-examine witnesses, produce documents, consult with counsel. (Section 3(g))

12. Receive notice of recommended disciplinary action or dismissal of complaint. (Section 4(b))

13. Request hearing before Ethics and Judicial Committee or make written submission to Ethics and Judicial Committee. (Section 5(a))

14. Receive Ethics and Judicial Committee's notice of date, time, and place of hearing. (Section 5(b))

15. Attend the Ethics and Judicial Committee hearing. (Section 5(b))

16. Receive notice of the Ethics and Judicial Committee's decision and explanation of appeals procedure. (Section 5(c))

17. Appeal Ethics and Judicial Committee's decision to Board of Directors. (Section 6(a))

18. Receive Board's notice of date, time, and place of hearing; appear and present testimony or make written submission. (Section 6(c))

19. Receive notice of Board of Directors' decision on appeal. (Section 6(g))

20. Receive notice of Ethics and Judicial Committee's decision on remand (if any) with explanation of appeals procedure. (Section 6(e))

21. Receive copy of CEC notice of noncompliance with conditions of probation. (Section 7(a))

22. Receive notice of Ethics and Judicial Committee's review as to noncompliance with probation and right to appear and/or make written submission. (Section 7(a)(1))

23. Receive Ethics and Judicial Committee's decision as to noncompliance with probation; right to appeal to Board of Directors if result is stricter disciplinary action. (Section 7(a)(2))

24. Submit request for termination of suspension to Ethics and Judicial Committee. (Section 7(b))

25. Receive notice of proposed determination of noncompliance with "Good Standing" conditions if based on evidence extrinsic to request for termination. (Section 7(b)(1))

26. Receive Ethics and Judicial Committee decision to terminate or extend suspension. (Section 7(b)(3))

Investigator's Responsibilities

1. Conduct objective unbiased investigation. (Section 3(b))

2. Give respondent and complainant opportunity to submit a statement of position or other evidence bearing on the charges. (Section 3(b))

3. Give respondent opportunity to respond to adverse evidence developed. (Section 3(b))

4. Transmit investigative file, with no recommendation, to CEC. (Section 3(c))

5. Be available if hearing takes place to clarify the contents of investigative file. (Section 3(c))

Board of Directors' Responsibilities

1. If no appeal is taken, receive copy of final decision of Ethics and Judicial Committee. (Section 6(a))

2. Receive notice of appeal from respondent. (Section 6(b))

3. If appeal is taken, receive record of proceedings of Ethics and Judicial Committee. (Section 6(b))

4. Notify respondent of date, time, and place of consideration of appeal. (Section 6(c))

5. Hear and make decision on appeal. (Section 6(d))

6. Notify the respondent of its decision. (Section 6(g))

7. Forward a copy of a final decision to the Ethics and Judicial Committee, the Chapter President, the CEC and the complainant (if any). (Section 6(g))

APTA Ethics and Judicial Committee: Approved, Board of Directors: November 1999; Last Amended, Board of Directors: March 2004 [BOD R03-04-11-23]

P-115

Guidelines: Professional Oath for Physical Therapists
HOD G06-04-23-19 [Initial HOD 06-00-32-12]

Whereas, The Code of Ethics, Guide for Professional Conduct, and Standards of Practice set forth principles and guidelines for professional behaviors;

Whereas, The profession has defined core values of accountability, altruism, compassion/caring, excellence, integrity, professional duty, and social responsibility;

Whereas, It is the responsibility of all academic and clinical faculty, clinical instructors, and professional mentors to actively promote to physical therapist students the importance of professionalism;

Whereas, An oath serves to enhance the commitment of the physical therapist professional to the patient, client, and themselves; and

Resolved, That the American Physical Therapy Association supports the use of a professional oath for students in accredited physical therapist education programs and for licensed physical therapists.

The evolution of physical therapy, accompanied by external factors, has intensified the focus and emphasis on ethics.

Applying Ethics to Real World Situations

by *Aaron* Dalton

A roundtable discussion offers suggestions on ways PTs can address ethical dilemmas in their daily activities.

Roundtable Participants

Participating in *PT Magazine*'s ethics roundtable were:

Linda Arslanian, PT, DPT, MS
Director of Rehabilitation Services,
Brigham & Women's Hospital

Carol Davis, PT, EdD, MS, FAPTA
Professor, Associate Director/Curriculum,
University of Miami School of Medicine

Gail Jensen, PT, PhD, FAPTA
Creighton University,
Department of Physical Therapy

Nancy Kirsch, PT, PhD
Associate Professor, University of Medicine
and Dentistry of New Jersey

Ruth Purtilo, PT, PhD, FAPTA
Professor and Director of Ethics Initiative,
MGH Institute of Health Professions

Laura ("Dolly") Swisher, PT, PhD
Assistant Professor, University of South Florida,
School of Physical Therapy

Susan Sisola, PT, PhD
Professor Emeritus, Doctor of
Physical Therapy Program,
College of St. Catherine

Herm Triezenberg, PT, PhD
Physical Therapy Program Director, Chair,
School of Rehabilitation and Medical Sciences,
Central Michigan University

Mary Ann Wharton, PT, MS
Curriculum Coordinator and Associate Professor,
Department of Physical Therapy,
Saint Francis University

Denise Wise, PT, PhD
Chair, Assistant Professor,
Department of Physical Therapy,
The College of St Scholastica in Minneapolis

The topics of ethics and values have attracted much attention recently, both within and outside of the health care communities. On the national stage, the results of November's presidential election generated debate and discussion about "moral values" and the roles that they may play in both political and non-political arenas. In health care generally, hotly debated issues involving ethics and values include stem cell research, cloning, HIPAA and patient confidentiality, informed consent, health care allocation, organ donation, patient autonomy, fetal screening, pain management techniques, caring for uninsured or underinsured patients, for-profit versus non-profit health care services, minority health disparities, clinical competence, sexual misconduct and abuses, financial conflict of interest, and more.

Many of these topics, along with others, also are being discussed within the profession of physical therapy. APTA's Vision Statement 2020 weaves the thread of ethics and integrity into a broader fabric when it states, "Guided by integrity, lifelong learning, and a commitment to comprehensive and accessible health programs for all people, physical therapists and physical therapist assistants will render evidence-based service throughout the continuum of care and improve quality of life for society."[1]

Many view this heightened interest in ethics as a positive development. "It reflects a maturity in our professional identity and concurrently in our professional educational focus," says Ruth Purtilo, PT, PhD, FAPTA, professor and director of ethics initiative at MGH Institute of Health Professions in Boston. "We have grown to a level where ethics is recognized as a central resource for preparing our students to become professional and civic leaders. The greater interest in ethics also comes from a renewed interest in professionalism in physical therapy and across the health professions spurred by a health care environment that has forced us to look at ourselves more closely. We must reckon with how we fit into the current environment and how we differ from 'businesses' that are driven strictly by economic and market forces. The question is: How do we remain true to our basic identity as purveyors of an essential human service?"

To shed some light on these issues, *PT Magazine* gathered 10 of the profession's leading ethical thinkers, practitioners, and educators to explore the ways in which ethics applies to everyday physical therapy practice.

PT Magazine: *How often do ethical situations arise in everyday practice?*

Sisola: Essentially, what folks are telling us is that ethical situations happen in clinical practice every day.

Davis: It's not that it hasn't always happened every day; it's that the immediacy and the consequences of not acting ethically now seem to be more dangerous and harmful to good care.

Jensen: The other issue embedded in this discussion is that *ethical* reasoning and decision-making is part of *clinical* reasoning and decision-making. It should not be seen as something separate.

Swisher: PTs have different degrees of ability when it comes to recognizing ethical issues. Some are very good at recognizing ethical issues in the health care environment, while others are not yet as tuned in to these issues.

Applying Ethics to RealWorld Situations

PT Magazine: How can the profession help the remaining few "tune in" to ethical practice issues?

Swisher: We need more dialogue in the clinic. People should discuss the ethical issues that they encounter. It would help to have different kinds of peer review of clinical practice to pick up on ethical questions that might go unnoticed by a member of the practice.

Arslanian: We have grown up as a profession. In an employer-employee situation, individual PTs [may] assume that their employer is looking out for their professional ethical responsibilities. To rely on the organization to be the safeguard of ethical practice just isn't cutting it anymore. [Some] PTs don't even recognize that their practice environment is undermining their ability to practice ethically.

Sisola: As the role of the PT has expanded, the potential for ethical issues has broadened as well. One issue involves the role of the PT in providing equipment to patients. As institutions look for ways to stay viable, PTs sometimes can become involved in marketing equipment in ways that may violate ethical boundaries. We need to stop and consider: Is the marketing practice overtaking the PT's obligation to the best interests of the patient?

PT Magazine: How can PTs recognize when a clinical situation calls for an ethical decision?

Purtilo: One way you can recognize a situation that may call for an ethical solution is when you get a sinking feeling in the pit of your stomach. It just doesn't feel right. It stops you.

Wise: People realize they are in an ethical dilemma when they see that their choices are not black-and-white. PTs who practice 8 hours per day are likely to encounter such ethical challenges once or even several times per day.

Davis: When a situation with an ethical component arises, it stops me. I have to ask myself "What do I do?"

Jensen: That's where the value and importance of clinical management comes in to support these front-line discussions.

Swisher: We can't see ourselves as a "Lone Ranger." We should not look passively to our administration to take care of ethical problems. We can participate at an organizational level. When we have case presentations, for example, we can routinely include ethical issues. It will bring these topics before people who don't necessarily have them on their radar screens. We can have in-service days during which we ask each other how we can recognize ethical issues and reach good solutions. One disadvantage of all this is that it takes time.

> *One way you can recognize a situation that may call for an ethical solution is when you get a sinking feeling in the pit of your stomach. It just doesn't feel right.*
>
> —Ruth Purtillo, PT, PhD, FAPTA

Arslanian: Saying that we need to look to the practice administration to give us the means and support to ensure we're practicing ethically puts people between a rock and a hard place. A physician would argue that she/he is responsible for practicing ethically in any environment. Being a professional is about being an individual professional regardless of the practice environment.

Davis: The question is: How do we support moral courage in adults and encourage people to act with that courage? If there is a culture of expectation for adults to act courageously and morally, then it is easier for them to do so. I understand Gail to be saying that administrators have a responsibility to set up that culture of moral expectation through cases, through questioning, and through student involvement, so that the person who acts ethically does not feel alone but instead feels inspired by his culture and colleagues to do what he feels is ethically right.

Arslanian: We have to try to engender an ethical culture, but I don't want PTs to think that anyone else can or should assume responsibility for their professional behavior. If PTs find themselves in a situation hostile to the ethical practice of physical therapy, it's their professional responsibility to spend some time evaluating whether they can change the culture. If not, they have an obligation to remove themselves from that situation. If I could give one take-home message to

continued on page 44 ▶▶▶

Applying Ethics to RealWorld Situations

continued from page 42

anyone, I would say that the marketplace for physical therapists has shifted dramatically. PTs are in the driver's seat, and they can spend time evaluating whether their practice environment will support these ethical practices.

Triezenberg: I agree strongly. PTs are part of the medical culture that we're talking about. We're not just blowing in the wind or victims of it. We have a major responsibility when we get involved in any organization to change it and make it better in any way we can.

PT Magazine: How do the ethical concepts we've been discussing relate to the question of PT professionalism?

Arslanian: The concept of professionalism comes down to an individual professional adhering to standards, codes, and behaviors arrived at by consensus by the profession. If the profession's consensus is that we will never let financial consideration drive how we treat a patient, then I'm obliged to follow that consensus. If I encounter a hostile environment that precludes or punishes me if I refuse to practice in a way that puts finances ahead of my patients' needs, then I have a decision to make: I either need to work as best I can to change that culture, or I am obliged by professional duty to leave.

PT Magazine: The concept of ethics might seem formal and abstract to some PTs. What is the value of formal ethical models, and how can PTs apply these models to their clinical situations? How can we bring the practice of ethics "down to earth"?

Jensen: Listening to the patient's values and preferences is really part of the ethical decision-making process and part of evidence. The evidence is not just in the literature, it's right there with the patient's values.

Davis: Patient values have to be the foundation of all ethical decisions. The context that the patient brings to the

Patient values have to be the foundation of all ethical decisions.

—Carol Davis, PT, EdD, MS, FAPTA

encounter with the clinician serves as the foundation for setting all priorities. So often, ethical decision making in a clinical setting is not a yes/no decision. It's "What do I first? Do I do this? Do I wait?" The ethic of care goes beyond benevolence. It goes beyond a contract between the patient and the therapist. Ethical practice really has to do with cultural sensitivity, with the PT recognizing the unique situation present in each patient encounter and then carefully weighing all of the details of that encounter in order to act specifically as an advocate for that particular patient. That's the ideal.

Wise: When we treat a patient, we base our intervention on the characteristic of our individual patient's needs. We accommodate that. That's what the focus needs to be on with the ethics—getting into that caring relationship and making the best decisions for the patient based on the situation. It's not relativism; it's just looking at the whole picture.

Arslanian: To look at these ethical issues from a political perspective and a professional society perspective, we can take as an example what medicine did with the gag rule that HMOs had in place for many years. The profession of medicine, specifically the American Medical Association, lobbied against the gag rule. They did that only after a critical mass of physicians agreed that their relationship with their patients was being undermined and that their professional and ethical responsibility was being sabotaged because of contractual and legal barriers that HMOs were imposing. They finally pushed back, said "this is unethical," and lobbied against gag rules. We can learn from that. Until you get a critical mass of PTs who recognize their obligation as

APTA Code of Ethics

(HOD 06-00-12-23)

Preamble

This Code of Ethics of the American Physical Therapy Association sets forth Principles for the ethical practice of physical therapy. All physical therapists are responsible for maintaining and promoting ethical practice. To this end, the physical therapist shall act in the best interest of the patient/client. This Code of Ethics shall be binding on all physical therapists.

Principle 1

A physical therapist shall respect the rights and dignity of all individuals and shall provide compassionate care.

Principle 2

A physical therapist shall act in a trustworthy manner towards patients/clients, and in all other aspects of physical therapy practice.

Principle 3

A physical therapist shall comply with laws and regulations governing physical therapy and shall strive to effect changes that benefit patients/clients.

Principle 4

A physical therapist shall exercise sound professional judgment.

Principle 5

A physical therapist shall achieve and maintain professional competence.

Principle 6

A physical therapist shall maintain and promote high standards for physical therapy practice, education and research.

Principle 7

A physical therapist shall seek only such remuneration as is deserved and reasonable for physical therapy services.

Principle 8

A physical therapist shall provide and make available accurate and relevant information to patients/clients about their care and to the public about physical therapy services.

Principle 9

A physical therapist shall protect the public and the profession from unethical, incompetent, and illegal acts.

Principle 10

A physical therapist shall endeavor to address the health needs of society.

Principle 11

A physical therapist shall respect the rights, knowledge, and skills of colleagues and other health care professionals.

Adopted by the House of Delegates June 1981; last amended June 2000.

professionals to advocate for their collective and individual patients, you won't get a critical mass that will push back, lobby, and advocate for those kinds of changes that are specific to our practice and for the benefit of society. Our issues aren't about gag rules. They're about 60 days of care and other barriers.

Jensen: With professional associations, we have to look not at our self-interest, but at the ethical and societal needs we need to advocate for as a moral community. That's the definition of our profession.

Arslanian: We have to demonstrate a commitment that is consistent with the best interests of society at large. If you can't find an ethical reason for how it's going to benefit society, then it's not going to enhance our credibility as autonomous professionals.

Purtilo: On the subject of ethical models, I want to remind the readers of *PT Magazine* that some models might be difficult to apply to realworld situations. Models are attempts to express in concrete terms difficult concepts and theories. In this regard, they are no different from any other models in clinical education. To suggest that they are is to falsely set them apart. Like all other models, ethical models continue to be refined. We are getting better at understanding what needs to be brought into our ethical models in order to cross the Rubicon between theory and practice. As we increase our understanding of the ways in which ethics relates to other aspects of practice, our ethical models also will continue to evolve.

Swisher: Some of us on the APTA Ethics and Judicial Committee—Carol, Linda, Susan, Nancy and I—put together a little ethical decision-making model—the Realm-Individual Process-Situation (RIPS) Ethical Analysis Model—that was a way to [examine] an ethical problem. We were gratified by how people took to this. The point was to look at a situation and figure out whether it was an individual, societal, or organizational problem. People are looking for pragmatic models, but, by the same token, the model doesn't really *solve* anything. It doesn't really provide new information, but it brings together some important elements.

Sisola: This is an opportunity to challenge PTs to identify their level of skill and comfort in recognizing and working with ethical issues in the same way that we assess other areas of clinical competence: Was ethics a prominent part of your education? How much of your continuing education is devoted to ethical practice? Should we challenge people to recognize that this is something we need to do continually throughout our career? Learning about ethical practice is not something that we do once and say, "Now I've got it and I don't need to pay attention to this any longer." This must be part of our ongoing professional development.

Kirsch: When I teach ethics, especially to postprofessional students, the first question they ask is "You're going to try to teach me to be ethical? Can you really do this?" By the end of the class, they've realized that I've taught them how to incorporate ethical decision making into clinical practice and they're great at doing it. The problem is that we are not socialized to this type of education throughout our entire professional education.

Wharton: There is more of an effort to instill ethical problem-solving throughout the entry-level curriculum, but I see the discomfort in some

Applying Ethics to RealWorld *Situations*

continued on page 48 ▶▶▶

For More Information

APTA offers many resources dealing with ethics and professionalism. Among them are the following, available at www.apta.org, under "About APTA":

Code of Ethics (HOD 06-00-12-23)
Contains principles for physical therapists. (See "Code of Ethics")

APTA Guide for Professional Conduct
Serves physical therapists in interpreting the Code of Ethics, in matters of professional conduct.

Professionalism in Physical Therapy: Core Values
Seven core values that define the critical elements that comprise professionalism.

Standards of Ethical Conduct for the Physical Therapist Assistant (HOD 06-00-13-24)
Sets forth standards for physical therapist assistants.

Ethics and Judicial Committee Compendium of Interpretations and Opinions
Contains statements on various ethical issues.

Ethics and Judicial Committee Opinions
The Ethics and Judicial Committee occasionally issues ethics opinions in response to requests from APTA members or other interested parties.

Procedural Document on Disciplinary Action (BOD 11-99-05-11)
Procedure to process claims that a member of the Association has violated the Association's Code of Ethics or Standards of Ethical Conduct for the Physical Therapist Assistant.

APTA Risk Management Resources

faculty members to include ethics as part of patient-client management or administrative decision making. It's probably because they are not confident with teaching ethical decision-making.

Sisola: Perhaps we can use the recent heightened awareness of professionalism to begin advocating for ongoing education in ethics as part of being a professional. This should be a goal wherever we fit into the continuum, whether as a new grad who has had a reasonable introduction to ethics, or someone who has been in practice for 20 years and didn't have any formal education in ethics but is willing to learn.

Swisher: To quote Ruth Purtilo, "Ethics is what happens when you stub your toe on the walk down the moral path of life." The more we can offer people the opportunity to reflect on real problems, the better off we will be.

PT Magazine: If you could give one piece of advice to the physical therapy profession or to an individual physical therapist about practicing ethically, what would you say?

Kirsch: As autonomous practitioners, ethical decision-making is an integral part of clinical decision-making. One cannot be separated from the other.

Wharton: Along with autonomous practice comes the obligation to practice ethically.

Swisher: It's the nature of the human condition that anything we could do with people will involve ethical issues. There always are concerns over whether or not we are doing the right thing.

Jensen: We have embraced the term "reflective practitioner"—it is in many of our APTA educational documents—but reflection also should lead to deliberate action. We've talked about that with our discussion of moral courage.

Arslanian: The good thing about exercising moral courage is that as we evolve into a truly autonomous profession, we are beginning to generate power among us. A strong consensus enables us as individuals to be more effective in going out on a limb and taking on the tough situations, such as being in an environment that [challenges] our responsibility to practice ethically. Being more cognizant that there is strength in numbers and that the consensus statements of our profession are consistent with ethical professional practice makes it easier to confront and deal with those factors that compromise our ethical practice. The more we talk about this, emphasize our obligations as autonomous professionals, and see the mission of meeting the needs of society as empowering, the more credible we will become. It's a win-win situation, but the most important thing is that it ends up being in the best interests of our patients.

Wise: My advice is that you only find what you look for. Challenge yourself. Find these issues and apply ethical concepts to every decision you make. People will find that ethics is something they can do on a daily basis—indeed, that they *have* been doing on a daily basis and just haven't realized it. They just have to start looking for it.

Davis: We need to think beyond the boundaries of APTA. It's not just members of APTA who are expected to practice according to the code of ethics. That's a best practice standard to which everyone is held accountable. We need to get chapter ethics committees engaged, get the newsletters involved with talking

> *As autonomous practitioners, ethical decision-making is an integral part of clinical decision-making. One cannot be separated from the other.*
>
> —Nancy Kirsch, PT, PhD

Applying Ethics to RealWorld Situations

continued from page 46

about ethics, get the word out to ACCEs and into clinics. Many PTs still are not members of APTA. It is really important to help them work them work through problem-solving practice.

Triezenberg: The practice of physical therapy is an ethical act. Our actions are within a specific system. So we need to be part of those who can change the environment of the system. We have a responsibility to make the system better for our patients. As physical therapists, we don't tend to get involved in the boards and the committees that make a lot of the decisions that have ethical implications, so we feel like we are being neglected in the decision-making process. I believe, however, that we can have a place at the table if we choose to take it.

Arslanian: Sometimes we dwell on those who aren't keeping up, but we should

turn and celebrate the fact we have as many people as we do out there changing our practice and profession.

Swisher: We haven't put our exemplars out there, either. There are incredible stories of PTs who exemplify ethical practice.

Davis: Our society is moving steadily forward on these issues. We have a sensitivity to moral issues and value-based decisions on which we will not go backwards—ever.

Sisola: I would encourage clinicians to be open to a variety of ways of learning about ethics and improving the practice of ethics in their clinical life. Going to a continuing education session and listening to a lecture isn't necessarily the way we learn best. Perhaps ethical practice also is learned in the community, talking with others, or discussing ethical situations with your colleagues. Who is the person in your clinical community you feel comfortable calling

up and discussing ethical issues when they occur? Do you have such a resource? If not, how can you find one? Are there ways you are continuing to learn [about ethics] on regular basis? Mentors within APTA certainly can help.

Purtilo: My advice is that if you walk into each situation thinking "What is the most caring response?" you are already half way to an ethical decision. You have lots of resources: call each other, use different models. There is reason for optimism, because a lot of us out there are committed to ethical practice. **PT**

Aaron Dalton is a freelance writer.

Reference

1 APTA Vision Statement for Physical Therapy 2020. Available at www.apta.org/About/aptamissiongoals/vision-statement. Accessed January 5, 2004.

Research Report

The Identification of Ethical Issues in Physical Therapy Practice

Background and Purpose. The purpose of this study was to identify (1) current ethical issues facing physical therapists and (2) ethical issues that may be faced in the future by physical therapists. **Subjects and Methods.** The Delphi technique was used as the research design for the study. The panel of experts for the study were selected from lists submitted by past and present members of the Judicial Committee of the American Physical Therapy Association. A series of three questionnaires were sent to the members of the panel. Following the Delphi technique, the first questionnaire contained broad questions designed to elicit a wide range of responses. The second and third questionnaires were then developed from the information received in the preceding questionnaire. **Results.** The results of the first question of the study identified 10 current ethical issues as consensus choices by the panel and 3 issues as near-consensus. The panel responses to the second question identified 4 future ethical issues. A combined list of current and future contained 16 issues in physical therapy. **Conclusion and Discussion.** The 16 issues addressed ethical considerations in different areas of physical therapy practice: 6 issues involving patient rights and welfare, 5 professional issues, and 5 issues relating to business and economic factors. Thirteen of these issues have not been discussed in previous physical therapy literature and would be suggested topics for future study. [Triezenberg HL. The identification of ethical issues in physical therapy practice. *Phys Ther.* 1996;76:1097–1106.]

Key Words: *Delphi technique; Ethics; Physical therapy profession, professional issues.*

Herman L Triezenberg

dentification and examination of the ethical issues facing a profession is an important activity[1] and is considered a mark of professionalism. During the past 20 years, there has been an increased interest in ethical issues. With this increase in interest, there has been a concurrent increase in publications relating to medical ethics. Much of this literature has related to medicine and nursing.[2] Only in the last few years have other health professions begun to address the ethical issues specific to their professions. The need for these other health professions to address their unique ethical issues has become more urgent as these professions have expanded their scope of responsibilities, placing practitioners into positions in which ethical decisions must frequently be made.

In recent years, the profession of physical therapy has increased its autonomy in decision making and has expanded its role in patient care.[3] These changes can be seen by examining the changes that have been made in the practice acts of nearly every state to give physical therapists some degree of autonomy in practice. This increase in autonomy has increased the ethical considerations for physical therapists and has served to focus more clearly the responsibility of physical therapists to identify and discuss ethical questions that arise in the practice of physical therapy. An example of this change can be observed by examining the increased role that physical therapists now have in the supervision of support personnel. Physical therapists are required to supervise a larger number and a more diverse group of assistants, aides, and related health care professionals. With this increase in the supervisory role come additional questions of authority, professional autonomy, responsibility, and quality of care. Other examples can be seen in the variety of business opportunities available to physical therapists. These business arrangements introduce a number of questions relating to patient autonomy, utilization of services, and equity in billing. Any change in practice creates a new set of ethical considerations.

In response to these recent changes in practice, there has been an increased interest in ethical issues facing physical therapists and in ethical decision making. Prior to 1970, there were only a handful of articles that broadly considered the responsibility of physical therapists to the physician and the patient.[4-8] The concepts of ethics described in these articles were represented in terms of appropriate professional behavior and etiquette rather than considerations of ethical decisions or issues.

These articles defined good professional behavior for that period in the history of physical therapy, but they did not address how to approach ethical decision making or what ethical issues are associated with the practice of physical therapy. The first *Code of Ethics* for the American Physical Therapy Association (APTA) was developed in 1935.[9] The establishment of a code as well as subsequent articles in the 1940s and 1950s,[4-8] however, indicated that the profession believed ethical behavior should be expected of its members. The responsibility of physical therapists to behave in an ethical manner was emphasized in subsequent literature.[9-16] This more recent literature identified physical therapists as professionals who were responsible for making ethical decisions[13,14,17,18] and who needed to understand the ethical principles involved in such decisions.[12] This perspective was presented by Guccione, in 1980, when he stated

> The need to identify and clarify ethical issues within a health profession increases as the profession assumes responsibility for those areas of direct patient care in its domain.... The physical therapist today, in defining the limits of his legal and professional autonomy, must examine the practice of his profession from an ethical point of view.[17(p1264)]

Purtilo, in 1979, also emphasized the changing role as she stated

> In short, nonphysician health professionals are involved in ethic decision-making processes and increasingly will be asked to participate in determining moral policy.[18(p1102)]

In 1980, Guccione[17] reported on a survey of 450 APTA members in New England in which he identified 7 primary and 11 secondary ethical issues in physical therapy. Identification of issues facing physical therapists helped to identify physical therapy as a profession with issues particular to itself and placed additional responsibility on the profession to address these issues. Guccione indicated in his conclusions that he wanted to establish priorities for action by APTA and encourage discussion, promote study, and direct education for physical therapists. No follow-up articles were written on

HL Triezenberg, PhD, PT, is Associate Professor and Chair, Department of Health Promotion and Rehabilitation, Central Michigan University, 134 Pearce Hall, Mt Pleasant, MI 48859 (USA) (herman.l.triezenberg@cmich.edu).

This study was approved by the institutional review board at Michigan State University.

This article was submitted September 19, 1995, and was accepted May 21, 1996.

any of the 7 primary issues identified by Guccione. These issues were

1. Establishing priorities for patient treatment when time or resources are limited.

2. Discontinuing treatment for noncompliant patients.

3. Continuing treatment with a terminally ill patient.

4. Continuing treatment to provide psychological support after physical therapy goals have been reached.

5. Determining professional responsibilities when a patient's needs or goals conflict with the family's needs or goals.

6. Deciding whether to represent certain necessary patient services in a way that would meet third-party payer limitations.

7. Maintaining a patient's or family's confidence in other health care professionals regardless of personal opinions.

Two of the secondary issues were considered in subsequent literature. The issues were (1) informing patients about limits of treatment or informed consent and (2) the duty of physical therapists to report misconduct by colleagues (ie, whistle blowing).

Articles that included discussion of ethical issues facing physical therapy were published in the 1980s and 1990s. The two issues that received the most attention were informed consent[18-20] and patient compliance.[11,19,21,22] Other issues that have been examined include the right to health care[18] and the treatment of patients with acquired immunodeficiency syndrome (AIDS).[23,24] During the 1980s and 1990s, however, there were still very few articles that addressed ethical issues in physical therapy.

This study was undertaken to assist in the process of identifying ethical issues that are important in the practice of physical therapy. The identification of important ethical issues facing physical therapists may provide a stimulus for increased discussion of those issues.

Methodology
The Delphi technique was chosen as the research method for this study. The Delphi technique is a commonly used method for determining consensus in social science research.[25-30] The Delphi method was developed in the early 1950s and was initially used in Future's research.[28-31] "Future's research" refers to research that attempts to predict future trends and outcomes. This technique consists of a series of questionnaires that are completed by a selected panel of experts. The purpose is to achieve consensus within a group of experts but to avoid the psychological distractions of group interaction.[25] There are typically three or four rounds of questionnaires, with the responses to each questionnaire providing the material for the development of the subsequent questionnaire.[29] The purpose of this process is to reach agreement among the group of experts on the specific statements.

The first questionnaire of the series is composed of broad questions that are intended to elicit open responses from the panel of experts. The composition of the questions in the second round are based on the responses of the panel members to the initial broad questions of the first questionnaire. The second questionnaire is intended to provide the panel with a compilation of the results of the initial questionnaire as well as questions to clarify the specific issues identified by the individual panel members. This questionnaire also provides the panel with a list of specific areas of consensus and areas of disagreement. The third questionnaire provides the panel with a compilation of the results of the second questionnaire and additional data on the opinions and comments of the other panel members. This questionnaire describes areas of agreement between the experts and also presents minority opinions. The third questionnaire provides the panel with an opportunity to make revisions and respond to the information presented from the results of the second questionnaire. If consensus is not obtained following the third questionnaire, then a fourth questionnaire would need to be constructed. Three questionnaires are usually considered sufficient, as little meaningful change usually takes place between the third and fourth rounds.[26]

The Delphi Panel of Experts
The choice of the panel of experts is an important step. In my study, the panel of experts was composed of 6 members. These experts were chosen by polling members of the Judicial Committee of APTA. Each member who had served on the Judicial Committee during the last 10 years was asked to identify five individuals who they considered to be experts in ethical issues for physical therapy. They were asked to write the names on a form provided and return this form to the investigator. Their responses remained anonymous. Of the 12 current or former Judicial Committee members contacted, nine responses (75%) were received. An individual was then selected for the panel of experts if he or she was identified by more than one Judicial Committee member as an expert. By use of this method, 6 individuals were identified as experts and included on the panel. All 6 of the potential panel members consented to participate in the study.

The final composition of the panel was quite diverse, with representation from the East, West, South, and Midwest regions of the United States. There were four male and two female panel members. This gender ratio does not reflect the current composition of the physical therapy profession. According to statistics provided by APTA, the physical therapy profession is approximately 76% female and 24% male.[32] Five of the panel members were physical therapists with extensive backgrounds in clinical practice. Four of these five physical therapists possessed advanced academic degrees. Three of the six panel members had academic appointments. All members of the panel have had additional experience in ethical issues relating to physical therapy as speakers, instructors, authors, or as members of state or national judicial committees.

The Delphi Instrument

The initial questionnaire of the Delphi instrument used in this study was composed of five questions. For the purpose of this report, I will focus on the first two of these questions. The first two questions dealt with present and future ethical issues facing physical therapists. The questionnaires for the second and third rounds of the Delphi instrument contained a compilation of the data received in the preceding questionnaire and requested that the panel consider their earlier responses in light of the additional information.

The first two questions of the initial questionnaire consisted of the following broad statements:

1. List the ethical issues that you feel are currently most important for physical therapists to address.

2. List any other ethical issues that you feel will become important for physical therapists within the next 10 years.

Each question was designed to elicit an open response in which the panel members could write as much or as little as they felt necessary.

The initial statements were then compiled and divided into groups of similar statements. The statements identified were supported by differing numbers of panel members. Some statements were supported by all the panel members, and some statements were supported by only one panel member.

The next step in the process was to determine the degree of consensus within the panel on the statements made. Questionnaire B presented the panel members with the statements of the other panel members and asked them to respond to these statements. This questionnaire was designed to allow for clarification of the specific issues and to develop statements that accurately represent the various issues. It was intended to give panel members information on the views of the other members of the panel to assist them in responding to further questions. Consensus was sought on the issues listed. The purposes of questionnaire B, therefore, were

1. To obtain clarification on the issues.

2. To obtain agreement on the content of the statements.

3. To obtain consensus on the issues derived from the first questionnaire.

4. To identify any issues that were omitted from the results of the first questionnaire.

The first two questions of questionnaire B reflected the same two questions contained in questionnaire A. For question 1, each of the 23 statements of ethical issues were listed as well as the statements made by the panel members in each of these 23 topic areas. The panel members were then asked to

1. Agree or disagree with the statement.

2. Suggest changes to clarify the statement.

3. Identify any panel statements that did not fit under this topic area.

4. Rephrase the panel statements that did not fit to clarify their distinctiveness from the ethical issues as written.

The same procedure was followed for question 2, which dealt with the eight future ethical issues.

Questionnaire C was developed based on an analysis of the information received in questionnaire B. This questionnaire was designed to allow the panel to reach consensus on which statements to include in a listing of ethical issues facing physical therapy and of practice issues that have ethical ramifications.

Question 1a of questionnaire C listed the consensus choices and asked the panel members to confirm their choice or make changes as necessary. Question 1b listed the statements that were chosen by the majority of the panel members and provided the panel members with the statements made by the panel members in questionnaire B. The panel members were asked to accept or reject these statements and to provide any comments they felt necessary. The same procedure was followed in question 1c with the issues that were rejected by the

- The inequity of the provision of health services within the current health care system
- The determination of appropriate utilization and supervision of personnel other than physical therapists (eg, physical therapist assistants, physical therapy aides, certified athletic trainers) in the treatment of patients referred for physical therapy
- The involvement of physical therapists in business relationships that limit professional autonomy or have the potential for financial abuse
- The overutilization of physical therapy services
- The qualification of physical therapists as the entry point into the health care system
- The delineation of professional expertise and practice in relationship to other health care providers
- The accountability of physical therapy education programs to develop in physical therapy students the skills needed as professionals
- The identification of what constitutes informed consent for physical therapy evaluation and treatment
- The protection of the patient's right to confidentiality in interactions with therapists, personnel under the supervision of therapists, and physical therapy students
- Justifiability of fees charged for services and reasonable rate of return
- Defining the proper ethical limits of intervention: When doing everything possible may not be in the best interests of the patient
- Truth in advertising
- Fraud in billing
- Sexual abuse by physical therapists
- The treatment or nontreatment of patients with acquired immunodeficiency syndrome by physical therapists
- Maintaining of clinical competency by physical therapists
- Compliance of physical therapists with the need for supportive documentation for services and charges rendered
- Resolving the conflicts that sometimes occur between what is permitted by law and what is not permitted by the *Code of Ethics*
- The lack of research evidence to support clinical practice techniques
- The lack of cultural diversity within the physical therapy profession
- Adhering to the ethical guidelines for the use of human subjects in clinical research
- The endorsement of equipment or products in which the physical therapist has a financial interest
- The use of ethics and the disciplinary process to achieve personal gain

Figure 1.
Initial list of current ethical issues from questionnaire A, question 1.

majority of the panel members in questionnaire B. This process was also followed in question 1d with new questions that were introduced by the panel members in questionnaire B.

Question 2 of questionnaire C dealt with future ethical issues. The same procedure was followed for question 2 as was outlined for question 1 of questionnaire C.

Results
The participation of the six chosen panel members in the three rounds of the study was good throughout the study. In the first round, all six panel members completed the questionnaire and responded to all questions. This provided the investigator with a large variety of responses from which to develop the second round of questions. The second questionnaire was the longest of the three questionnaires given to the panel, and it required the panel members to consider the responses of the other panel members in determining their answers to the questions. Five of the six panel members completed the second questionnaire. The third questionnaire was less complex than the second questionnaire. This questionnaire asked the panel members to either agree or disagree with the statement of issues presented in rounds 1 and 2. Five of the six panel

members responded to the third questionnaire. The results of the study presented in this article provided information in the two topic areas of current ethical issues in physical therapy and future ethical issues in physical therapy.

Current Ethical Issues
The first portion of this study identified current ethical issues in physical therapy. The panel members were given the broad directive in question 1 of "List the ethical issues that you feel are currently most important for physical therapists to address." This open-ended question allowed the panel members to identify a wide variety of ethical issues.

The question resulted in a total of 41 responses by the panel members. The number of issues indicated by the individual panel members varied from four to nine issues. Some issues were included by all panel members, and some issues were only listed by one member. From the list of 41 statements of ethical issues, 23 unique issues were identified. The 23 statements of current ethical issues are listed in Figure 1.

The 23 ethical issues that were identified in the initial round of the study were the starting point for determining a list of consensus ethical issues facing physical therapy. In the next two rounds of the Delphi study, the panel members were asked to consider this list of ethical issues while also considering the statements of the other panel members. They were asked to modify the statements if they felt it would clarify the issue. They were also instructed to add additional statements if they felt a new statement was needed. At the completion of three rounds of the study, a positive consensus was achieved on 10 of the original 23 statements. Three of the statements were also considered near-consensus items. An item was considered a near-consensus item if only one panel member dissented. There was also negative or near-negative consensus on 6 of the 23 statements. Of the remaining 4 statements, there was a majority vote to accept 2 statements and a majority vote to reject 2 statements.

The results obtained after three rounds of questionnaires had identified 10 statements as consensus choices and 3 statements as near-consensus choices. These 13 statements are listed in Figure 2. A fourth round for this question was not considered necessary because 19 of the 23 statements were at or near consensus and the final 4 statements did not show substantial change between the second and third questionnaires.

Future Ethical Issues

The second goal of this study was the identification of ethical issues that are likely to face physical therapists in the future. In questionnaire A, the panel was asked to list additional ethical issues that could become important issues for physical therapists within the next 10 years. The panel members identified 12 statements as future ethical issues. Eight specific issues were identified from the 12 statements of ethical issues. Three of the six panel members also stated that all of the issues identified as current issues would be likely to remain in the future. One panel member stated, "I don't expect the issue to change substantially in the next 10 years, and I doubt that many of the current issues will be totally resolved in the next 10 years, either." The 8 original statements of the future ethical issues are listed in Figure 3.

The results of the second round of the study achieved consensus on four of the statements of future ethical issues. The third round of the Delphi study did not provide any change in the results obtained from the second round. The three rounds of questionnaires identified the four consensus future ethical issues, which are listed in Figure 4. A fourth round was not considered necessary as the responses of the panel did not show any changes between the second and third questionnaires.

The responses of the panel members to the first two questions of this study, relating to current ethical issues

and future ethical issues, resulted in the 16 distinct ethical issues that are listed in Figure 5. These 16 ethical issues have been included in a list as important issues facing physical therapists and constitute the final results of this study. I have combined both current and future ethical issues in the final list because a majority of the panel members felt that current ethical issues will remain in the future and future issues must be dealt with today. The distinction between future ethical issues and current ethical issues was not clear, and it seemed appropriate to combine all of the ethical issues into one composite list.

Discussion

The 16 issues identified in this study dealt with a wide variety of topics relating to different aspects of physical therapy practice. Further examination of these issues suggested three classifications of issues. For the purpose of discussion, the 16 issues have been divided into the following groups: (1) issues that relate to patient rights and welfare, (2) issues associated with professional responsibility and role, and (3) issues involving business relationships and economic considerations.

Dividing the issues into specific categories helps to focus the discussion on areas of general concern and to understand the relationships between various issues. There is necessarily some overlap of categories, as an issue in one category may also affect another category of issues. An example of this overlapping of categories is that a professional issue may also have an impact on patient welfare. The issues have been assigned to their specific category based on my determination as to what constituted the primary focus of that issue. This classification has been done for the purpose of discussion and with the understanding that there could be other groupings of these issues that are equally as valid.

Patients' Rights and Welfare

Issues were included in this category of issues if the primary focus of the concern related directly to the therapist interaction with the patient and involved the individual rights of the patient. Six issues were identified as belonging to this classification (Fig. 6). These issues focus on personal interaction and human rights and deal with informed consent, confidentiality, sexual and physical abuse, social characteristics, and personal relationships. Of the ethical issues identified in this section, the issue of the patient's right to informed consent has been most frequently discussed in physical therapy literature.[19,20,33,34] The ethical implications of this issue were examined by Coy[19] and Purtilo,[20] and the issue was discussed from a legal perspective by Banja and Wolf[33] and Scott.[34] Guccione also identified the issue of informed consent as a secondary issue in his 1980 study.[17] The only other issue from this category that has been discussed in the physical therapy literature is the

Consensus Choices

- The determination of the appropriate level of training, utilization, and supervision of supportive personnel other than physical therapists who assist in the delivery of physical therapy treatments
- The overutilization of physical therapy services
- The identification of the factors that constitute informed consent
- The protection of the patient's right to confidentiality in interactions with therapists, personnel under the supervision of therapists, and physical therapy students
- The justification of appropriate fees charged for the services rendered by physical therapists
- The maintenance of truth in advertising
- The identification and prevention of sexual misconduct (abuse) with patients by physical therapists
- The maintenance of clinical competence by physical therapists
- The adherence to ethical guidelines for the use of human subjects in clinical research
- The endorsement of equipment or products in which the physical therapist has a financial interest

Near-consensus choices

- The involvement of physical therapists in business relationships that have the potential for patient exploitation
- The identification and elimination of fraud in billing for physical therapy services
- The responsibility of physical therapists to provide adequate physical therapy services to all patients according to their need for care without regard to the patients' personal or social characteristics

Figure 2.
Final list of ethical issues identified by panel of experts in questionnaire C, question 1.

- The response of physical therapists to environmental issues of pollutants and health hazards associated with specific treatment modalities
- Discriminating in employment opportunities within physical therapy private practices
- The duty of physical therapists to report misconduct in colleagues
- Defining the limits of personal relationships within the professional setting
- How to address the issue of encroachment of other disciplines into the practice of physical therapy
- The utilization of treatment techniques without research to verify the degree of effectiveness
- The use of advertising in physical therapy practice
- The sexual and physical abuse of patients by physical therapists or those supervised by physical therapists

Figure 3.
Initial list of future ethical issues identified by panel members in questionnaire A, question 2.

issue of providing services without consideration of a patient's social characteristics. This issue was discussed by Sim and Purtilo[24] relative to the treatment of patients with AIDS. The remaining issues in this category have not yet been considered in the physical therapy literature. This omission includes the important issues of physical and sexual abuse, confidentiality, and the limits on personal relationships. The implications of these issues on the welfare and rights of patients are great and suggest a need for immediate discussion and study.

Professional Issues

The second category of issues was designated as professional issues. The issues in this category dealt primarily with policies that affect the delivery of physical therapy services and with physical therapists' interactions with other health professionals. The five issues identified as belonging to this classification are overutilization of services, maintaining clinical competence, supervision of personnel, the environment, and reporting misconduct

of others (Fig. 7). The only issue of this group that has been discussed in the physical therapy literature is the reporting of misconduct by colleagues, which was addressed by Banja[10] in 1985. In that article, Banja presented a clear description of the ethical principles and issues associated with whistle blowing.

Guccione,[17] in his 1980 study, identified as secondary issues three of the five issues that were classified as professional issues in the current study. The ethical issues identified in both Guccione's study and the current study related to (1) the use of support personnel, (2) the reporting of misconduct by colleagues, and (3) the responsibility of therapists to maintain clinical competence. Professional issues that have not been discussed include overutilization of services, utilization of support services, and maintenance of competence and standards. These are important issues that have a major impact on our relations with other organizations and professions. The recent examination of the health care industry has

- The responsibility of physical therapists to respond to the environmental issues of pollutants and health hazards associated with physical therapy treatment
- The duty of physical therapists to report misconduct in colleagues
- The need for therapists to define the limits of personal relationships within the professional setting
- The sexual and physical abuse of patients by physical therapists or those supervised by physical therapists

Figure 4.
Final list of future ethical issues identified by panel of experts in questionnaire C, question 2.

- The overutilization of physical therapy services
- The identification of the factors that constitute informed consent
- The protection of the patient's right to confidentiality in interactions with therapists, personnel under the supervision of therapists, and physical therapy students
- The justification of appropriate fees charged for the services rendered by physical therapists
- The maintenance of truth in advertising
- The identification and prevention of sexual and physical abuse of patients by physical therapists or those supervised by physical therapists
- The maintenance of clinical competence by physical therapists
- The adherence to ethical guidelines for the use of human subjects in clinical research
- The endorsement of equipment or products in which the physical therapist has a financial interest
- The determination of the appropriate level of training, utilization, and supervision of supportive personnel other than physical therapists who assist in the delivery of physical therapy treatments
- The involvement of physical therapists in business relationships that have the potential for patient exploitation
- The identification and elimination of fraud in billing for physical therapy services
- The responsibility of physical therapists to provide adequate physical therapy services to all patients according to their need for care without regard to the patients' personal or social characteristics
- The responsibility of physical therapists to respond to the environmental issues of pollutants and health hazards associated with physical therapy treatment
- The duty of physical therapists to report misconduct in colleagues
- The need for therapists to define the limits of personal relationships within the professional setting

Figure 5.
Final list of current and future ethical issues identified by panel of experts.

brought many of these issues into policy discussions and decisions. It is important that physical therapists engage themselves in those discussions and consider the policy changes from an ethical as well as an economic point of view. To assist in determining the appropriate ethical position for the profession of physical therapy through these changing times, we need further study and discussion of the ethical implications of the policies being considered.

Business and Economics

The third category of issues related to business relationships and economic factors. For an issue to be included in this category, its primary focus had to be related to financial considerations. The five issues in this category dealt with appropriate fees, advertising, endorsement of equipment, exploitive business relationships, and fraud in billing (Fig. 8). These are all issues that determine how physical therapists conduct themselves in relation to the business aspects of the profession. The fair and appropriate use of resources is an important consideration for all health care providers. The current discus-

sions at the national level on the containment of health care costs emphasized the importance of the examination of these issues by individual health professions. In this examination, it is again important to identify and discuss the ethical considerations as well as the financial issues.

None of the issues identified in this category have been discussed from an ethical perspective in the physical therapy literature. Guccione[17] did not identify any of the issues listed in this category as either primary or secondary issues. There has been an absence of formal discussion on the important ethical issues relating to business interaction. This appears to be an area that has great potential and need for exploration and study.

Limitations

My study was designed to stimulate and help clarify the discussion of ethics within the profession of physical therapy. The results of this study should be viewed in the context of the study's limitations. The first limitation was the small size of the panel of experts and whether they

- The identification of the factors that constitute informed consent
- The protection of the patient's right to confidentiality in interactions with therapists, personnel under the supervision of therapists, and physical therapy students
- The identification and prevention of sexual and physical abuse of patients by physical therapists or those supervised by physical therapists
- The adherence to ethical guidelines for the use of human subjects in clinical research
- The responsibility of physical therapists to provide adequate physical therapy services to all patients according to their need for care without regard to the patients' personal or social characteristics
- The need for therapists to define the limits of personal relationships within the professional setting

Figure 6.
Issues relating to patients' rights and welfare.

- The overutilization of physical therapy services
- The maintenance of clinical competence by physical therapists
- The determination of the appropriate level of training, utilization, and supervision of supportive personnel other than physical therapists who assist in the delivery of physical therapy treatments
- The responsibility of physical therapists to respond to the environmental issues of pollutants and health hazards associated with physical therapy treatment
- The duty of physical therapists to report misconduct in colleagues

Figure 7.
Issues of professional role and responsibility.

were representative of all experts. To choose a panel, it was necessary to outline specific procedures prior to the study. These procedures were then followed throughout the study. This process identified a panel of six experts. This is a relatively small panel size but not necessarily a problem for a Delphi study. The primary problem associated with a small panel is that the number of issues that are identified would be limited to the experiences of the small number of panel members. This could lead to some important issues being overlooked. The panel should represent a broad constituency and diverse opinions.

The six-person panel used in this study appeared to represent a large portion of the physical therapy community, but it is still likely that some issues may have been overlooked due to the small size of the panel. As described earlier, the panel consisted of four men and 2 women. This gender ratio does not accurately reflect the population of physical therapists in the United States, which is 76% female and 24% male.[32] This discrepancy could result in a bias toward issues of concern to male therapists and less emphasis on issues that have greater impact on female therapists. It would therefore be prudent not to consider this study as all-inclusive or to limit the discussions of ethical issues in physical therapy to only the ethical issues identified in this study. Important ethical issues could have been overlooked by the panel of experts participating in the study.

Another limitation was the focus on the development of general statements about ethical issues. These represen-

tations removed the contextual information from the issues in an attempt to create more generic statements that reflect many specific instances. Because ethical action takes place in specific situations in which the particular context defines the ethical issue, this removal of context creates the risk of making these statements of issues too generic to be useful or meaningful. To address that limitation, the purpose of the study needs to be considered. The purposes of this study were to identify ethical issues that warrant further analysis and to stimulate discussion. The initial step in this process needed to be a broad one that could initiate additional study. The broad statements of the ethical issues identified in this study need to be understood as representing constellations of similar specific issues, which then need to be separated by further studies. This study was useful in identifying these broad issues but did not address specific cases. The results of the study also suggest the need for a series of more focused studies on the particular broad issues that could then identify the specific forms the issue may take. That type of study would provide a way to examine the particular cases and stories associated with the issue. The process for coming to an understanding about the ethical components of our practice requires many steps, and this study should be viewed as only one of the steps toward that understanding.

Recommendations and Conclusion

Within each of the three categories, I believe that there is an identified need for further study. Areas of inquiry that could provide important additional information

- The justification of appropriate fees charged for the services rendered by physical therapists
- The maintenance of truth in advertising
- The endorsement of equipment or products in which the physical therapist has a financial interest
- The involvement of physical therapists in business relationships that have potential for patient exploitation
- The identification and elimination of fraud in billing for physical therapy services

Figure 8.
Issues involving business relationships and economic factors.

include (1) a comprehensive examination of the broad issues identified in the study to identify the specific instances and problems, (2) a broad study of clinicians to identify additional ethical issues that may have been omitted in this study and to identify the importance of these issues in practice, and (3) a study to examine the methods and substance of the current teaching of ethics within physical therapy curricula, and (4) a series of studies to examine the effects of various teaching methods on the moral development of physical therapy students. Each of these areas of future study has great potential for adding to the understanding of ethical thought and action in physical therapy practice.

In order to broaden the discussion of ethics within physical therapy, a comprehensive study was needed to identify the ethical issues that are important to the current practice of physical therapy. This study was undertaken to fulfill that need. The ethical issues presented in Figure 5 provide us with a list of important ethical issues that warrant examination. The Delphi method used in this study provides a high degree of confidence that the 16 issues identified in this study are ethical issues of some importance to physical therapy practice. A panel of experts have agreed that these issues should be included as a part of a list of important ethical issues facing physical therapy. Although there may be other ethical issues that were overlooked in this study, I believe that the 16 issues listed provide a good starting point for the study of ethical issues facing physical therapists. Some additional goals of this study were to generate greater discussion of ethical issues and to promote additional study of the specific issues that were identified.

Ethical decision making and ethical action have long been an important component of professional development. Discussion of ethical issues relating to physical therapy, however, has been limited in the physical therapy literature. This deficit needs to be addressed as physical therapy develops as an autonomous profession. The integrity and diligence with which a profession examines its unique ethical issues, understands its ethical interactions, and develops methods for educating its students will largely determine the moral position of that profession. Physical therapists have begun that process, but additional study is needed to understand and clarify the issues relating to the practice of physical therapy. Increased dialogue among physical therapists and further study will help us chart the best moral course through the many changes facing our profession.

References

1 Purtilo RB, Cassel CK. *Ethical Dimensions in the Health Profession.* Philadelphia, Pa: WB Saunders Co; 1981.

2 Veatch RM, Sollitto S. Medical ethics teaching: report of a national medical school survey. *JAMA.* 1976;235:1030–1033.

3 Burch E, Mathews J, eds. *Practice Issues in Physical Therapy.* Thorofare, NJ: Slack Inc; 1989:5–28.

4 Hardenbergh H. Ethics for the physical therapist: from the point of view of the medical practitioner. *Phys Ther Rev.* 1946;26:231–233.

5 Haskell O. Essentials of professional ethics in physical therapy. *Phys Ther Rev.* 1949;29:231–233.

6 Marton T. Ethics. *Phys Ther Rev.* 1950;30:178.

7 McLoughlin CJ. Ethics and the physical therapy technician. *Phys Ther Rev.* 1941;21:203.

8 Arey LB. Ancient precepts for the modern practitioner. *Phys Ther Rev.* 1951;31:10.

9 Purtilo RB. The American Physical Therapy Association's *Code of Ethics*: its historical foundation. *Phys Ther.* 1977;57:1001–1006.

10 Banja J. Whistle blowing in physical therapy. *Phys Ther.* 1985;65:1683–1695.

11 Guccione AA. Compliance and patient autonomy: ethical and legal limits to professional dominance. *Topics in Geriatric Rehabilitation.* 1988;3(3):62–73.

12 Purtilo RB. Understanding ethical issues: the physical therapist as ethicist. *Phys Ther.* 1974;54:239–243.

13 Purtilo RB. Reading *Physical Therapy* from an ethics perspective. *Phys Ther.* 1975:55:361–364.

14 Purtilo RB. Who should make moral policy decisions in health care? *Phys Ther.* 1978;58:1076–1081.

15 Purtilo RB. Ethics in allied health education: state of the art. *J Allied Health.* 1983;12:211–212.

16 Purtilo RB. Professional responsibility in physiotherapy: old dimensions and new directions. *Physiotherapy.* 1986;72:579–583.

17 Guccione AA. Ethical issues in physical therapy practice: a survey of physical therapists in New England. *Phys Ther.* 1980;60:1264–1272.

18 Purtilo RB. Structure of ethics in teaching physical therapy: a survey. *Phys Ther.* 1979;59:1102–1106.

19 Coy J. Autonomy-based informed consent: ethical implications for patient noncompliance. *Phys Ther.* 1989;69:826–833.

20 Purtilo RB. Applying the principles of informed consent to patient care. *Phys Ther.* 1984;64:934–937.

21 Clompton N, McMahon T. Patient compliance. *Clinical Management.* 1992;12(1):59–65.

22 Davis AJ. Clinical nurses' ethical decision making in situations of informed consent. *ANS Adv Nurs Sci.* 1989;11(3):63–69.

23 Hansen RA. The ethics of caring for patients with AIDS. *Am J Occup Ther.* 1990;44:239–242.

24 Sim J, Purtilo RB. An ethical analysis of physical therapists' duty to treat persons who have AIDS: homosexual patient as a test case. *Phys Ther.* 1991;71:650–655.

25 Chaney H. Needs assessment: a Delphi approach. *Journal of Nursing Staff Development.* 1987;3:48–53.

26 Couper MR. The Delphi technique: characteristics and sequence model. *Journal of Advances in Nursing Science.* 1984;7:72–77.

27 Goodman CM. The Delphi technique: a critique. *Journal of Advances in Nursing Science.* 1987;12:729–734.

28 Helmer O. *Looking Forward: A Guide to Future Research.* London, England: Sage Publications Ltd; 1983:134–157.

29 Rasp A. Delphi: a decision-maker's dream. *Nation's Schools.* 1973; 92(1):29–32.

30 Weatherman R, Swenson K. Delphi techniques. In: Handey SP, Yates JR, eds. *Futurism in Education.* Berkeley, Calif: Cutchan; 1974:97–112.

31 Weaver T. The Delphi forecasting method. *Phi Delta Kappan.* 1971;52(5):267–272.

32 Gender-Based Career Differences in Physical Therapy. In: *APTA Research Briefings.* 1995;2(1).

33 Banja JD, Wolf SL. Malpractice litigation for uninformed consent to patient care: legal and ethical considerations for physical therapy. *Phys Ther.* 1987;67:1226–1229.

34 Scott RW. Informed consent. *Clinical Management.* 1991;11(3):12–14.

● Invited Commentary

Triezenberg's study is a fine example of "descriptive ethics." Descriptive ethics uses the methods of empirical research to identify the perceived ethical issues facing practitioners or others in a given health professions group. The goal of descriptive ethics is to describe the factual basis of practice to better evaluate what ought to be encouraged in the profession. In that regard descriptive ethics is very much a part of the endeavor to create a more ethical environment for all involved in health care. The term "descriptive *ethics*" may be misleading to some, only insofar as most people think that ethics must concentrate directly on the right- or wrong-making characteristics of acts or the virtue of professionals. A more accurate distinction is to call the latter "normative ethics."

As Triezenberg notes correctly, the profession of physical therapy has been slow to generate data by which to judge the focus for ethicists, physical therapy practitioners, and policymakers in their efforts to help create ethical practices and policies relevant to the actual situations facing physical therapy.

Triezenberg's study makes a signal contribution in several specific ways. First, it further legitimizes physical therapy as a profession. As he notes in the article, one of the descriptors of a profession is that the group has ethical issues and they are taken seriously. Second, his study provides an opportunity for considered and informed discourse with other health care disciplines. In an era when strong winds are creating sometimes stormy seas in the health professions world, the necessity of identifying common values, issues, and ethical challenges takes on greater importance than when there are few waves of change. Data such as this study provides are

resources for survival as well as the ability to thrive in an unsettled moment.

A third contribution is that his and other such studies by physical therapists provide public statements about the ethical concerns physical therapists themselves are identifying as a focus for their reflection and action. This, in turn, allows for others to evaluate and correct the profession's self-perceptions. For instance, it is interesting that Triezenberg's panel of experts identified informed consent as a key issue for physical therapists. At the same time, some writers are questioning whether informed consent is an ideal method of enablement and communication for complex processes such as rehabilitation. At the very least, the fact that the physical therapy profession is aware of this mechanism and has named the issue for discussion signals that we are willing to be on the front lines of rethinking informed consent, if necessary.

There are also some caveats in this type of study. One caveat is embedded in the 19th century philosopher George E Moore's adage: "Is does not imply ought." In other words, simply identifying what *is* (perceived to be an ethics issue) does not *necessarily* lead to direct guidance about what (the ethical standards) *ought* to be. Put another way, although Triezenberg succeeds in delineating the group's key areas of ethical concern, the consensus of the group could be faulty, short-sighted, or otherwise unhelpful in determining how physical therapists can become more ethical in their practice. The worst outcome would be that readers will not allow room for error in the panel of experts' perceptions about what the most important ethical issues are or to limit further identification of new issues as they arise. A time-honored method of testing the accuracy of a small group's perception of the moral life is to measure their judgments against standards of the profession and larger society. Although even this is not foolproof (ie, there are unjust laws and misguided guidelines), it does serve as a system of checks and balances.

Triezenberg notes that the small number of subjects created a limitation. Although he is speaking from a research design perspective, the comment also could apply to the fact that wisdom about the moral life is not a private or even small-group-of-experts affair. One "higher standard" the experts and the profession as a whole have are a number of documents that bring together the best collective judgment of the profession over time. Our *Code of Ethics* and *Guide to Professional Conduct* are two such documents.

There is a possibility that what professionals identify as important ethical issues are not judged similarly by patients. Because our raison d'être is to provide good patient care, the ethical issues have significance only if patients are indeed benefited by our concerns with such issues. Sociologists and others have leveled the criticism against professionals that much of what we do is in our own *self*-interest rather than for the benefit of the patients we "profess" to be serving or the society that allows us privileges in exchange for our services. It would be a useful exercise to compare Triezenberg's identification of ethical issues with issues perceived by patients to present ethical dilemmas in the physical therapy context.

In spite of these few caveats about studies of this type, overall Triezenberg's study is a welcome and needed addition, enhancing the profession's awareness of its responsibilities to patients, the profession, and society. The more physical therapists can do to create a broad base of understanding about the ethical issues facing the profession, the more likely we are to enter the new millennium prepared to make a meaningful contribution.

Ruth Purtilo, PhD, FAPTA
Director
Center for Health Policy and Ethics
Creighton University
2500 California Plaza
Omaha, NE 68178

● Author Response

I want to thank Dr Purtilo for her review and thoughtful comments regarding my article "The Identification of Ethical Issues in Physical Therapy Practice." Her commentary serves as an additional conclusion to my study. Dr Purtilo clearly identifies both the potential contributions of this study and many additional questions that need to be investigated and actively discussed in the physical therapy community.

I wholeheartedly agree with Dr Purtilo's suggestion that we expand the discussion of these issues to include the perceptions of more than a small group of individuals nominated as experts in the area of professional ethics. The variety of practice settings and continual changes in our roles and responsibilities as clinicians provide many new and evolving issues. Discussion about the many faces of an ethical issue from differing clinical and individual perspectives could provide valuable insights to others on how one might approach similar situations; alternatively, such discussion can shed light on the ubiquity and complexity of ethical issues that arise in everyday practice. I hope that my study assists in stimulating and facilitating such discussion by identifying issues but does not limit the breadth and depth of consideration about these and other ethical issues in physical therapy.

I am also in strong agreement with Dr Purtilo's observation that we need to place the interests of the patient at the center of our concerns. Good patient care must guide our discussions of ethical issues. Yet it is in the exploration and defining of what is "good" or "best" care that many ethical issues and the moral foundation and commitments of our profession will emerge. To define what is good care, it is of utmost importance that patients are invited into, and engaged in, ongoing dialogue with physical therapists regarding their perceptions about and expectations of physical therapists in our clinical encounters with them. A patient's perspective of a situation may differ significantly from that of the clinician. We need to consider these differences of perspective in all discussions. This is an area of study that could provide interesting and invaluable information and guidance as we continue to shape a caring and exemplary rehabilitation profession.

In the final paragraph of her commentary, Dr Purtilo states: "The more physical therapists can do to create a broad base of understanding about the ethical issues facing the profession, the more likely we are to enter the new millennium prepared to make a meaningful contribution." Her statement exemplifies the purpose of this study and presents a challenge for the future. An understanding of our ethical issues and our day-to-day thinking and action will need to be based on the observations, thoughts, and stories of clinicians, patients, family members, and experts. This suggests the need for further study and discussion to prepare us to make the greatest contribution to our patients, health care, and society today and in the future.

Herman L Triezenberg, PhD, PT

Research Report

A Retrospective Analysis of Ethics Knowledge in Physical Therapy (1970–2000)

Background and Purpose. Purtilo, Guccione, and others have noted that increased clinical autonomy for physical therapists presents more complex ethical dilemmas. The body of literature examining physical therapy ethics, however, is relatively small and has not been analyzed. The primary purposes of this research were: (1) to use multiple perspectives to describe and analyze literature examining ethics in physical therapy from 1970 to 2000, (2) to develop a model to describe the evolution of knowledge of ethics in physical therapy during this period, and (3) to compare the proposed model with the evolutionary models proposed by Purtilo in physical therapy and by Pellegrino in bioethics. Sample. The sample consisted of peer-reviewed journal articles cited in the MEDLINE or Cumulative Index to Nursing and Allied Health Literature (CINAHL) databases between 1970 and 2000 or referenced in *Ethics in Physical Therapy*. Methods. A two-phase mixed quantitative and qualitative method was used to analyze publications. In the quantitative phase, the author sorted publications into a priori categories, including approach to ethics, author, decade, country of publication, role of the physical therapist, and component of morality. During the qualitative phase of the research, the author analyzed and sorted the publications to identify common themes, patterns, similarities, and evolutionary trends. These findings were compared with the evolutionary models of Pellegrino and Purtilo. Results. The 90 publications meeting inclusion criteria were predominantly philosophical, using the "principles" perspective; focused on the patient/client management role of the physical therapist; and addressed the moral judgment component of moral behavior. As predicted by Purtilo's model, the focus of identity evolved from self-identity to patient-focused identity, with increasing representation of societal identity. Recurrent themes included the need to further identify and clarify physical therapists' ethical dilemmas, the interrelationship between clinical and ethical decision making, and the changing relationship with patients. Discussion and Conclusion. Although knowledge of ethics grew steadily between 1970 and 2000, this retrospective analysis identified gaps in our current knowledge. Further research is needed to address the unique ethical problems commonly encountered in all 5 roles of the physical therapist; patient perspectives on ethical issues in physical therapy; variety in ethical approaches; factors affecting moral judgment, sensitivity, motivation, and courage; and cultural dimensions of ethical practice in physical therapy. [Swisher LL. A retrospective analysis of ethics knowledge in physical therapy (1970–2000). *Phys Ther.* 2002;82:692–706.]

Key Words: *Morality, Physical therapy profession, Professional ethics, Research.*

Laura Lee Swisher

O ver the last 30 years, physical therapists have sought a more autonomous clinical decision-making role within the health care system.[1,2] Leaders within physical therapy have repeatedly noted that increased autonomy brings more complex ethical dilemmas and responsibility.[3–7] Charles Magistro warned in 1989: "As physical therapists assume a more autonomous role in health care delivery, ethical judgments will play an increasingly important role in the gamut of clinical decisions a physical therapist will have to make."[3(p531)] Significantly, Magistro framed ethical decision making as part of clinical decision making. Building on Magistro's insights, Clawson described ethical decision making as a "component" of clinical decision making,[8(p14)] arguing that "physical therapists must try harder to assimilate ethical theory into their daily decision-making."[8(p11)]

Recent studies in physical therapy expertise support the notion that moral knowledge is embedded in the fabric of everyday physical therapy decision making.[9,10] Ethical decision making and moral virtue are dimensions of clinical expertise rather than separate steps in the process of providing physical therapy. A physical therapist, for example, who encounters signs of physical abuse during the examination of a patient faces a problem that is both clinical and ethical. Because ethical issues are embedded within clinical encounters, each health care profession encounters different ethical dilemmas and problems. Ruth Purtilo,[5,6] the first to focus attention on the unique nature of physical therapists' ethical dilemmas, identified the need to determine the ethical issues encountered by physical therapists.

Despite increasing recognition of the ethical dimensions of physical therapy practice, Guccione's 1980 report on a survey of ethical issues in physical therapy practice indicated little progress in this area of study, and he observed that the "ethical dimension of actual clinical practice is not well-documented in the literature."[7(p1265)] In the same report, he noted that "[t]he need to identify and clarify ethical issues within a health profession increases as the profession assumes responsibility for those areas of direct care in its domain."[7(p1264)] Guccione issued this warning:

> The educational implication of this data is inescapable: in order to meet all the challenges of clinical practice, physical therapy students must be taught how to make ethical as well as clinical judgments. To prepare future clinicians less adequately could jeopardize the integrity and the autonomy that physical therapy as a health profession has so arduously worked to achieve.[7(p1271)]

Nearly 2 decades later, Triezenberg observed, "During the 1980s and 1990s, however, there were still very few articles that addressed ethical issues in physical therapy."[11(p1099)]

The limited attention given to ethical issues in the physical therapy literature poses particular problems in the current managed care environment. As professionals, I believe, physical therapists have historically placed fidelity to their patients as their first priority. Under managed care, however, physical therapists are asked to balance fiscal accountability with the professional obligation to fidelity.[12] When the managed care provider approves only 6 outpatient physical therapy visits for a 16-year-old after traumatic brain injury, the situation simultaneously presents a clinical and ethical dilemma. How can the patient achieve maximum rehabilitation potential? To what extent should the therapist advocate

LL Swisher, PT, PhD, is Assistant Professor, School of Physical Therapy, University of South Florida, MDC 77, Tampa, FL 33612-4766 (USA) (LSwisher@hsc.usf.edu).

This article was submitted August 17, 2001, and was accepted January 22, 2002.

for the patient? If the managed care company provides incentives for cost containment, the physical therapist may also have a dilemma between fidelity to the patient and economic self-interest or even organizational survival. Given the ethical dilemmas posed by managed care, Purtilo's and Guccione's concern that moral knowledge should keep pace with the increasing complexity and evolving professional autonomy of the physical therapy profession appears to be even more relevant.

Since the 1970s, physical therapy has continued to evolve in terms of professional autonomy (freedom and independence in making and implementing professional judgments).[13(p29)] However, it is legitimate to ask whether knowledge of ethics in physical therapy has kept pace with the increasing challenges delineated by Magistro,[3] Purtilo,[5,6] Guccione,[7] and others.[4,14,15] The answer to this question, in my view, requires an understanding of ethics as a discipline, the development of professional ethics in physical therapy, and the changing context of bioethics in the United States.

The discipline of ethics provides one perspective for understanding the evolution of physical ethics. The field of ethics typically divides the study of ethics into philosophical or normative ethics and descriptive or social scientific ethics.[16(pp6–7)] Philosophical ethics is concerned with what people ought to do and how they ought to conduct themselves (normative or prescriptive ethics), as well as the rational basis for these types of decisions (metaethics or analytic ethics). The philosophical approach to ethics embraces the deontological, utilitarian, care, virtue, and principles[17] approaches. Social scientific or descriptive ethics focuses on studying human ethical behavior with social scientific or empirical tools.[16(pp6–7)] The 2 ethical approaches also differ in purpose and goal. The goal of philosophical ethics is to prescribe action, to shed light on what "ought" to happen. The goal of social scientific or descriptive ethics, however, is to explore what "is."[16] The ethical problem of truth telling highlights the differences between the 2 approaches. In social scientific ethics, a psychologist or social scientist might analyze the influence of social and contextual factors in telling the truth (What is the prevalence of not telling the truth in specific contexts, and what factors affect whether people tell the truth?). Philosophical ethics, however, is concerned with prescribing human action (Under what conditions is one obligated to tell or not to tell the truth?) and with moral judgments about truth telling (It is always right to tell the truth, or not telling the truth has negative consequences.).[16(pp5–7)]

Recently, a number of ethicists have called for an approach that brings together the philosophical and social scientific perspectives. Nelson noted, "The common picture of the relationship between bioethics and the social sciences oversimplifies the relationships between the moral, the empirical, and the conceptual."[18(p13)] Similarly, Zussman observed that both philosophical and social scientific approaches have normative and empirical dimensions: "The best work in both disciplines should recognize the different ways in which they each join normative reflection and empirical description."[19(p7)] To make an ethical decision requires normative commitments and factual information. As Nelson and Zussman implied, the traditional model of ethics that rigidly separates facts from values represents a limited model of ethical behavior.

The unidimensional nature of ethical behavior implied by either a strictly philosophic or social scientific ethic points to the need for a multidimensional model of ethical behavior to blend normative and empirical elements. Working from a psychological perspective, James Rest[20] developed the Four Component Model of Moral Behavior. Rest's model contends that ethical behavior involves at least 4 psychological components: ethical sensitivity (recognizing and interpreting situations), moral judgment (making a decision about right or wrong and determining a course of action), moral motivation (putting ethical values before other values), and moral courage (persevering against adversity).[20] He emphasized that the components are not steps but psychological processes that may overlap and occur simultaneously.

In describing the evolution of bioethics, Pellegrino[21] has also identified this blending of the philosophical and social scientific. According to Pellegrino, the metamorphosis of bioethics embraces 3 time periods, with each having its own unique thread and language: the era of proto-bioethics, the era of philosophical bioethics, and the era of global bioethics. Pellegrino stated, "In the proto-bioethics period [1960 to 1972], the language of human values predominated; in the era of bioethics philosophically construed [1972 to 1985], it was the language of philosophical ethics; and in the era of bioethics globally construed [1985 to present], the social and behavioral sciences have gained greater prominence."[21(p74)] Pellegrino noted that the period of philosophical ethics relied heavily on the ethical approach called "principlism"[17] (or the "four principles approach"). The principles perspective uses the philosophical concepts of common morality as the basis for making decisions: autonomy, beneficence, nonmaleficence, and justice. Ultimately, the focus on philosophical ethical principles was not adequate to the complexity of psychosocial, economic, sociological, legal, cultural, religious, and organizational factors involved in moral dilemmas. Pellegrino contended that attention to each of the 3 threads (human values, philo-

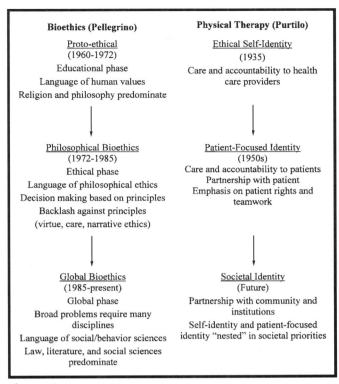

Bioethics (Pellegrino)

Proto-ethical
(1960-1972)
Educational phase
Language of human values
Religion and philosophy predominate

Philosophical Bioethics
(1972-1985)
Ethical phase
Language of philosophical ethics
Decision making based on principles
Backlash against principles
(virtue, care, narrative ethics)

Global Bioethics
(1985-present)
Global phase
Broad problems require many
disciplines
Language of social/behavior sciences
Law, literature, and social sciences
predominate

Physical Therapy (Purtilo)

Ethical Self-Identity
(1935)
Care and accountability to health
care providers

Patient-Focused Identity
(1950s)
Care and accountability to patients
Partnership with patient
Emphasis on patient rights and
teamwork

Societal Identity
(Future)
Partnership with community and
institutions
Self-identity and patient-focused
identity "nested" in societal priorities

Figure 1.
Periods of ethics in medicine (Pellegrino[21,23]) and physical therapy
(Purtilo[22]).

sophical ethics, and social and behavioral sciences) is critical in the emerging interdisciplinary synthesis of global bioethics because moral problems are inherently multidimensional.[21(pp84–85)]

Purtilo[22] has described the evolution of professional ethics in the physical therapy profession as the "seeds" of care and accountability adapting to the changing social environment. In contrast to Pellegrino's focus on the language and methods used in each period, Purtilo's model focuses on the commitments (care) and duties and responsibilities (accountability) inherent in professional relationships. During the period of self-identity (beginning with the 1935 American Physical Therapy Association Code of Ethics), professional ethics, in Purtilo's opinion, focused on establishing commitment and accountability to other health care professionals. In the period of patient-focused identity (1950s to the present), according to Purtilo, ethics focused on "establishing a true partnership with patients as persons"[22(p1115)] against a social backdrop of increasing emphasis on patients rights and teamwork in health care. Purtilo described an emerging future period, the period of societal identity, as blending the 2 previous seasons. According to Purtilo, the primary ethical task of the new period of societal identity would be to "establish the moral foundations for a true professional partnering with the larger community of citizens and institutions."[22(p1116)] Figure 1 com-

pares Purtilo's 3 periods of physical therapy ethics[20] with Pellegrino's 3 periods of bioethics.[21,23]

The primary purposes of my research were: (1) to use multiple perspectives to describe and analyze the literature examining ethics in physical therapy from 1970 to 2000, (2) to develop a model to describe the evolution of knowledge of ethics in physical therapy during this period, and (3) to compare the proposed model to the evolutionary models proposed by Purtilo in physical therapy and by Pellegrino in bioethics. The multiple perspectives used to analyze and describe the literature examining ethics in physical therapy included ethical approaches, issues and topics, components of moral behavior, role of the physical therapist, and evolutionary period. Figure 2 presents a diagrammatic representation of the model of analysis used in this study.

Method

Sample

The sample consisted of peer-reviewed journal articles cited in the MEDLINE[24] or Cumulative Index to Nursing and Allied Health Literature (CINAHL)[25] electronic database indexes between 1970 and July 2000 and relevant peer-reviewed journal articles published or referenced in the 2-volume set, *Ethics in Physical Therapy.*[26] For the purposes of this study, the term "physical therapy ethics" meant explicit reflection on right or wrong behavior in performing the professional role of the physical therapist. There is some debate as to whether the terms "ethics" and "morality" may be distinguished. Those who distinguish ethics from morality note that ethics involves systematic or conscious rational reflection.[16,27,28] Morality refers to the complex of personal and social rules and values that guide human conduct.[16(pp2–3),27(p12),28(p5),29(p3)] To add to the confusion, the adjective forms of these terms are often used interchangeably.[16(p2),29(p3)] Because the topic of interest of my study was the body of knowledge that consciously reflects on right and wrong behavior in the professional role of the physical therapist, the term "ethics" was most appropriate for this task. Although some people distinguish between the adjectives "ethical" and "moral," the terms are used interchangeably throughout the text.

Inclusion criteria were: (1) English-language article; (2) publication in a peer-reviewed journal between 1970 and July 2000; (3) physical therapy ethics as an explicit major subject, topic, or key word; (4) primary target audience of physical therapy professionals or rehabilitation professionals, including physical therapists; and (5) referenced or published in MEDLINE, CINAHL, or *Ethics in Physical Therapy.* Because the overall purpose of the study was to examine advances in knowledge of ethics in physical therapy in the United States, the

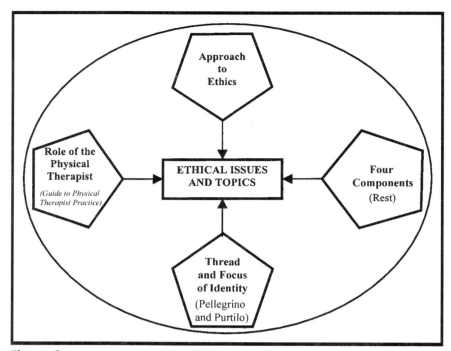

Figure 2.
Model for analysis.

descriptive techniques to identify the number of publications by author, country of publication, and journal of publication. I then categorized publications into a priori categories, including ethical approach, decade, component of morality, physical therapy period (focus of identity), bioethics period (thread), and primary role of the physical therapist as described in the *Guide to Physical Therapist Practice*[31] (patient client management, administration, critical inquiry, education, consultation). To determine periods according to the evolutionary models of Purtilo and Pellegrino, each article was classified as representing Purtilo's self-identity, patient-focused identity, or societal identity and Pellegrino's thread of values, philosophical ethics, or social science. Although I performed numerous data sorts from a variety of perspectives, the discussion in this article is limited to the elements described in the purpose statement and illustrated in Figure 2. Following entry of data onto a computer spreadsheet, the SPSS[32] statistical software program* was used to compute descriptive statistics.

One data sort involved categorizing each publication according to component or morality using Rest's Four Component Model.[20] Because some overlap exists among moral sensitivity, moral judgment, moral motivation, and moral courage, the determining factor in classification was the purpose of the article. For example, Coy[33] described the use of the principle of autonomy in making decisions about informed consent. Although the discussion of informed consent might also help the therapist recognize and interpret situations involving informed consent (moral sensitivity), the primary intention of the publication was to discuss the ethical foundation for making decisions about informed consent (moral judgment). Publications that focused on more than one component were classified as addressing multiple components. The article "Understanding Ethical Issues: The Physical Therapist as Ethicist" by Purtilo[5] looked at both moral judgment and moral sensitivity and fit into this category.

Qualitative analysis generally followed the format of Miles and Huberman[34(p9)] in assigning codes, making notes, sorting, and sifting to identify themes. During this phase of the research, I clarified descriptive results and identified

sample excluded routine publication of professional codes of ethics, standards, or position statements and non–peer-reviewed journal articles. Additional exclusion criteria were: (1) non-English language, (2) major topic not related to physical therapy ethics, (3) non–physical therapy target audience, (4) letters to the editor, or (5) editorials.

Procedure

During the summer of 2000, a literature search was conducted using the terms "physical therapy" and ethics-related terms (eg, "ethics," "morality," "morals," "autonomy," "confidentiality," "informed consent," "moral reasoning," "moral judgment," "justice," "paternalism," "care," "duty," "responsibility," "discrimination," "attitudes," "values") for the specified time periods. The search used multiple terms because of the lack of agreement on the terms "ethics" and "morality," the paucity of literature using the key word "ethics," and the desire to include appropriate publications from all approaches. Regardless of terminology, publications that did not consciously reflect on ethics were excluded from the sample. Because the CINAHL electronic database did not begin until 1982, the CINAHL index was searched by hand for the years 1970 through 1982.

A two-phase mixed quantitative and qualitative research method[30] was used to analyze publications. I made notes on each publication related to the descriptive categories and qualitative codes. In the quantitative phase, I used

* SPSS Inc, 233 S Wacker Dr, Chicago, IL 60606.

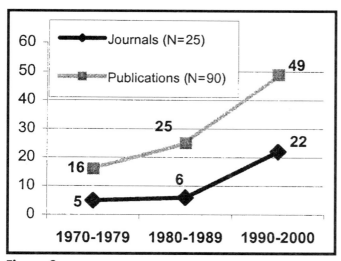

Figure 3.
Number of publications and journals in each decade (not cumulative over the decades).

Table 1.
First Authors With Multiple Publications in the Sample[a]

Author (Country of Residence)	Number	Percentage
Ruth Purtilo (United States)	15	16.67
Julius Sim (United Kingdom)	10	11.11
Rosemary Barnitt* (United Kingdom)	5	5.56
Sandy Elkin (New Zealand)	4	4.44
Eugene Michels (United States)	3	3.33
John Banja* (United States)	2	2.22
Claudette Finley (United States)	2	2.22
David Thomasma* (United States)	2	2.22
Herman Triezenberg (United States)	2	2.22
First authors of single publications	45	50.00
Total	90	99.99

[a] Asterisk indicates author is not a physical therapist.

themes, patterns, and similarities within the publications. For example, I used a number of different a priori categories to sort the publications by issue or topic. These categories included philosophical principles (autonomy, justice, beneficence, veracity, confidentiality, and informed consent), setting, and focus of relationships. Documents that did not fit into the existing categories were analyzed to develop final categories. After determining issues for each article, the data were sorted into 3 decades and analyzed to determine topical themes for each decade.

Because one purpose of my study was to analyze evolutionary trends in the physical therapy literature on ethics in the United States, publications that focused on topics unique to settings outside the United States were excluded from that portion of the analysis. Nine of the 90 publications fell into this category. Publications in foreign journals or written by authors outside of the United States were not automatically excluded from the study because I felt that the reader in the United States could apply the information to a different setting. For example, Haswell[35] addressed changes in informed consent procedures for manual therapy of the cervical spine in Australia. Although the details of Australian policies may or may not be relevant to practice in the United States, the ethical dilemmas are not entirely different. In brief, at least some ethical issues in physical therapy transcend national boundaries.

Results

Ninety articles[†] published in 25 peer-reviewed journals between 1970 and July 2000 met the inclusion criteria. The total number of authors (including second to sixth authors) was 83. Figure 3 illustrates the number of

[†] References 3–11,14,15,33,35–112.

publications and journals in each decade and indicates a significant increase in number of publications and journals during the most recent decade.

Physical therapists served as first author of most publications (78.2%). Nine authors served as first author of half of the publications, and 3 authors (Purtilo,[5,6,36–48] Sim,[49–58] and Barnitt[59–63]) were first author of 33.3% of all publications (Tab. 1). Of the 25 journals in this sample, *Physical Therapy* published the highest number (n=36 or 40%).

Approach

Sorting publications into the 2 a priori categories (philosophical and social scientific) based on the ethical approach used indicated that 43.2% used a philosophical approach and 33.3% used a social scientific approach (Tab. 2). An analysis of the remaining publications produced 3 other approaches. The third category, professional/historical documents, included published conference addresses and historical reviews. Examples of the professional/historical category were the Mary McMillan Lectures of Ruth Wood[14] and Eugene Michels[64] and descriptions of the historical development (eg, code of ethics). The fourth emergent category (theoretical) contained publications that developed a theoretical model linking physical therapy practice and ethics. For example, Jensen et al[9] developed a model of physical therapy expertise that embraced moral virtue. Sim[56] compared models of health based on their ability to provide a foundation for ethical decision making. A final category of approach used legal concepts to interpret a policy or law. As indicated by Table 2, the philosophical approach was the most common in the first 2 decades studied. However, the percentage of articles using a social scientific approach increased with each decade, and there

Table 2.
Ethics Approach[a]

Approach	1970–1979 (n=14)	1980–1989 (n=24)	1990–2000 (n=43)	1970–2000 (n=81)
Philosophical	6 (42.9%)	11 (45.8%)	18 (41.9%)	35 (43.2%)
Social scientific	3 (21.4%)	6 (25.0%)	18 (41.9%)	27 (33.3%)
Professional/historical	5 (35.7%)	6 (25.0%)	0	11 (13.6%)
Law/policy interpretation	0	1 (4.2%)	1 (2.3%)	2 (2.5%)
Theoretical	0	0	6 (14.0%)	6 (7.4%)

[a] Values represent the number (percentage) of publications within the specified time periods (excludes publications with a focus specific to settings outside the United States).

Table 3.
Issues and Topics Listed by Corresponding Author

Issue or Topic	Authors
Ethical role, responsibilities, obligations	Magistro,[3] Singleton,[4] Richardson,[10] Wood,[14] Purtilo,[41] Sim and Purtilo,[49] Sim,[53] Michels,[64] Bellner,[67] Thomasma,[68] Hogshead[69]
Historical	Purtilo,[45] Elkin and Anderson,[70] Robinson,[71] Paynter,[72] Kline[73]
Moral decision-making process	Purtilo,[5] Clawson,[8] Jensen et al,[9] Sim,[56] Barnitt and Partridge,[61] Edwards,[66] Elkin and Anderson,[70] Thomasma and Pisanechi[74]
Identification of ethical issues	Purtilo,[6] Guccione,[7] Triezenberg,[11] Barnitt,[59,63] Barnitt and Partridge[61]
Ethical principles	
Autonomy	Giffin,[15] Coy,[33] Purtilo,[36] Sim[55,57] Kuczewski,[75] Meier and Purtilo,[76] Bruckner[77]
Informed consent/truth telling	Coy,[33] Haswell,[35] Purtilo,[36] Sim,[55,57] Barnitt,[63] Kuczewski,[75] Elkin and Anderson,[78] Delany,[79] Banja and Wolf,[80] Michels,[81,82] Ramsden,[83] Banja[84]
Confidentiality	Sim,[50] Elkin and Anderson[78]
Justice (see also discrimination)	Purtilo[38,40,41,43]
Research ethics	Purtilo,[37] Sim,[54,57,58] Barnitt and Partridge,[62] Bonder,[85] Michels,[81,82] Warren[86]
Relationship to patient	Bellner,[67] Thomasma,[68] Paynter,[72] Meier and Purtilo,[76] Bruckner,[77] Ramsden,[83] Padilla and Brown,[87] Elkin and Anderson,[88] DeMayo,[89] Gartland[90]
Interprofessional relationships	Purtilo,[47,48] Paynter,[72] Elkin and Anderson,[88] Thompson,[91] Teager[92]
Ethics education	Purtilo,[6,39] Barnitt,[60] Triezenberg,[93] Finley and Goldstein,[94] Davis[95]
Conflict of interest/"double agent"	Bruckner,[77] White,[96] Richardson,[97] Finley[98]
Patients' rights	Purtilo,[42] Sim,[50] Ramsden,[83] Elkin and Anderson,[99] Scott[100]
Allocation of resources/reimbursement	Giffin,[15] Purtilo,[38,40,41,43,44] Sim,[51] Richardson[97]
Legal Issues	Purtilo,[36] Elkin and Anderson,[78,88] Delany,[79] Banja and Wolf,[80] Banja,[84] Scott,[100] Barrett,[101] Hayne[102]
Health care organization, policy, system	Giffin,[15] Purtilo,[38,40,41,43,44,46–48] Mattingly,[65] Thomasma,[68] Bashi and Domholdt,[103] Emery[104] Darnell and Fitch[112]
Discrimination, bias, prejudice	
Race	Haskins et al[105]
Age	Nicholas et al,[106] Barta Kvitek et al[107]
Gender	Raz et al,[108] Kemp et al[109]
Sexual harassment	DeMayo,[89] McComas et al[110]
Disability	Sim,[52] White and Olson[111]
Culture	Padilla and Brown[87]

were equal percentages of articles from the philosophical and social scientific perspectives from 1990 to 2000. The theoretical approach did not appear until the most recent time period.

Within the 43.2% of publications in which the authors used a philosophical approach, there were a variety of ethical perspectives: principles, virtue ethics, care-based or case study approaches, or combination approaches. Although it was not possible to categorize each publication, most authors (n=21 or 60% of the philosophical category) used a principles approach. In the entire sample of 90 articles, one author used a care perspective,[65] one author used a virtue perspective,[66] and one author used a narrative perspective.[61]

Issue or Topic

Table 3 lists the publications in the sample by issue or topic. Full elaboration of findings from the analysis of each topic category is beyond the scope of this article. For the purposes of this article, discussion focuses on themes within each decade and 3 selected topical themes as they developed across the entire time period: identification of ethical issues, relationship between clinical and ethical decision making, and relationship to patients or clients. These 3 themes are highlighted because they presented recurrent patterns or questions in physical therapy ethics during this 30-year period.

Topical themes of the decade 1970–1979 were establishing the role of the physical therapist as ethical decision-maker, informed consent, research ethics, teaching physical therapy ethics, and the historical context of physical therapy ethics. From 1980 to 1989, authors focused on themes of applying philosophical principles to ethical problems, justice in resource allocation, informed consent, and the ethical responsibility of autonomous practice. Themes for the most recent period (1990–2000) included managed care and scarce resources, prejudice and discrimination, and the evolving relationship between physical therapists and patients. This theme of the evolving relationship was seen in new theoretical models of the physical therapist role, in concern over the effects of managed care, in reflection over the effects of discrimination, and in new notions of the therapist's relationship to the patient.

In each decade, at least one publication delineated the need to further identify or clarify the types of ethical issues encountered by physical therapists. During the 1970s, Purtilo observed that allied health care workers encounter unique ethical issues, noting that "the specific ethical questions which arise vary from field to field according to the particulars of their roles."[6(p14)] Guccione, in 1980, identified 4 groups of ethical concerns: "choice to treat, obligations deriving from the patient-therapist contract, moral obligation and economic issues, and a physical therapist's relationship with other health professionals."[7(p1267)] In 1996, Triezenberg[11] reported on a Delphi study of ethics experts that identified current and future ethical issues in physical therapy. In a 1998 study of occupational therapists' and physical therapists' ethical dilemmas in the United Kingdom, Barnitt[59] found different themes in the ethical dilemmas of the 2 groups. While physical therapists were concerned about resource limitations and effectiveness of treatment, the ethical dilemmas of occupational therapists focused on dangerous patient behavior and unprofessional staff behavior. However, type of ethical dilemmas also differed by setting. A previous study by Barnitt[63] showed that "truth telling" presented ethical dilemmas for both occupational therapists and physical therapists. Barnitt and Partridge's[61] subsequent study of occupational therapists' and physical therapists' moral reasoning further reinforced the importance of the context of ethical dilemmas.

A second recurring theme in the literature was the interrelationship between clinical and ethical decision making. As previously discussed, a number of the authors recognized that clinical decisions have associated ethical ramifications. Across the 3 decades, there was an increasing recognition that ethical decisions are an integral part of clinical decision making. Purtilo observed: "Increased skill in making ethically sound decisions begins by being able to recognize which components have a moral quality to them."[5(p242)] During the period 1980 to 1989, Magistro,[3] Singleton,[4] and Wood[14] each spoke of the ethical demands that changes in clinical roles would bring. Reinforcing the thoughts of Clawson,[8] Haswell observed in the most recent decade that "ethical decision making must take place as a component of clinical decision making."[35(p151)] Similarly, the theoretical models developed during the 1990s by Jensen et al[9] and Sim[56] emphasized the inextricable relationship between clinical and ethical decision making.

A third recurring theme in the literature was that of changing relationships with patients. Responding to the emphasis on informed consent and the patient's right to know, Ramsden,[83] in 1975, recognized the need to discard traditional hierarchical relationships with patients. Ramsden stated, "Suggested here is that the traditional authority must be replaced by a shared decision-making process between patient and practitioner."[83(p137)] The work of Purtilo demonstrated a constant reframing of relationships, posing autonomy as a "valid moral standard" that is nevertheless "not sufficient"[113(p321)] and subordinate to empowerment of the patient.[114] Similarly, Meier and Purtilo[76] suggested a model of mutual respect similar to friendship in relating to patients. Bellner[67] developed the notion of profes-

Table 4.
Component of Moral Behavior[a]

Component	1970–1979 (n=14)	1980–1989 (n=24)	1990–2000 (n=43)	1970–2000 (n=81)
Moral sensitivity	6 (42.9%)	6 (25.0%)	18 (41.9%)	30 (37.0%)
Moral judgment	3 (21.4%)	17 (70.8%)	22 (51.2%)	42 (51.9%)
Moral motivation	1 (7.1%)	0	1 (2.3%)	2 (2.5%)
Moral courage	0	0	0	0
Multiple components	4 (28.6%)	1 (4.2%)	2 (4.7%)	5 (8.6%)

[a] Values represent the number (percentage) of publications within the specified time periods (excludes publications with a focus specific to settings outside the United States).

Table 5.
Role of the Physical Therapist[a]

Role	1970–1979 (n=14)	1980–1989 (n=24)	1990–2000 (n=43)	1970–2000 (n=81)
Patient/client management	4 (28.6%)	10 (41.7%)	25 (58.1%)	39 (48.1%)
Critical inquiry	3 (21.4%)	3 (12.5%)	2 (4.7%)	8 (9.9%)
Administrator	2 (14.3%)	1 (4.2%)	4 (9.3%)	7 (8.6%)
Education	2 (14.3%)	1 (4.2%)	5 (11.6%)	8 (9.9%)
Consultant	0	0	0	0
Multiple roles	3 (21.4%)	9 (37.5%)	7 (16.3%)	19 (23.5%)

[a] Values represent the number (percentage) of publications within the specified time periods (excludes publications with a focus specific to settings outside the United States).

Table 6.
Evolutionary Periods of Pellegrino and Purtilo[a]

Evolutionary Periods	1970–1979 (n=14)	1980–1989 (n=24)	1990–2000 (n=43)	1970–2000 (n=81)
Pellegrino's periods				
Values	1 (7.1%)	3 (12.5%)	1 (2.3%)	5 (6.2%)
Philosophical ethics	12 (85.7%)	20 (83.3%)	26 (60.5%)	58 (71.6%)
Social scientific	1 (7.1%)	1 (4.2%)	16 (37.2%)	18 (22.2%)
Purtilo's periods				
Self-identity	6 (42.9%)	1 (4.2%)	0	7 (8.6%)
Patient-focused Identity	6 (42.9%)	17 (70.8%)	24 (55.8%)	47 (58%)
Societal identity	2 (14.3%)	6 (25%)	19 (44.2%)	27 (33.3%)

[a] Values represent the number (percentage) of publications within the specified time periods (excludes publications with a focus specific to settings outside the United States).

sional responsibility deriving from the community, calling for a more interactive model of relationship with patients. Kuczewski[75] proposed a process model of informed consent to include family. Sim[56] elaborated the limitations of the disease model, exploring models of health more conducive to sound ethical decision-making. Against this backdrop, other authors[15,47,68] explored the negative effects of managed care on the relationship between physical therapists and patients.

Four Components of Morality
As indicated in Table 4, in a majority of publications in the sample (51.9%), authors emphasized moral judg-

ment. The focus on moral judgment was greatest during the decade 1980–1989 when 70.8% of publications dealt with moral judgment. In a few publications, authors addressed moral motivation, and no publication focused on moral courage.

Role of the Physical Therapist
Most authors either explicitly or implicitly emphasized the patient/client management, critical inquiry, educator, or administrative roles of the physical therapist (Tab. 5). In almost half (48.1%) of the publications, authors focused on the patient/client management role. None directly addressed the consultant role. Across the

Table 7.
Descriptive Model of the Evolution of Knowledge of Ethics in Physical Therapy[a]

Elements	1970–1979	1980–1989	1990–2000
Approach	Philosophical* Professional/historical	Philosophical	Philosophical and social scientific (equal numbers)
Component of moral behavior	Moral sensitivity	Moral judgment	Moral judgment
Issues and topics	Historical context Physical therapist as ethical decision-maker Teaching ethics Research and informed consent	Applying principles to physical therapy problems Justice in resource allocation Informed consent Ethical responsibility of autonomous practice	Managed care and scarce resources Discrimination and prejudice Relationship between physical therapist and patient/client Theoretical models of physical therapy embracing ethics
Role of the physical therapist*	Patient/client management Critical inquiry Administrator Educator	Patient/client management Critical inquiry	Patient/client management Educator Administrator Critical inquiry
Identity (Purtilo)	Self-identity and patient-focused	Patient-focused	Patient-focused (growing societal)
Thread/language* (Pellegrino)	Philosophical ethics	Philosophical ethics	Philosophical ethics Social scientific ethics
Recurring themes	Need to identify the ethical issues encountered by physical therapists Close relationship between clinical and ethical decision making Changing relationship with patient (from hierarchical to mutual models)		

[a] Asterisk indicates patterns of focus listed in descending order of frequency from most frequent to least frequent.

30-year time period, Purtilo[41,42,44,46] repeatedly emphasized the importance of the role of the physical therapist as policymaker and the necessity to "become involved in the formation, review, and refinement of health policy at the institutional, local, regional, and national levels."[41(p33)]

Evolutionary Periods (Purtilo and Pellegrino)
Overall, the majority of the sample represented Purtilo's patient-focused identity (58%) and Pellegrino's philosophical ethics thread (71.6%). However, as indicated in Table 6, there were differences among the decades.

As predicted by Purtilo, publications from the self-identity focus gradually decreased and totally disappeared by 1990 in the United States. During the period of self-identity, Purtilo[5] and Thomasma and Pisanechi[74] established the ethical decision-making role of the physical therapist and emphasized the unique nature of the ethical problems encountered by the physical therapist. The patient-focused perspective was most heavily represented in the decade of the 1980s. For example, Coy[33] and Sim[55,57] discussed the concept of informed consent. The societal focus progressively increased, reaching its highest proportion in the 1990s. Mattingly's[65] discussion of the mother-fetal dyad from a policy systems perspective and the myriad reflections on the impact of managed care[15,46,47] are representatives of the societal focus.

Like Purtilo's patient-focused identity, Pellegrino's philosophical thread was more influential during the first 2 decades. While Davis'[95] discussion of the affective aspects of education provides an example of Pellegrino's period of values, the sociological perspective on cultural aspects of patient education by Padilla and Brown[87] and numerous descriptive studies represent the third social scientific period. Although the philosophical thread was still dominant during the period 1990 to 2000, the social scientific thread reached its peak during this period. This general direction of development supports Pellegrino's pattern and coincides with results obtained in examining ethical approaches.

Descriptive Model of the Evolution of Knowledge of Ethics in Physical Therapy
Table 7 provides a descriptive framework based on the findings of this study and summarizes the changing patterns of focus of physical therapy literature on ethics over the period 1970 to July 2000.

Discussion and Conclusion
In my retrospective study, I analyzed literature on ethics in physical therapy between 1970 and 2000. Over the 3 decades covered by the study, there was an increase in the number of articles and social scientific studies. Results suggested that knowledge of ethics in physical therapy was predominantly philosophical in approach, from the principles perspective, written by a limited

number of authors, focused on the patient/client management role of the physical therapist, and addressed the moral judgment component of moral behavior. As predicted by Purtilo's model, the focus of identity in these publications evolved from one of self-identity to patient-focused identity, with increasing representation of societal identity. Although the focus of articles changed over the 3 decades, 3 recurrent themes across the entire 30 years were: (1) the need to further identify and clarify physical therapists' ethical dilemmas, (2) the interrelationship between clinical and ethical decision making, and (3) the changing relationship of therapists with their patients.

My analysis of the publications generally supported Pellegrino's idea of movement from philosophical approaches toward the social scientific approach. However, there were differences between the evolutionary patterns of bioethics and physical therapy ethics. Pellegrino[23] had described the 1980s as a period of "anti-principlism" in medical ethics, indicating a move away from principles toward a variety of other approaches. For example, medicine and nursing applied developmental approaches to moral reasoning.[115–118] Other disciplines tried non-principle types of approaches to ethics: care, virtue, case-based, and narrative. Although there was an increase in articles based on the social scientific approach, only 3 authors used alternative philosophical approaches—one from a care perspective,[65] one from a virtue perspective,[66] and one from a narrative perspective.[61]

One of the themes across all 3 decades was that of increasing mutuality and movement away from hierarchical models of physical therapists' relationships with patients. However, no publication in the sample addressed the perspective of the patient or client on ethical issues in physical therapy. Responding to Triezenberg's[11] study, Purtilo stated:

> There is a possibility that what professionals identify as important ethical issues are not judged similarly by patients. Because our raison d'être is to provide good patient care, the ethical issues have significance only if patients are indeed benefited by our concerns with such issues. Sociologists and others have leveled the criticism against professionals that much of what we do is in our own *self*-interest rather than for the benefit of the patients we "profess" to be serving or the society that allows us privileges in exchange for our services. It would be a useful exercise to compare Triezenberg's identification of ethical issues with issues perceived by patients to present ethical dilemmas in the physical therapy context.[119(p1108)]

In studying research ethics, Barnitt and Partridge[62] found that research participants experienced concerns or disappointment about their involvement in that research. Similar studies with physical therapists' patients and clients could provide greater insight into ethical aspects of physical therapy. Dialogue with patients could also provide important information about cultural dimensions of ethical dilemmas,[22] an area largely unexplored in this sample except in the context of discrimination.

My findings highlight some gaps in the existing physical therapy knowledge base. Although there were an increasing number of studies focusing on ethical issues, few studies attempted to define the ethical issues physical therapists routinely encounter. Indeed, I found only 5 publications of this nature authored by Guccione,[7] Triezenberg,[11] Barnitt,[59,63] and Barnitt and Partridge.[61] This lack of clarifying studies may provide evidence that, in answer to Purtilo and Guccione, knowledge of ethics may not have kept pace with increasing clinical autonomy. In combination with the steady growth of descriptive studies, the lack of studies specifying the unique ethical dilemmas faced by physical therapists may also support the need for a theoretical framework to guide further research. Because of the complex nature of articles dealing with ethical issues seen in practice, particularly autonomous practice, the possibility exists that some articles were missed.

Results of this study should be interpreted within the context of its limitations. The sample contained only peer-reviewed literature. Although *PT Magazine* published a series of ethics articles from 1993 to 1996, these articles were not included in the study because the journal is not peer reviewed. A second limitation relates to the categories of analysis and process of classification. A priori categories for analysis were derived from the fields of ethics, medicine, psychology, and physical therapy. However, quantitative and qualitative analysis involved considerable interpretation by the author. It is possible that a different researcher might reach other conclusions based on the same data. An additional limitation relates to the sample and inclusion criteria. The particular databases and search strategies used in this research also may have influenced these results. Because the focus of this research was on physical therapy literature, the search did not identify a study of moral reasoning by Brockett et al[120] indexed in a social science database or publications with key words related more globally to all rehabilitation providers.[113,114,120,121] Inclusion of editorials and perspective articles also might have yielded additional publications.

This article began by posing the question: Has ethical knowledge in physical therapy kept pace with the challenges of increasing professional autonomy? Although the body of knowledge of ethics in physical therapy grew steadily from 1970 to 2000, this retrospective analysis identified gaps in our current knowledge and suggests directions for future exploration. Further research should address the unique ethical problems commonly encountered in all 5 roles of the physical therapist; patient perspectives on ethical issues in physical therapy; variety in ethical approaches; factors affecting moral judgment, sensitivity, motivation, and courage; and cultural dimensions of ethical practice in physical therapy. Adequately addressing gaps in our knowledge of ethics will require both philosophical and social scientific research. Because ethical action is a complex multidimensional[20] process that is embedded within clinical encounters,[8,9] research into physical therapy ethics might benefit from a multidimensional framework to guide inquiry.

The model of ethics discussed in this article could serve as an appropriate theoretical guide for future ethics research and education because it is a multidimensional model that integrates philosophical and social scientific approaches. This model could be used to develop 4 different sets of questions to research in physical therapy ethics. The first set of questions would focus on moral sensitivity. What are the ethical issues that physical therapists routinely encounter? What ethical issues are frequently overlooked by physical therapists? How does organizational context or setting influence recognition or interpretation of ethical issues? A second set of research questions would focus on moral judgment. What type of moral reasoning do physical therapists use? Does gender, religion, or culture influence moral judgments? What should a physical therapist do in response to frequently encountered ethical dilemmas? What level of informed consent is necessary before spinal mobilization or other interventions? The following questions address moral motivation: (1) Do physical therapists' view of the professional role cause them to advocate for their patients? and (2) What organizational, contextual, or policy factors act as barriers or resources to ethical behavior? In researching moral courage, one might explore the following areas: (1) Who are moral exemplars in physical therapy? (2) What are the qualities of moral exemplars? (3) What factors influence some therapists to overcome obstacles to moral behavior? and (4) What are the important implementation skills in situations of adversity?

The model of ethics discussed in the article also could assist in integrating the normative and social scientific aspects of ethical questions in physical therapy. For example, the results of my study suggest that autonomy has been extensively explored as a philosophical principle in physical therapy. However, we have little data about the unique problems that physical therapists or their patients encounter with regard to autonomy. This type of research ultimately could provide data for normative judgments about patient autonomy. Proot et al[122] studied nursing home residents' experience of autonomy. Describing their model as "changing autonomy," they identified 3 dimensions of autonomy (self-determination, independence, and self-care), and they delineated factors that facilitate and constrain patient autonomy in this setting. Similar research could help physical therapists to understand the myriad of factors that influence patient autonomy in a variety of settings and contexts. This type of research also could provide valuable information to guide decisions about the content and emphasis of curricular content in professional education.

A major purpose of my study was to identify evolutionary trends in the literature on ethics in physical therapy from 1970 to 2000. Results of this research indicate that knowledge of ethics in physical therapy changed in approach, topics, and focus of identity during this time period, with an increase in social scientific study and in societal focus. During the most recent decade, social scientific publications achieved a balance with the previously dominant philosophical publications. However, few studies blended the 2 approaches. The model of ethics discussed in this article could provide a framework to guide research on ethics in physical therapy by blending philosophical and social scientific approaches and providing a broad framework to integrate normative and empirical investigation. The results of my study point to the need for further research in the area of physical therapy ethics and perhaps suggest that ethics research could benefit from a research agenda similar to the Clinical Research Agenda for Physical Therapy[123] developed by the American Physical Therapy Association to address clinical questions. Given the close relationship between clinical and ethical decision making, research in the ethical role of the physical therapist is a necessary complement to questions within the Clinical Research Agenda for Physical Therapy. This type of research agenda could ensure that knowledge of ethics in physical therapy continues to grow, builds on previous knowledge, and responds to the needs of the profession.

References

1 Rose SJ. Editor's note: Gathering storms. *Phys Ther.* 1989;69:354–355.

2 Rose SJ. Editor's note: Our body of knowledge revisited. *Phys Ther.* 1989;69:297–298.

3 Magistro CM. Clinical decision-making in physical therapy: a practitioner's perspective. *Phys Ther.* 1989;69:525–534.

4 Singleton MC. Independent practice—on the horns of a dilemma. a special communication. *Phys Ther.* 1987;67:54–57.

5 Purtilo RB. Understanding ethical issues: the physical therapist as ethicist. *Phys Ther.* 1974;54:239–242.

6 Purtilo RB. Ethics teaching in allied health fields. *Hastings Cent Rep.* 1978;8(2):14–16.

7 Guccione AA. Ethical issues in physical therapy practice: a survey of physical therapists in New England. *Phys Ther.* 1980;60:1264–1272.

8 Clawson AL. The relationship between clinical decision making and ethical decision making. *Physiotherapy.* 1994;80:10–14.

9 Jensen GM, Gwyer J, Shepard KF, Hack LM. Expert practice in physical therapy. *Phys Ther.* 2000;80:28–43.

10 Richardson B. Professional development, 2: professional knowledge and situated learning in the workplace. *Physiotherapy.* 1999;85:467–474.

11 Triezenberg HL. The identification of ethical issues in physical therapy practice. *Phys Ther.* 1996;76:1097–1107.

12 Morreim EH. *Balancing Act: The New Medical Ethics of Medicine's New Economics.* Washington, DC: Georgetown University Press; 1995.

13 Bebeau MJ, Born DO, Ozar DT. The development of a professional role orientation inventory. *Journal of the American College of Dentists.* 1993;60:27–33.

14 Wood R. Twenty-Third Mary McMillan Lecture: Footprints. *Phys Ther.* 1989;69:975–980.

15 Giffin A. Coping with the prospective payment system (PPS): ethical issues in rehabilitation. *Issues on Aging.* 2000;23(1):2–8.

16 Thiroux JP. *Ethics: Theory and Practice.* 5th ed. Englewood Cliffs, NJ: Prentice-Hall; 1995.

17 Beauchamp TL, Childress JF. *Principles of Biomedical Ethics.* 4th ed. New York, NY: Oxford University Press; 1994.

18 Nelson JL. Moral teachings from unexpected quarters: lessons for bioethics from the social sciences and managed care. *Hastings Cent Rep.* 2000;30(1):12–17.

19 Zussman R. The contributions of sociology to medical ethics. *Hastings Cent Rep.* 2000;30(1):7–11.

20 Rest JR. Background: theory and research. In: Rest JR, Narvaez D, eds. *Moral Development in the Professions: Psychology and Applied Ethics.* Hillsdale, NJ: Lawrence Erlbaum Associates; 1994:1–26.

21 Pellegrino ED. The origins and evolution of bioethics: some personal reflections. *Kennedy Institute Ethics J.* 1999;9(1):73–88.

22 Purtilo RB. Thirty-First Mary McMillan Lecture: A time to harvest, a time to sow: ethics for a shifting landscape. *Phys Ther.* 2000;80:1112–1119.

23 Pellegrino ED. The metamorphosis of medical ethics: a 30-year retrospective. *JAMA.* 1993;269:1158–1162.

24 MEDLINE [database online]. Bethesda, Md: National Library of Medicine Medlars Management; 2000. Updated October 2000.

25 Cumulative Index to Nursing and Allied Health Literature [database online]. Gardendale, Calif: Updated October 2000.

26 *Ethics in Physical Therapy.* Vols 1 and 2. Alexandria, Va: American Physical Therapy Association; 1998.

27 Purtilo RB. *Ethical Dimensions in the Health Professions.* 3rd ed. Philadelphia, Pa: WB Saunders Co; 1999.

28 Hinman LM. *Ethics: A Pluralistic Approach.* 2nd ed. Philadelphia Pa: Harcourt Brace College Publishers; 1998.

29 Shaw WH. *Social and Personal Ethics.* Belmont, Calif: Wadsworth Publishing Co; 1993.

30 Tashakkori A, Teddlie C. *Mixed Methodology: Combining Qualitative and Quantitative Approaches.* Applied Social Research Methods Series, vol 46. Thousand Oaks, Calif: Sage Publications; 1998.

31 *Guide to Physical Therapist Practice.* 2nd ed. Alexandria, Va: American Physical Therapy Association; 2001.

32 *Statistical Program for the Social Sciences, Version 10.0.5.* Chicago, Ill: SPSS Inc; 1999.

33 Coy J. Autonomy-based informed consent: ethical implications for patient noncompliance. *Phys Ther.* 1989;69:826–833.

34 Miles MB, Huberman AM. *Qualitative Data Analysis: An Expanded Sourcebook.* 2nd ed. Thousand Oaks, Calif: Sage Publications; 1994.

35 Haswell K. Professional issues: informed choice and consent for cervical spine manipulation. *Australian Journal of Physiotherapy.* 1996;42:149–155.

36 Purtilo RB. Applying the principles of informed consent to patient care: legal and ethical considerations for physical therapy. *Phys Ther.* 1984;64:934–937.

37 Purtilo RB. Reading "physical therapy" from an ethics perspective. *Phys Ther.* 1975;55:361–364.

38 Purtilo RB. Justice in the distribution of health care resources: the position of physical therapists in the United States and Sweden. *Phys Ther.* 1982;62:46–50.

39 Purtilo RB. Structure of ethics teaching in physical therapy: a survey. *Phys Ther.* 1979;59:1102–1106.

40 Purtilo RB. Justice in the distribution of health care resources: the position of physical therapists, physiatrists, and rehabilitation nurses. *Phys Ther.* 1982;61:1594–1600.

41 Purtilo RB. Whom to treat first, and how much is enough? Ethical dilemmas that physical therapists confront as they compare individual patients' needs for treatment. *Int J Technol Assess Health Care.* 1992;8:26–34.

42 Purtilo RB. Professional responsibility in physiotherapy: old dimensions and new directions. *Physiotherapy.* 1986;72:579–583.

43 Purtilo RB. The right to health care: ideal or imperative? *Phys Ther.* 1979;59:728–732.

44 Purtilo RB. Saying "no" to patients for cost-related reasons: alternatives for the physical therapist. *Phys Ther.* 1988;68:1243–1247.

45 Purtilo RB. The American Physical Therapy Association's code of ethics: its historical foundations. *Phys Ther.* 1977;57:1001–1006.

46 Purtilo RB. Who should make moral policy decisions in health care? *Phys Ther.* 1978;58:1076–1081.

47 Purtilo RB. Managed care: ethical issues for the rehabilitation professions. *Trends in Health Care Law Ethics.* 1995;10(1–2):105–108, 118.

48 Purtilo RB. Interdisciplinary health care teams and health care reform. *J Law Med Ethics.* 1994;22:121–126.

49 Sim J, Purtilo RB. An ethical analysis of physical therapists' duty to treat persons who have AIDS: homosexual patient as a test case. *Phys Ther.* 1991;71:650–655.

50 Sim J. Confidentiality and HIV status. *Physiotherapy.* 1997;83:90–96.

51 Sim J. Ethical issues in the management of persistent vegetative state. *Physiother Res Int.* 1997;2(2):7–11.

52 Sim J. Physical disability, stigma, and rehabilitation. *Physiotherapy Canada.* 1990;42:232–238.

53 Sim J. Ethical considerations in physiotherapy. *Physiotherapy.* 1983;69:119–120.

54 Sim J. Methodology and morality in physiotherapy research. *Physiotherapy.* 1989;75:237–243.

55 Sim J. Professional issues: informed consent and manual therapy. *Manual Therapy.* 1996;1(2):104–106.

56 Sim J. The concept of health. *Physiotherapy.* 1990;76:423–428.

57 Sim J. Informed consent: ethical implications for physiotherapy. *Physiotherapy*. 1986;72:584–587.

58 Sim J. The ethics of single-system (n=1) research. *Phys Ther*. 1974;54:239–243.

59 Barnitt R. Ethical dilemmas in occupational therapy and physical therapy: a survey of practitioners in the UK National Health Service. *J Med Ethics*. 1998;24:193–199.

60 Barnitt R. Deeply troubling questions: the teaching of ethics in undergraduate programmes. *Br J Occup Ther*. 1993;56:401–406.

61 Barnitt R, Partridge C. Ethical reasoning in physical therapy and occupational therapy. *Physiotherapy Research International*. 1997;2: 178–194.

62 Barnitt R, Partridge C. The legacy of being a research subject: follow-up studies of participants in therapy research. *Physiotherapy Research International*. 1999;4:250–261.

63 Barnitt R. Truth telling in occupational therapy and physiotherapy. *Br J Occup Ther*. 1994;57:334–340.

64 Michels E. Nineteenth Mary McMillan Lecture. *Phys Ther*. 1984;64: 1697–1704.

65 Mattingly SS. The mother-fetal dyad and the ethics of care. *Physical and Occupational Therapy in Pediatrics*. 1996;16(1/2):5–13.

66 Edwards JK. Enid Graham Memorial lecture: Personal values—professional ethics. *Physiotherapy Canada*. 1987;39:319–323.

67 Bellner AL. Senses of responsibility: a challenge for occupational and physical therapists in the context of ongoing professionalization. *Scand J Caring Sci*. 1999;13:55–62.

68 Thomasma DC. The ethics of managed care: challenges to the principles of relationship-centered care. *J Allied Health*. 1996;25: 233–246.

69 Hogshead HP. Responsibility: a modality for the next decade. *Phys Ther*. 1974;54:588–591.

70 Elkin S, Anderson L. Ethics and physiotherapy: an introduction. *New Zealand Journal of Physiotherapy*. 1998;26(3):9–12.

71 Robinson P. Objectives, ethics and etiquette. *Physiotherapy*. 1994; 80(A 100 Years Suppl):8A-10A.

72 Paynter B. Our ethical code: an historical survey. *New Zealand Journal of Physiotherapy*. 1990;18(1):7–11.

73 Kline IC. Ethical considerations in the practice of physical therapy. *Prog Phys Ther*. 1970;1:332–338.

74 Thomasma DC, Pisanechi JI. Allied health professionals and ethical issues. *J Allied Health*. Summer 1977:15–19.

75 Kuczewski MG. Reconceiving the family: the process of consent in medical decision making. *Hastings Cent Rep*. 1996;26(2):30–37.

76 Meier RH III, Purtilo RB. Ethical issues and the patient-provider relationship. *Am J Phys Med Rehabil*. 1994;73:365–366.

77 Bruckner J. Physical therapists as double agents: ethical dilemmas of divided loyalties. *Phys Ther*. 1987;67:383–387.

78 Elkin S, Anderson L. How much to disclose: health information and the physiotherapist. *New Zealand Journal of Physiotherapy*. 1999;27:27–32.

79 Delany C. Professional issues: should I warn the patient first? *Australian Journal of Physiotherapy*. 1996;42:249–255.

80 Banja JD, Wolf SL. Malpractice litigation for uninformed consent: implications for physical therapists. *Phys Ther*. 1987;67:1226–1229.

81 Michels E. Research and human rights, part 1. *Phys Ther*. 1976;56: 407–412.

82 Michels E. Research and human rights, part 2. *Phys Ther*. 1976;56: 546–552.

83 Ramsden EL. The patient's right to know: implications for inter-personal communication processes. *Phys Ther*. 1975;55:133–138.

84 Banja J. Whistle blowing in physical therapy. *Phys Ther*. 1985;65: 1683–1695.

85 Bonder BR. Planning the initial version. *Physical and Occupational Therapy in Pediatrics*. 1989;9(1):15–42.

86 Warren MP. Personal ethical responsibility. *Physiotherapy*. 1982;68: 355–356.

87 Padilla R, Brown K. Culture and patient education: challenges and opportunities. *Journal of Physical Therapy Education*. 1999;13(3):23–30.

88 Elkin S, Anderson L. Challenges within professional relationships: a case scenario. *New Zealand Journal of Physiotherapy*. 1999;27(2):15–17.

89 DeMayo RA. Patient sexual behaviors and sexual harassment: a national survey of physical therapists. *Phys Ther*. 1997;77:739–744.

90 Gartland G. Essentials of ethics in clinical practice: a communications perspective. *Physiotherapy Canada*. 1987;39:179–182.

91 Thompson M. Relationships between physiotherapists and doctors. *Physiotherapy*. 1979;65:176–178.

92 Teager DP. Referral. *Physiotherapy*. 1983;69:49–50.

93 Triezenberg HL. Teaching ethics in physical therapy education: a Delphi study. *Journal of Physical Therapy Education*. 1997;11(2):16–22.

94 Finley C, Goldstein MS. Curriculum survey: ethical and legal instruction—a report from the APTA Department of Education and the APTA Judicial Committee. *Journal of Physical Therapy Education*. 1991;5(2):60–4.

95 Davis CM. Affective education for the health professions: facilitating appropriate behavior. *Phys Ther*. 1981;61:1587–1593.

96 White JA. Managing care: the ethical dilemma. *Physical Therapy Case Reports*. 1998;1:213–215.

97 Richardson D. To treat or not to treat: PVS or is he? *Physiotherapy Research International*. 1997;2(2):1–6.

98 Finley C. Gift-giving or influence peddling: can you tell the difference? *Phys Ther*. 1994;74:143–148.

99 Elkin S, Anderson L. Ethics and physiotherapy: the Code of Health and Disability Services Consumers' Rights. *New Zealand Journal of Physiotherapy*. 1999;27(1):17–20.

100 Scott R. The Patient Self-Determination Act of 1990: are health care providers meeting their legal duties owed to patients? *Issues on Aging*. 1997;20(2):17–19.

101 Barrett P. Codes of ethics and the Commerce Commission. *New Zealand Journal of Physiotherapy*. 1990;18(1):11–13.

102 Hayne CR. Safe . . . sure? *Physiotherapy*. 1978;64:10–13.

103 Bashi HL, Domholdt E. Use of support personnel for physical therapy treatment. *Phys Ther*. 1993;73:421–436.

104 Emery MJ. The impact of the prospective payment system: perceived changes in the nature of practice and clinical education. *Phys Ther*. 1993;73:11–25.

105 Haskins AR, Rose-St Prix C, Elbaum L. Covert bias in evaluation of physical therapist students' clinical performance. *Phys Ther*. 1997;77: 155–168.

106 Nicholas JJ, Rybarcyzkk B, Meyer PM, et al. Rehabilitation staff perceptions of characteristics of geriatric rehabilitation patients. *Arch Phys Med Rehabil*. 1998;79:1277–1284.

107 Barta Kvitek SD, Shaver BJ, Blood H, Shepard KF. Age bias: physical therapists and older patients. *J Gerontol.* 1986;41:706–709.

108 Raz P, Jensen GM, Walter J, Drake LM. Perspectives on gender and professional issues among female therapists. *Phys Ther.* 1991;71: 530–540.

109 Kemp KI, Scholz CA, Sanford TL, Shepard KF. Salary and status differences between male and female physical therapists. *Phys Ther.* 1979;59:1095–1101.

110 McComas J, Hebert C, Giacomin C, et al. Experiences of student and practicing physical therapists with inappropriate patient sexual behavior. *Phys Ther.* 1993;73:762–770.

111 White MJ, Olson RS. Attitudes toward people with disabilities: a comparison of rehabilitation nurses, occupational therapists, and physical therapists. *Rehabil Nurs.* 1998;23:126–131.

112 Darnell RE, Fitch DH. External review in quality assurance. *Phys Ther.* 1980;60:559–563.

113 Purtilo RB. Ethical issues in teamwork: the context of rehabilitation. *Arch Phys Med Rehabil.* 1988;69:318–322.

114 Purtilo RB, Meier RH III. Team challenges: regulatory constraints and patient empowerment. *Am J Phys Med Rehabil.* 1993;72:327–330.

115 Duckett LJ, Ryden MB. Education for ethical nursing practice. In: Rest JR, Narvaez D, eds. *Moral Development in the Professions: Psychology and Applied Ethics.* Hillsdale, NJ: Lawrence Erlbaum Associates; 1994: 51–69.

116 Self DJ, Wolinsky FD, Baldwin DC Jr. The effect of teaching medical ethics on medical students' moral reasoning. *Acad Med.* 1989;64:755–759.

117 Self DJ, Olivarez M. The influence of gender on conflicts of interest in the allocation of limited critical care resources: justice vs care. *J Crit Care.* 1993;8:64–74.

118 Rest JR, Narvaez D, Bebeau MJ, Thoma, SJ. *Postconventional Moral Thinking: A Neo-Kohlbergian Approach.* Hillsdale, NJ: Lawrence Erlbaum Associates; 1999.

119 Purtilo RB. Commentary on: Triezenberg HL. The identification of ethical issues in physical therapy practice. *Phys Ther.* 1996;76: 1097–1108.

120 Brockett M, Geddes EL, Westmoreland M, Salvatori P. Moral development or moral decline? a discussion of ethics education for the health care professions. *Med Teach.* 1997;19:301–309.

121 Sim J. Respect for autonomy: issues in neurological rehabilitation. *Clin Rehabil.* 1998;12(1):3–10.

122 Proot IM, Crebolder HFJM, Abu-saad HH, et al. Facilitating and constraining factors on autonomy: the view of stroke patients on admission into nursing homes. *Clin Nurs Res.* 2000;9:460–478.

123 Clinical Research Agenda for Physical Therapy. *Phys Ther.* 2000; 80:499–513.

Whistleblowing & Problem Solving:
A 5-STEP APPROACH

By Claire Coyne

When a PT, PTA, or student witnesses what may be illegal or unprofessional conduct, what should he or she do? This 5-step model may help.

Consider these dilemmas:

❖ A physical therapist (PT) discovers that a colleague is submitting false insurance claims.

❖ A graduate PT practicing in his first clinical setting becomes concerned that some interventions are not meeting best practice standards as he understands them.

❖ A physical therapy student in her first clinical affiliation witnesses an aide providing physical therapy services without proper supervision.

What should they do?

Although few health care professionals want to be placed in such positions, situations do arise in clinical settings that warrant taking action. Challenges that PTs, physical therapist assistants (PTAs), and students may encounter in clinics include the provision of substandard care, interventions being provided by unqualified personnel, inadequate supervision, and questionable billing practices.

"Whistleblower" is the popular term for someone who reports wrongdoing (by a co-worker, employer, or other person or company) to a person in a position of authority or publicly. In a legal sense, it usually means someone who observes or learns of illegal activity, or at least activity believed to be unlawful, and reports it either to 1) a supervisor in the organization in which the whistleblower is employed or 2) a government agency with responsibility to investigate or enforce laws regarding the alleged wrongdoing. Sometimes, a whistleblower is someone who simply testifies truthfully in a legal hearing or other proceeding.

APTA's Code of Ethics, Principle 9, states, "A physical therapist shall protect the public and the profession from unethical, incompetent, and illegal acts." The interpretation of this Principle in Section 9.1(C) of the Guide for Professional Conduct says, "A physical therapist shall report any conduct that appears to be unethical, incompetent, or illegal."[1]

However, APTA's Ethics and Judicial Committee (EJC) pointed out in a recent decision that "Section 9.1(C) of the GPC is intentionally vague as to the identity of the person or body to whom a physical therapist should report." It adds, "The EJC believes that, where reporting is called for, the physical therapist should use mature judgment in deciding to whom to report....The EJC does not believe that any one-size-fits-all approach to the question would be appropriate or feasible....The decision to whom to make a report should be based on all the relevant circumstances and guided by the aim to make the world of physical therapy a better place for those it serves. The decision should be guided also by attention to who is in the best position to rectify the unethical, incompetent, and/or illegal behavior in question."[2]

According to APTA's Committee on Risk Management and Member Benefits, PTs who find themselves in problem situations can take specific steps on behalf of patients—and the profession—to effect positive change. This action often can be taken in a constructive and nonconfrontational fashion.

Presented below is a 5-step model for PTs, PTAs, and students who may find themselves in a situation in which they believe whistleblowing may be an option.

Step One: Self-Analysis

The very first step a potential whistleblower needs to take after witnessing questionable behavior is to "conduct a self-analysis," says Kathy Lewis, PT, MAPT, JD, current committee chair and associate professor in the graduate program in physical therapy at Wichita State University. "Ask yourself: Is this action permissible but simply different than one I would take? Is it actually meeting the minimum standard of care? Is it ethical?"

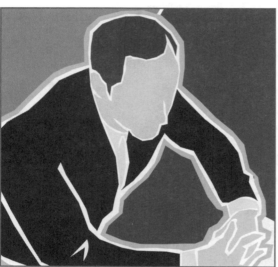

Cathy Thut, PT, MBA, director of physical medicine at Baylor Medical Center at Irving (Texas), notes that "there are good practices and there are 'best practices.' While a given treatment may not be the standard 'best practice,' it can nevertheless be an appropriate course of action." She offers an example: "In some cases, we are missing a piece of the puzzle on a patient's diagnosis. For instance, we may have a patient with other complicating diagnoses who presents with a wound. We have questions as to whether there is adequate blood flow to the area. We don't want to do sharp debridement when we question whether or not there is good circulation. In this case, we will err on the side of conservative treatment." A student in this situation, however, may feel that the team isn't being aggressive enough and thus not providing adequate care. The stu-

dent is simply "not seeing the full case," Thut explains.

The EJC opinion reinforces the message that a potential whistleblower must examine the facts before proceeding. It states, "The existence of an ethical duty under GPC 9.1(C) is dependent on the character and strength of the evidence that misconduct has occurred or is occurring....A physical therapist does not have an ethical obligation to report wrongdoing unless he/she has sufficiently reliable evidence of misconduct."[2]

> "Ask yourself: Is this action permissible but simply different than one I would take? Is it actually meeting the minimum standard of care? Is it ethical?"
>
> –Kathy Lewis, PT, MAPT, JD

Step Two: Discuss

If the self-analysis does not resolve the PT's discomfort with the situation, an appropriate second step may be to talk to the individual responsible for providing the intervention, Lewis suggests. "Just have a professional chat and say, 'I notice that you are doing such-and-such. I'm wondering how you decided on that plan of care,'" she says. The resulting dialogue may well resolve the PT's concerns.

Even when the PT is confident that improper conduct has occurred, it may be appropriate to speak to the other individual. The EJC opinion states, "A physical therapist sometimes may carry out his/her ethical obligation simply by calling the improper conduct to the attention of the offending physical therapist."[2]

Lewis concedes that this step can be a difficult one to take. "We don't properly

educate students about giving constructive criticism," she notes. "We need to do a better job. This type of training needs to be enhanced in the physical therapy curriculum."

Step Three: Approach a Supervisor

If the PT's concerns still are not resolved, or if the problem is such that direct interaction with a colleague isn't appropriate (such as in an impaired provider situation, in which a PT suspects a colleague is working with patients while under the influence of drugs or alcohol), he or she should approach a supervisor. The focus at all times must be kept strictly on patient care. "In all whistleblowing situations, it is very important to focus on improving quality of care, rather than on making accusations or causing conflict," Lewis stresses. Any meeting should be scheduled in confidence. "Don't discuss this with other colleagues," she says. "It is imperative to maintain confidentiality throughout the process. You do not want to cause unnecessary harm to a person's reputation."

When a PT approaches a supervisor about an aspect of care, the supervisor's response may be, "That's how we do things here and these are the reasons why." And that process may indeed be serving patients well. "Don't jump to conclusions based on one or two interactions," Thut cautions.

Some situations, however, are not ambiguous. "A PT may witness an aide providing inappropriate services without PT supervision," says Joy Sterneck, PT, MHA, 1997-2002 chair of the Committee on Risk Management and Member Benefits. "Or a PTA is asked to perform an initial evaluation. These actions clearly are not within the purview of accepted standards of practice."

The EJC opinion advises a PT to use "mature judgment" in deciding to whom to report the matter, being guided by the underlying purpose to protect the public. The opinion states, "A physical therapist might have to communicate to some per-

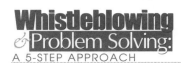

Whistleblower Protections

Federal and state whistleblower laws form a bit of a "crazy quilt" of overlapping laws that require extensive research to determine protections for a specific situation. Many laws against employment retaliation are designed to protect employee whistleblowers as well. Laws addressing specific crimes such as sexual misconduct, child abuse, and elder abuse also may contain provisions protecting the person who reports the crime from retaliation.

There also are federal and state statutes that protect whistleblowers, as well as "common law" provisions developed over time by the courts. It is appropriate to consult a knowledgeable lawyer to determine strategy and available protection.

Federal

The False Claims Act dates back to the Civil War. It was rejuvenated in 1986 during the Reagan Administration, with amendments added strengthening its provisions and incorporating whistleblower protections. The Act applies to persons making false statements to the government in order to receive money or to have the government make payments on one's behalf.

The Corporate and Criminal Fraud Accountability Act of 2002 contains historic protections for corporate whistleblowers, including a 90-day statute of limitations permitting whistleblowers to seek federal court relief if the US Department of Labor (which handles these cases) does not resolve a case within 180 days.

State

Most states have some sort of statutory or common law "whistleblower" or anti-retaliation laws. Those states that have explicit statutory protections for whistleblowers include: California, Connecticut, Delaware, Florida, Hawaii, Louisiana, Maine, Michigan, Minnesota, Montana, New Hampshire, New Jersey, New York, North Carolina, Ohio, Oregon, Rhode Island, Tennessee, and Washington.

The following states and the District of Columbia have recognized a public policy exception to the "employment at will doctrine," providing some protection to employee whistleblowers: Alaska, Arizona, Arkansas, California, Colorado, Connecticut, Florida, Hawaii, Idaho, Illinois, Indiana, Iowa, Kansas, Kentucky, Louisiana, Maine, Maryland, Massachusetts, Michigan, Minnesota, Missouri, Montana, Nebraska, Nevada, New Hampshire, New Jersey, New Mexico, North Carolina, North Dakota, Ohio, Oklahoma, Oregon, Pennsylvania, Rhode Island, Tennessee, Texas, Vermont, Virginia, Washington, West Virginia, Wisconsin, and Wyoming.

Source: www.whistleblowerlaws.com

son within his/her organization having authority over the person directly responsible for the problematic behavior."

Regardless of whether the actions are questionable or clearly inappropriate, the potential whistleblower must document carefully what he or she witnesses. "It is necessary to document observations over time," Lewis stresses, "and to consult resources such as the *Guide to Physical Therapist Practice* to determine if the action being witnessed is adequate and acceptable." Those interviewed for this article agreed that the Guide is a valuable resource to help determine what is appropriate practice.

Potential whistleblowers must weigh the possible effects of taking action and keep in mind that careers can be injured or ruined through this process. Lewis recalls how a name of a physician was brought up during a professional meeting years ago, and one attendee commented, "I believe he is being investigated for Medicare fraud." Lewis says the other attendees were shocked. "This is not the type of information to mention casually during a meeting," she stresses. "Even if the doctor was under investigation," it did not mean that he was guilty of the charges. PTs must take extreme care in determining what situations are worthy of whistleblowing, particularly to an agency outside of the PT's facility.

Step Four: Go Up the Ladder

Once the PT has exhausted avenues for reporting problems within the department, it may be time to seek the counsel of those higher up. "In a facility, you are going to have a departmental supervisor; that person has a supervisor. Run it up the ladder. If necessary, talk to the medical director of the department," Thut advises.

"Fix it before you report it outside," Lewis cautions. "A lot of problems can be dealt with internally." Because patient care situations are likely to involve individuals, or, at most, one department's practices, the facility itself may best be able to address the issues involved. "If the goal is quality of care, you need to look at the internal structure first," Lewis stresses.

Step Five: File a Complaint

In many cases, when a PT reports a problem internally and works with those in charge at a given facility to address it, the issue can be resolved. Many disagreements stem from differences of opinion regarding quality of care and appropriate treatment. These often are resolved through internal quality control procedures. In those relatively rare cases in which internal options have been exhausted, however, and a problem threatening patient well-being is identified and not resolved, the appropriate next step is to file a complaint with an outside agency such as a state licensing board.

To do so, the whistleblower must put his or her own name out in public. While some facilities may offer options for anonymously registering internal complaints, individuals filing reports with licensing boards must identify themselves.

continued on page 47

continued from page 44

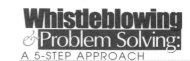

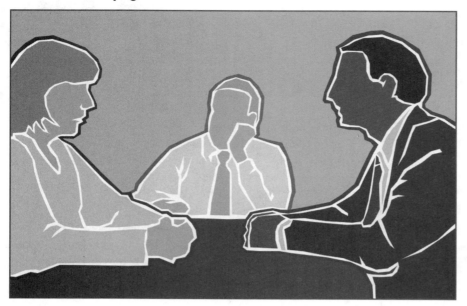

"In a facility, you are going to have a departmental supervisor; that person has a supervisor. Run it up the ladder. If necessary, talk to the medical director of the department."

–Cathy Thut, PT

Although this can be an uncomfortable step to take, it is a necessary one when patient care is being compromised, Lewis says: "You need to be willing to stand up for your profession."

The EJC opinion states, "In some situations, the appropriate party to whom to report misconduct undoubtedly would be the physical therapist licensing agency. The EJC imagines that the licensing agency most likely would be the appropriate party to whom to report misconduct if the behavior in question involved violations of provisions of the physical therapy practice act or implementing regulations."[2]

Lewis, who has served on the licensing board of the state of Kansas, again stresses the need for documentation. "In order to get protection so that someone cannot in turn sue you for defamation of character or invasion of privacy, you must submit a 'good faith' report, which means that you provide the board with enough facts so that it appears that there is indeed a wrongdoing."

"Different states handle claims differently, but they all request some form of written information and ask that you state the facts in your name," she reports. "This helps to avoid frivolous or vindictive actions." Specific data are crucial to the filing of any report. "When you fill out a report for an external agency, you want to include specific times and dates—that this occurred on this date," Lewis explains. "The only information you must leave out is the patient name, to protect confidentiality."

Students

Physical therapist student who are faced with troublesome situations during a clinical affiliation must deal with a unique set of challenges, because their position is particularly vulnerable. "If a student blows a whistle regarding a certain facility, do they have to leave that clinical affiliation and begin looking for another one? Will that delay graduation and getting a job?" Sterneck asks.

The Best Defense Is Prevention

Facilities may be able to reduce the likelihood of whistleblower actions by taking well-thought-out preventive steps like the ones listed below, offered by Carol Schunk, PT, PsyD, Portland, Oregon.

Take every report or complaint seriously. "Research shows that, in most cases, whistleblowers do not do so to be vindictive or to turn in a facility to collect money. They usually do it because they have exhausted every other means, and no one has paid proper attention to them. In that respect, whistleblowing is a preventable occurrence. If someone brings a problem or a concern to your attention, give it credence."

Follow up. "When you do pay attention to a staff member's complaint, and you say you will investigate the situation and get back to them, make sure you do so. Follow up with them in a timely manner."

Never make excuses. "Don't try to mask a situation, or claim that, 'That's not what the regulation says' when someone registers a valid complaint. Look into it, work on resolving it, and report back to the staff member."

Create a team environment. "Be up front about your policies with the team. Say, 'This is what we're doing about confidentiality and about other issues, but sometimes it is hard to interpret the regulations. We are doing the best we can, but we might have to make changes along the way. If you see anything that you question, make sure you come to me.'"

Provide avenues of approach. "Be public about who individuals can go to if they spot a problem or have a question. Make sure they always have an avenue for internal reporting."

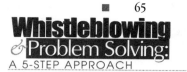

She suggests that the student first approach the clinical instructor (CI). "If you see something happening that is putting the patient at risk because a standard is not being met, or supervision is not within APTA guidelines for supervision, then it's time to take action."

Like a practicing PT, the student should seek counsel from a number of sources. "If the answer to the student's question about an inappropriate procedure is, 'That's how we document here,' or 'That's how we use our aides (or assistants) here,' then the student should report the problem to the university's academic coordinator of clinical education (ACCE)," Sterneck says.

Lewis, who spoke recently to the National Student Conclave on risk management, agrees that students need to speak with the CI when they encounter inappropriate situations, such as when they are asked to perform a function that is beyond their scope of training, or are asked to delegate to an aide a function that they don't believe is proper. "Students do not have to agree to do something that isn't appropriate," she comments. "If they don't get a satisfactory result from the CI, they have the right to report to the ACCE at their university." Lewis notes that it also may be best to notify the school when a problem is first identified, to keep the institution aware of the situation. Once the student reports an unresolved problem to the ACCE, that person can serve as an intermediary with the clinic.

Such situations are troubling for the school as well, which doesn't necessarily want to sever an ongoing relationship with an affiliating clinic. However, Lewis is blunt: "We [universities] cannot operate from fear. By sending students to a facility where you have determined that things are not OK, you are implying that whatever is going on there is acceptable. Students will model after what you do and don't do. We can't complain about a facility, yet still send them to it."

Local universities are familiar with state laws applying to whistleblower situations. Whistleblower protection laws do exist (see sidebar), but liabilities factor into the situation as well. "If a student sees a problem and doesn't report it, he or she could be held liable if another whistleblower calls attention to the situation," Thut cautions. "In the eyes of the law, ignorance is not bliss." **PT**

Claire Coyne is a freelance writer.

References

1. APTA Guide for Professional Conduct. Available at www.apta.org/pt_practice/ethics_pt/pro_conduct. Accessed December 9, 2002.
2. Ethics and Judicial Committee Opinion 4/12/02 [Topic: Preserving Confidences: Physical Therapist's Reporting Obligation with Respect to Unethical, Incompetent, or Illegal Acts]. Available at www.apta.org/PT_Practice/ethics_pt/ejc_opinion_4_12_02. Accessed December 19, 2002.

A Time to Harvest, a Time to Sow: Ethics for a Shifting Landscape

Ruth B Purtilo, PT, PhD, FAPTA

Ruth B Purtilo, known to many physical therapist students and clinicians through her numerous publications in the area of ethics, has influenced the delivery of health care nationally and internationally. Throughout her long career, she has educated us about the moral issues and courses of direction that guide us in our daily lives as health care professionals.

Dr Purtilo has been a visiting professor or named lecturer to more than 30 different colleges and universities worldwide. Her publications, primarily on ethics in health care, include 8 books and more than 70 articles and chapters.

In addition to being involved in APTA, Dr Purtilo has served as President of the American Society of Law, Medicine, and Ethics and was a founding member of the Society of Bioethics Consultation. She is a member of many other professional organizations, including the American Association of Bioethics, the American Philosophical Association, the Society for Health and Human Values, and the World Confederation for Physical Therapy.

Dr Purtilo has been recognized by APTA as a recipient of the Golden Pen Award, the Helen Hislop Award for Outstanding Contributions to Professional Literature, and a Catherine Worthingham Fellowship.

[Purtilo RB. Thirty-First Mary McMillan Lecture: A time to harvest, a time to sow: ethics for a shifting landscape. *Phys Ther.* 2000;80:1112–1119.]

Ruth B Purtilo

I am deeply gratified by the great honor of this lectureship. I know that every McMillan lecturer before me has felt humbled in his or her attempt to honor the legacy of Mary McMillan, and I share in their humility today as I stand before you.

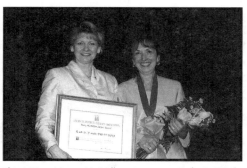

Thirty-First Mary McMillan Lecturer, Ruth B Purtilo (right), accepts award from APTA President Jan K Richardson.

My husband, Vard Johnson, was my most constant encouragement over the months as this lecture did begin to take shape. Thank you, Vard, for all the ways you honor the work of this profession and have commemorated this moment with me already.

In talking to several McMillan lecturers about their experience, I learned that each lecturer prepared for this day a little differently. I began last fall by setting a schedule to read every previous McMillan lecture. They were wonderful! But by January I was terrified. I realized I had nothing to say that had not already been said—and better.

Then one day I read a quote from the great Nebraska plains novelist, Willa Cather, who wrote in *O Pioneers!*: "There are only two or three human stories and they go on repeating themselves as fiercely as if they had never been told before."[1] I realized that there are some important human stories in physical therapy that bear repeating and that my job today is to help remind you of some of them related to our ethical foundations. I hope to say something that will be *worthy* of your remembering in order to tell future generations!

So, to the Nebraska Chapter of the American Physical Therapy Association (APTA) who nominated me, which itself was quite a process, to the many colleagues and friends who wrote letters of support, to the selection committee, to the APTA staff who attended to every detail, and now to you who came today, thank you for this grand opportunity to be a voice to the stories.

Jan Richardson told me that the selection committee thought it fitting to focus on the ethics of our profession as we begin a new millennium. The turn of a millennium does create a natural pause in human history, a "comma" inserted into time. It is a time to look back on what was and to welcome the arrival of a new season in human history.

Dag Hammarskjöld probably was having an evening that felt like the end of one millennium and knew he would awaken to a new one when he wrote in *Markings*:

> Night is drawing nigh.
> For what has been–thanks,
> For what shall be–yes![2]

For what has been–thanks, comma, and for what shall be–yes! In those natural "commas" during our headlong rush through life, something wonderful happens! Fresh air blows into our spirit so that reflection and creativity can thrive. Therefore, having made it through a winter that midway coughed us out on the other side of Y2K, bodies and computers more or less intact, it is a fitting, fresh-air time to prepare the soil and begin the ethical planting for future generations.

RB Purtilo, PT, PhD, FAPTA, is Director, Center for Health Policy and Ethics, Creighton University, 2500 California Plaza, Omaha, NE 68178 (USA) (rpurtilo@creighton.edu).

The Thirty-First Mary McMillan Lecture was presented at PT 2000: The Annual Conference and Exposition of the American Physical Therapy Association; June 14, 2000; Indianapolis, Ind.

What *do* we need to include in a millennial ethics that will yield a "yes" from our professional progeny and assure society's acceptance of us as professionals? The good news is that in any period of a profession's task to grapple with its ethics, there are only 2 time-tested strains of seeds to sow: (1) the seed of care and (2) the seed of accountability. The seed of *care* sends the essence of a profession's commitment deep into the soil of society. *Accountability* sprouts ethical duties and responsibilities so that society has a basis of measuring what it reasonably can expect from the profession. These 2 strains—due care and accountability—are the "staple crops" of professional ethics. The only tending a profession needs to give to these enduring strains is to be sure they will adapt to the social conditions—the peculiarities—of a given time and place: what I call *the social landscape.*

Webster's dictionary tells us that a landscape is "the aggregate landforms of a region."[3] I live in a part of the world where the condition of the physical landscape can make a difference in the world's well being. Flooded wheat fields in Nebraska will drive up bread prices in Macon, Georgia, and pasta prices in Milan. If the good topsoil in the nation's breadbasket blows away, a drought will ensue and people in Tennessee, Thailand, or Timor may feel it. At the same time, year after year farmers and others realize the world's largest harvests, partially as a result of responding knowledgeably to a landscape that is yielding to powerful external forces.

Just as US heartland farmers must know the conditions of the soil for their seeds to take root and grow, so must we become intimately familiar with the human community in which we offer our professional services. Aristotle called ethics "practical philosophy," its methods simply tools for developing "habits of thought" for reflection on complex and changing social realities. Ethical insights are not sequestered in our minds or sealed in the heavens. Forget navel-gazing or stargazing for answers! The tools of ethics are designed for sifting through muddy details of everyday life, examining them for why, to whom, and how we must show care and be accountable.

Today I will describe 2 major seasons or periods in physical therapy's history when we correctly "read" the social landscape and could conclude with confidence that society was ready for us to plant the seeds of our professional ethic. These 2 seasons of physical therapy's ethical identity are the *Period of Self-Identity* and the *Period of Patient-Focused Identity*. In the Period of Self-Identity, we established the moral foundations for a true professional relationship with physicians and other health care professionals. In the Period of Patient-Focused Identity, we established the moral

> **Due care and accountability are the "staple crops" of professional ethics.**

foundations for a true professional relationship with our patients and clients.

I will devote the final minutes of this lecture to a proposition that as our self-identify and our patient-focused identity continue to mature today, we are approaching a third season in a seriously shifting social landscape that appears unfamiliar to us who are accustomed to focusing primarily on the physical therapist's relationships with professional teammates or individual patients. I am calling this emerging season physical therapy's *Period of Societal Identity*. In this most recent period, our task will be to establish the moral foundations for a true professional partnering with the larger community of citizens and institutions.

These 3 periods do not have discreet endpoints in which the stubble of the first successful harvest is cleared for the next planting. The contribution of each previous period is required to provide the appropriate conditions for the next to be added.

The First Season: The Period of Self-Identity
Physical therapy's formal ethical identity formation commenced in 1935 with the issuance of *The American Physiotherapy Association Code of Ethics and Discipline.*[4] At that time, physical therapists lived in a mountainous terrain where physician lords, mostly benevolent and duty-bound men, ruled from on high. All other health care groups were similar to serfs (who knew no other model for relationship with the lords) and skillfully worked the lord's health care fields toward their common goal of good patient care.

In 1935, a group of physiotherapists convened in Atlantic City and drafted a "Code." Today, when I read the document to physical therapist students, many are amazed. No wonder! Listen:

1a. Diagnosing, stating the prognosis of a case and prescribing treatment shall be entirely the responsibility of the physician. Any assumption of this responsibility by one of our members shall be considered unethical.

1b. The patient shall be referred back to the physician for periodical examinations.

2b. [re: Announcements:] A statement that the work is medically supervised should appear in the announcement.[4]

. . . and so on. Both literally and figuratively, the physical therapist promised to stand up when the physician came into the room. And look cheerful. All the time.

That now seems so, well, "retro!" But let's look closely at what was happening. Notice that the patient is not the explicit focus of these statements. The items in this code, sown like apple seeds across the lord's landscape, is about the physical therapists' relationship to physicians! That bold, bright generation of physical therapists, all women, declared, "We're here! And this is what you can expect from us." Furthermore, as codes have as their function to be public statements, they were also saying, "The land we are working is *society's soil*—it doesn't belong to you physicians!" As Carl Rodgers would say, we had "individuated!"

I submit that their timing was perfect. These therapists had read, correctly, a shifting social landscape that was enduring a worldwide depression and would, a few short years later, feel the corrosive effects of a world war and the challenges of social reconstruction following it, as well as face the global ravages of the polio epidemic. Indeed, the entire social terrain of the western world would force physicians down from the mountaintops to labor shoulder to shoulder with nurses and whoever else would share the crushing burden of health care in these extreme circumstances. They found physical therapists ready. Because physical therapy had planted a professional ethical identity, however new and fragile and however constrained its arena of accountability may seem today, its members were positioned to move from serfdom to strong moral partnership.

Sociologists[5] tell us that in this period the health care team was born, and we were positioned to help provide comprehensive coordinated care for a population of patients that could benefit more from a *team's* services than anything we might have offered on our own. Over the next quarter of a century, our heightened professional standing in the health professions would spring not only from an increasing area of expertise, but also from our place at the negotiating tables of policy, because through our code and team activities we were present and proved we could be morally accountable for the success (or lack of success) of our specific contributions on the health care team.[6] Thanks to those awesome women in 1935, we were able to take the first steps toward whom we could become. They helped us heed the words inscribed on the ancient Delphic oracle: "KNOW THYSELF" (before taking on the rest of society)!

The Second Season:
The Period of Patient-Focused Identity

Whereas the ethical task of the first period was to take our place among other health care professionals, the task of the long second period (from the 50s to the present) has been to show care through establishing a true partnership with patients as persons.

The most significant social landscape shift in this period was the introduction in 1957 of "informed consent" into the legal fabric of the physician-patient relationship and its subsequent spread to all clinical and human studies environments.

This mechanism itself partially came about as a result of a post-World War II landscape strewn with new thinking about the scope of individual rights. New rights were articulated through the United Nations Declaration of Human Rights, the US Civil Rights Movement, Medicare and Medicaid legislation, the American Hospital Association Patient's Bill of Rights, and the constitutional right to privacy, to name some. In this rights-intensive territory, the individual's interests became the ideological, political, and economic *standard of policy* so that health care professionals had only to follow what was happening in the rest of society to give patients a stronger voice in decisions affecting them. In fact, patients would meet us more than halfway in our journey from a paternalistic model to a partnership (and, eventually, advocacy) model.

An additional significant aid was the team notion I described in the discussion of our self-identity period. Its emphasis on equal standing among members helped to create an ethos that was more inclusive.

But with all of these factors at play—informed consent mechanisms, rights language, team models—still our initial attempts to make patients decision-making partners were clumsy. In the old mountainous kingdom, patients had been passive recipients. Unfortunately, team members, long accustomed to taking the lordship model as normative, often transferred lordship behavior to the whole health care team. All too often, patients (correctly) experienced it as a team gang-up on them. I remember one glaring example from my experience as a young therapist. A patient assigned to me was 16-year-old John, who had become partially paraplegic when a tree house he was building for his young sister collapsed on him. His ideas about his rehabilitation goals put him at odds with just about all of us. One day, I earnestly told him that he, too, was a key component of the rehabilitation team, so he really must be more cooperative. He just as earnestly replied, "Yeah, you're the players, and I'm the football."

Learning how to partner, let alone advocate, took all of us laboring together. I, like many in this audience, took my own tentative steps in the new, freer, plains landscape: The first APTA paper I ever presented, scared to my toes and grateful that only a handful of people showed for this 7:10 AM session on the last day of conference, was on informed consent. (I had just begun to study ethics and wanted to share this with my colleagues). Within 5 minutes into the presentation, several people had walked out, presumably to go find something more relevant to listen to. My professional "big sister," Catherine Perry Wilkinson, stayed the whole time, though she had already heard me practice that talk aloud in our room at least a dozen times. And afterward, 2 young men who had also stayed to the end came up. The short, taut-muscled, dark wavy-haired one with twinkly eyes told me, "Keep working on this issue! It will help us treat patients with respect, and that is the most important thing we can do." He introduced himself as Charles Magistro. The other guy, softer, rounder, kept nodding in agreement. Before he turned to leave, he said, "Oh sorry, the name's Gene. Gene Michels." Their affirming words sent me skipping all the way back to my room—and ethics studies!

They were right about informed consent, though I, myself, didn't know how right at the time. In fact, it is taking many years for this tender new seedling to root down in the furrows that had been prepared for it by the larger society. Today, it has a prominent place in our *Standards of Practice for Physical Therapy* and other major documents. (It was featured on the front page of the nation's newspapers on Monday, and it continues to be a focus of medical and policy journal articles, especially in regard to its role in clinical research).

Our transformation to a patient-centered identity required attention in other areas as well. Our *Code of Ethics* continued to be our most visible public statement. In the early 1970s, I became the youngest—and greenest—member of the APTA Ethics Committee (then called the Judicial Committee, recently renamed the Ethical and Judicial Committee). There, I joined toilers who were working to weed out of the *Code of Ethics* the emphasis on the size and content of an ad a physical therapist could place in the yellow pages of the telephone directory. The overriding ethical dilemma we struggled with seemed to be: When are capital letters morally permissible?

For all our good work, our efforts were but one season of uprooting, planting, and cultivating new ethical guidelines, each in its own time when the societal soil was ready. Those who have followed since my 1970s experience have continued the process of refining our *Code of Ethics, Standards of Practice for Physical Therapy*, and *Guide to Physical Therapist Practice*[7] and our educational guidelines and research documents toward more patient-focused advocacy.

> **Our task will be to establish the moral foundations for a true professional partnering with the larger community of citizens and institutions.**

So, to all of these contributors, too, on behalf of us all, "thanks!"

During the early years of this second season, physical therapy also took the risk of embracing a formally trained "ethicist." My interest in ethics was generated by my own clinical practice and heightened by questions from my wonderful physical therapist students at Boston University. Adelaide McGarrett, who had already taken the risk of hiring a young, ponytailed instructor just back from Africa and intent on now saving the rest of the world with physical therapy, encouraged me. I entered graduate studies with trepidation, afraid that theology and philosophy would be too daunting for someone in a physical therapist uniform. My suspicions were quickly confirmed: I had at least heard of God, but in my first week, when a young fellow student relayed what he had discovered in his fourth reading of Wittgenstein, I remember thinking, "I don't even know how to *spell* Wittgenstein!"

But there was a far more overriding fear, too. As I wrestled with God, Wittgenstein, Nietzche, and Kant, I felt I was losing my connection with physical therapy, the profession I loved. How would physical therapists understand what an "ethicist" could contribute, when I wasn't certain myself? Sure enough, in one of my first invited physical therapy talks during my ethics studies, I was introduced as an "ethnicist" and shortly after that as a "Methodist-in-training!" One day, I tearfully poured out my anxiety to Nancy Watts. She drew herself up to maybe 8 feet tall and replied in an authoritative, but caring, voice, "Don't think for a moment we will *ever* let you go, Ruth." Nancy herself never let me go, and for her—and many others'—support at key moments, I am deeply grateful. I want to share just a couple other examples.

Carol Davis, that young 60s radical who stood up in the House of Delegates to say we should take political positions on key issues (some of us thought we had met Angela Davis in a blond wig), called me every day to encourage me when my mother was dying from cardiac failure during the same weeks I had to complete my dissertation. And one especially low day before comprehensive exams when I felt myself "going down the tubes," I called Colleen Kigin. She told me to switch on my TV. We sat for the next 2 hours, ears to respective telephone receivers, watching together "The Incredible Shrinking Woman," who, of course, does go down the drain—and survives! Finally, as a new "certified" ethicist teaching my first physical therapy ethics course at the newly opened MGH Institute of Health Professions, I was visited by 2 of the brightest graduate students I would ever work with, Bette Ann Harris and Lee Nelson. They just wanted to be sure I *really* had intended to include Martin Buber's torturous, impossible-to-understand *I & Thou*[8] in the required reading section. When I said, "Yes, it's about respect," Bette Ann finally replied, hesitatingly, "Well, if *that's* what he's trying to say . . ." Both have since gone on to become exemplars of what he was trying to say. Oh, and I've since dropped Buber from my reading list. Too torturous.

Why share these snippets of my own experience with you at such a moment as this? Because I am certain these colleagues and others were not quite sure where I would fit in the end. However, they were so much in the practice of expressing care and making another accountable for what was important to that person that they were able to direct support and encouragement my way when I needed it the most. What more is the ethics of physical therapy all about than this?

I joyfully thank the whole constellation of bright lights that guided me through that forest and back home to this profession, this moment, at this podium. It was a great gift you gave to me, just as it is when you give to patients, clients, students, and others.

I have since happily given up my role as the sole formally trained physical therapist ethicist. Younger people with fresh approaches constitute an impressive team with whom I count it a great privilege to partner, to mentor, and to be mentored by. Together with everyone here, we are learning that the basic tenets of our professional ethics (based on a strong self-awareness and patient-focused loyalty) are instilling themselves deep into the grain of our collective being. And none too soon.

The Third Season:
The Period of Societal Identity

I suggested at the outset of this lecture that our present task is to become full partners with society. Why try to make such a partnership? Because the larger community of citizens and its institutions no longer will accept any other alternative. Either we fully partner or be routed out like the last millennium's dead stalks. One would have to admit that the health care system has handed quite a full plate to society as the new millennium begins. For example:

- the Human Genome Project with its promise to render transplantation obsolete and face-to-face encounters with health care professionals a topic for historical novels—why make a trip to the doc-

tor's office or physical therapy clinic when you can send a nail clipping or lock of hair?,
- megtables and agripharmaceuticals—why make a trip to the pharmacy when genetically implanted medications can be served up in your corn or maple syrup?,
- 100-g babies and 100-year-old grandmas racing for the same therapist's attention,
- robots in the surgical suite,
- CPR—that's Computerized Patient Records—and electronic medical data surveillance,
- 12,000+ people in persistent vegetative states in US long-term care facilities—and increasingly cared for in their loved ones' homes, and
- Molly, Dolly, and the specter of online ordering of cabbage-patch-perfect babies.

Physical therapy, with all *its* new innovations, is in the same seedbag of new possibilities. And there is deep criticism that some of these new seeds of "opportunity," marketed as "progress" may serve society's values best by being left in the silos, unsown.

This criticism often pinpoints the health care professions' highly personalized and individualized approach to patient care as the basis of the problem. Both our technology and the professional skilled personnel who provide the services are targeted. The criticism goes something like this: The post-World War II period yielded an impressive harvest of individual rights and values, but those shoots were sown so heedlessly to create our present health care empire that their roots now threaten to strangle other important values in the larger community.

The one phrase that most fully captures the criticism is: "You cost too much. The price is too high." One aspect of this "price," though not the only important one, is money. I want to say something about money. Not only are we being pinched financially regarding future *expansion* of physical therapist services and educational programs. Note our recent scrape with the 1997 Balanced Budget Act: It was clear and convincing evidence that some US policy-making bodies, especially business and government, want to snip off the seedpods of our current personalized patient practices in an attempt to diminish our propagation and thereby decrease the money society pays us for the services we are already offering. We call our charges "just remuneration"; society's institutions of business and government call them insurance premium hikes, higher taxes. Citizens often respond that health care today is just a "rip-off."

Still, I am often astonished to encounter unwillingness among my physical therapy colleagues to do the homework needed to argue *convincingly* to society that it is getting a great value for our services. We can be convincing through the use of evidence-based outcomes data and other aggregate data that could counter superficial criticism about various interventions we offer to individual patients. These data can be buttressed with stories of individual cases. But our loyalty to individual patients' cases and old familiar approaches seem to leave us unprepared at times to enter into critical policy decisions because we so distrust all decisions based on pooled, aggregate data. This resistance renders us guilty of making an idol of the individual—and, in the end, cheating the very patients we propose to serve.

We need reliable data and rigorous documentation to support when and why our present practices are merited. We need to let lay fallow those practices that have not been submitted to careful review for their effectiveness and cost-efficiency. Such accountabilities on our part will put costs to society into the larger perspective of what it is sacrificing if cuts are made on a more superficial analysis of our contributions. They will also prepare us for a considered response to critics of specialization, doctoral-level preparation, and clinical residencies because, in the eyes of the larger community, these trends are self-interested with the potential simply to make physical therapist services and education "more expensive."

At the same time, we must pay attention not to rush and uproot our time-tested strain of patient-focused identity because we see land-leveling machinery in the distance. It is one thing to accurately arrange data about our practices to bring information into an aggregate form that allows us an effective voice as a partner with society; it is another to let our basic identity be plowed under to make way for something entirely different. One recent article in the medical literature proposed that the best path the professions can follow today is to be a nonbiased "broker" between the traditional patient orientation of professional ethics and the duty to do whatever it takes to cut costs.[9]

We can do better. We can diligently nest the ideals of the profession into the very center of society's priorities. I have 2 brief, basic suggestions regarding how this can be accomplished, and I know you will be able to add others.

First, we can use our strong self-identity to remind society what a health care profession—and the profession of physical therapy specifically—is designed to do. There is absolutely no time for any more whimpering about not knowing exactly who we are. We do know. We know enough. A health care profession is designed to address the health care needs of individuals who can benefit from professional services. Accordingly, from this understanding of self, physical therapists must demand appropriate care for all patients who can

I am talking about making cultural competence as nonnegotiable a graduation requirement—and tested for as rigorously—as competence in pathokinesiology.

benefit more from physical therapy interventions than from those of any other group or by any other means, *then* partner with society to find the resources to make this possible.

Second, we can use what we have learned from our successes in developing a patient-focused identity to make a compelling case for how we can work with society to ensure that a well-defined area of basic patient needs can be met in the new season. We are making some important strides in this area. For example, in 1999, APTA urged PT Team, APTA's 17,000-member grassroots network, to partner with patients in supporting key legislation.[10] Together, arms linked, they could contact members of Congress to sponsor bills to redress the shortcomings of some health plans that had cut physical therapist services that were essential to those patients' appropriate care. That is the right idea.

But taken alone, no one approach is sufficient. For example, attempts to contain costs must not be affirmed if they are implemented simply for additional profit to be realized. As I am sure you know, some current cost-containment measures are needlessly trimming people from eligibility for basic care, especially among working poor people, minorities, and children. We can form coalitions with socially marginalized groups, and with organizations created to help give them voice, to let them know it goes against the essence of a profession to trim people before trimming unnecessarily large margins of profit, trimming administrative overstaffing, or trimming lethargy regarding old practices. If we are complicit in accepting or welcoming the unnecessary pruning of people whose suffering could be prevented or ameliorated, but whose well-being goes unattended for want of physical therapist services, we should drop our claim to professional status now, while we can still walk out of the emerging landscape under our own power. This is about the seed germ—the essence—of our "professing" identity, and all the privileges society has accorded us on that basis—and no other.

There is one prior task we have to accomplish if we are to be successful in meeting the new challenges, even in the 2 general ways I've suggested. We must first plant deeper respect for all people, no matter their color, sex, age, ethnicity, or other personal characteristics. When we do, it will make our claim more plausible when we argue for providing services to anyone who needs them.

As you know, this will be difficult because we are so diversity challenged in our profession. On the encouraging side, in recent years. the profession has learned some of the benefits of embracing diversity, so our numbers among ourselves do gradually look better. And our actions toward patients, subjects, students, and others also continue to show more genuine understanding of the gains all around when differences are appreciated as distinct gifts. Our language has improved thanks to Suzanne "Tink" Martin and others who have shown us how to incorporate nonbiasing terminology into our communications.[11] Our Vision Statement affirms "cultural sensitivity."

But we are not there yet. Just look at how PALE this audience is! Ninety-three percent of the physical therapists in APTA list themselves as "white." More than that speak English as their first language. If we compared ourselves proportionally with people likely to need our services in North America alone, fewer than a third of us in this ballroom should have that profile. And, of course, we are not equally culturally sensitive to all cultures. There is the enigma of the disability culture. How many physical therapists still find "disabled" and "normal" contradictory terms?

Our contribution of enrichment for the millennial landscape will have to include greater diversity within our own ranks at all levels, especially in leadership positions, and many additional changes in our attitudes and practices. A fundamental requirement for successful completion of our educational programs must be cultural competency. I am talking about making cultural competence as nonnegotiable a graduation requirement—and tested for as rigorously—as competence in pathokinesiology.

In short, societal critics today call us to a partnership that accepts constraint and makes prudent use of resources in the name of the common good of the human community. It is up to us to take society's concerns seriously under advisement, then accept only those conditions that honor true public spiritedness and fidelity to our promise. Our promise is to *show care* and *accept responsibility* for the well-being of *all* members who can benefit more from our services than anything else society can offer to prevent or ameliorate the suffering that our expertise allows us to address effectively. The very core of being professional demands it, and it is the key to survival in the new millennium.

Looking back, looking ahead, finding a propitious time for harvesting, uprooting, planting, and, again, harvesting. Dag Hammarsjköld beckoned us to be both thankful and full of anticipation as we survey the larger social landscape at any moment in time. And our experience with our own developing professional ethics is teaching us that there *is* an appropriate time for taking advantage of each new season. We have learned from the past that as we emerged, singing "Here we are!", we were able immediately to join a larger group of health care professional allies and fellow sowers. By being attentive to what constitutes good ethical practice, we were able to plant seeds of patient-centered professionalism into fertile soil. We have enjoyed the fruits of a society where the importance of the individual increasingly has been recognized and respected through laws, policies, and practices. As we go into the future, it is important to remember that each new moment is also a new beginning.

Any one of us here, as we look around this auditorium, probably recognizes people who were "there at the beginning" to help us understand what to be and do when faced with those 2 or 3 important human stories. Thirty-eight years ago, young Susie Isernhagen, Marty Feretti, and I stood in the front row in our shorts and halters on our first day of physical therapy classes, looking askance at each other. Jack Allison announced, noticing our furtive glances, "You will have to get used to working with each other before you can work with patients and go out into society! You are in for a grand adventure!" He was right.

I think if she were here, Mary McMillan would join us in saying, in a loud voice, "For ALL that has been— THANKS, inserting that comma into time, For ALL that can be—YES!"

References

1 Cather W. *O Pioneers!* 1913.

2 Hammarskjöld D. *Markings.* Sjöberg L, Auden WH, trans. New York, NY: Knopf; 1964. Originally published in Swedish as *Vägmärken.* Stockholm, Sweden: Bonniers; 1963.

3 Woolf HB, ed. *Webster's New Collegiate Dictionary.* Springfield, Mass: G & C Merriam Co; 1974.

4 *The American Physiotherapy Association Code of Ethics and Discipline.* Presented at the Fourteenth Annual Convention of the American Physiotherapy Association, Atlantic City, NJ, June 1935.

5 Brown T. An historical view of health care teams. In: Agich G, ed. *Responsibility in Health Care.* Boston, Mass: Reidel; 1982:603–778.

6 Purtilo RB. Ethical issues in teamwork: the context of rehabilitation. *Arch Phys Med Rehabil.* 1988;69:318–322.

7 *Guide to Physical Therapist Practice.* Rev ed. Alexandria, Va: American Physical Therapy Association; 1999.

8 Buber M. *I and Thou.* Magnolia, Mass: Peter Smith Publisher Inc; 1923.

9 Minogue B. The two fundamental duties of the physician. *Acad Med.* 2000;75:431–442.

10 Policy Briefs. *PT Magazine.* 1999;7(7):1–2.

11 Martin S. Language shapes thought. *PT Magazine.* 1999;7(5):44–46.

HABITS OF THOUGHT

By Ruth B Purtilo, PhD, PT, FAPTA

"An Instrument of Our Own Minds"

*Ethical analysis is a tool we can use to attain a desired goal—
in this case, high standards of professional morality.*

You recently may have seen, in a popular magazine, a cartoon that shows a man standing at a crossroads. A road sign points to "Medical Ethics" in one direction, "Legal Ethics" in another direction—and "Ethics Ethics" in yet another direction. The cartoonist probably was poking fun at the pervasiveness of "talk" about ethics in society today. But the cartoon reminded me of something very important: No matter which direction we take as professionals, we will be forced to address ethics. We will be required, at the very least, to reckon both with our profession's *Code of Ethics* and the reasonable expectations that our patients and our society have of us.

In this issue of *PT*, you are given an opportunity to explore an ethical issue that is confronting more health care professionals than ever before. Indeed, the health care professions are at a crossroads as they decide how to report and deal compassionately but firmly with professionals whose functioning is impaired as a result of substance abuse.

For a long time, the topic of substance abuse and its deleterious effects on the way professionals function was shoved to an inconspicuous spot on the side of the road, where it was rarely viewed as noteworthy and even more rarely attended to. Only in recent years have professional organizations and institutions worked to develop mechanisms for the identification, support, and, if necessary, discipline of professionals who are substance abusers.

What Is Ethics?

To help us think about this challenge from an ethics point of view, we must review

> U nlike physical therapy treatment modalities, ...ethical analysis is an instrument of our own minds. It is a disciplined way of thinking.

some basic working definitions and ideas regarding professional ethics.

First, what *is* ethics? *Ethics is both the study of morality and a means through which we can address the practical problems of morality.* In the study of ethics, we try to understand and uphold *morality,* which includes those ideals and guidelines that help a society live peacefully and harmoniously according to its most cherished values. A *problem* isn't always a negative thing. The definition of ethics could be rephrased this way: *Ethical analysis can be used to meet the challenges involved in protecting cherished moral values both of individuals and of communities.*

Ethical analysis may be viewed as a modality or a tool. Like physical therapy treatment modalities, ethical analysis is a means we can use to attain a desired goal—in this case, high standards of professional morality. Unlike physical therapy treatment modalities, however, ethical analysis is an instrument of

our own minds. It is a disciplined way of thinking ("habits of thought"). Some of the concepts we use in analyzing morality are concepts involving "duties," "rights," and "virtues." When important values related to our morality are challenged, we ask, "Who has a duty to protect the values in this situation? Why? What duty does it entail? Whose rights are at risk? Whose responsibility is it to make certain that harm is minimized and benefit is maximized?"

Ethical Analysis at Work

Suppose that during the past few months you have seen a drastic change in your colleague AB, who lately has a disheveled appearance and is unable to remember even simple things. Something clearly is wrong. Every time you approach AB about this, he says he is okay; however, several incidents in the last week have convinced you that he is putting patients at risk. One patient even took you aside and suggested that AB was "acting kind of strange," but the patient would not elaborate.

You strongly suspect AB has a substance abuse problem.

In addition to your concern for AB, what else is going through your mind? You probably are worrying about your own—and your other colleagues'—duty to make certain that patients are not harmed as a result of AB's behavior. You may be thinking about the patients' rights to safety and respect. You also may be thinking about AB's rights (and your own) if you decide to pursue the matter. Overall, you are analyzing this perplexing situation in terms of its deleterious effects on the well-being of your colleague, the people dependent on your colleague, the professional community, and the larger society. *You are engaging in ethical analysis.*

Four Steps of Ethical Analysis

An ethical analysis of a practical problem such as this one requires several steps:

1. *Gather relevant clinical and other facts so that you will be able to identify the specifics of the challenge ahead of you.* Find out as much as you can about AB's difficulty, a process you already have begun. Share your own observations with key people, such as other therapists. You may need to strike a delicate balance between protecting AB's confidentiality and finding out the facts. Explore the existing laws, policies, and other guidelines regarding persons who are impaired as a result of substance abuse. In other words, your first step is to *verify and document.*

2. *Identify key moral concepts and ideals.* As a physical therapist, AB has duties, among which are a) the duty not to harm patients, b) the duty to help patients, and c) the duty to meet patients' reasonable expectations. (In professional ethics, these duties are called *nonmaleficence, beneficence,* and *faithfulness* or *fidelity.*) As a potential "whistleblower," you have these same duties; however, you also owe a duty to your colleague AB not to cause him undue harm, and a duty of beneficence to society to protect it from people whose behavior may be harmful to others. Think about the various rights involved: the patients', yours, society's, and AB's. What is the extent and type of your moral responsibility in this situation? At this time, your task is to *assess and reflect.*

    You now realize you have an ethical dilemma—the type of situation in which you are caught "between the devil and the deep blue sea." If you act to protect one set of values, you will necessarily compromise another set of values. Protecting the patients' right to safety, for example, may compromise your colleague's ability to make a living, whereas protecting your colleague's confidentiality may com-

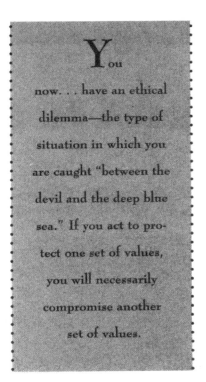

You now... have an ethical dilemma—the type of situation in which you are caught "between the devil and the deep blue sea." If you act to protect one set of values, you will necessarily compromise another set of values.

promise society's right to be protected from undue harm at his hands.

3. *Think about your options.* If you decide not to act, you may not be fulfilling your moral responsibility to protect patients and society from harm. If you *do* act, you are at risk of harming AB or putting yourself in jeopardy. Because you have completed steps 1 and 2, your commitment to upholding the high moral standards of the profession now must govern your judgment about whether and how to take action. These standards are important because they reflect cherished values both of society and of the physical therapy profession.

    The virtue of temperance will serve you well in your desire not to act rashly or cause undue harm. Think of "blowing the whistle" as a last-resort action to be used only when more conservative approaches—such as talking with AB about his substance abuse—have failed to alleviate the problem. *Your biggest challenge is to think creatively and expansively.*

4. *When you have taken all factors into account, you must carry out your plan.* To do less is to show complicity in the harm that may ensue. At the same time, your actions should be carried out with the goal of minimizing the harm to all affected parties. *To act takes courage.*

Ethics and Everyday Practice

The steps used in the ethical analysis of a situation involving a colleague who is a substance abuser may be applied to many other types of situations in everyday practice. In the months ahead, you no doubt will have an opportunity to do so. *PT*

Next month: **John Banja, PhD,** *reflects on fraud in physical therapy practice and research.*

Ruth B Purtilo, PhD, PT, FAPTA, *is Professor of Clinical Ethics, Creighton University Center for Health Policy and Ethics, Omaha, Neb. She received her bachelor's degree in physical therapy from the University of Minnesota-Minneapolis, practiced physical therapy in the United States and Swaziland, and worked as a physical therapy consultant with Project Hope in Colombia. She received a Master of Theological Studies degree in ethics from the Harvard Divinity School and a doctoral degree in ethics from the Harvard University Graduate School of Arts and Sciences, Cambridge, Mass.*

Dr Purtilo has been Henry Knox Sherrill Professor of Medical Ethics and Ethicist-in-Residence, Massachusetts General Hospital; Visiting Scholar in Medical Ethics, the Karolinska Institute, Stockholm, Sweden; Associate Professor of Community and Family Medicine, University of Massachusetts Medical School, Worcester; and Chairperson and Professor, Department of Medical Jurisprudence and Humanities, University of Nebraska College of Medicine, Omaha.

An international lecturer in biomedical ethics, Dr Purtilo has served as an ethics consultant to the US government and to other governmental agencies throughout the world. She is a fellow of the Hastings Center, a renowned ethics research center, and is a member of the board of directors of the American Society of Law and Medicine and Society for Bioethics Consultation. She was named a Catherine Worthingham Fellow of APTA in 1989.

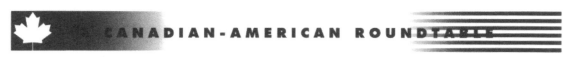

CANADIAN-AMERICAN ROUNDTABLE

Ethical Dilemmas in Practice:
BOTH SIDES OF THE BORDER

As managed care and health care reform revise health care delivery, resolving ethical dilemmas in physical therapy practice becomes increasingly critical. Six administrators, managers, and clinicians from the United States and Alberta, Canada, share their concerns with medical ethicist Ruth Purtilo.

To frame this discussion of nuts-and-bolts ethical issues in practice, Ruth Purtilo suggests that there are three levels of professional ethics:

Level 1—Actions and behaviors that are morally required and therefore not negotiable. If situations make it impossible to follow these morally required actions and behaviors, physical therapists as professionals in those situations automatically are practicing below the acceptable "ethical threshold."

Level 2—Actions and behaviors that may not be ethically or otherwise ideal but that are morally permissible. At this level, physical therapists have the option to consider their responsibilities to either "fix" these situations or accommodate them.

Level 3—Actions and behaviors that are morally prohibited. PTs are duty-bound both to avoid these actions and behaviors and to prevent them from occurring.

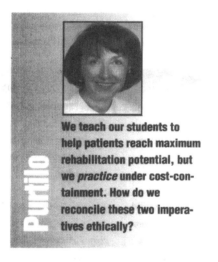

Purtilo

We teach our students to help patients reach maximum rehabilitation potential, but we *practice* under cost-containment. How do we reconcile these two imperatives ethically?

Purtilo: A number of dilemmas, new and old, face PTs practicing in the United States and Canada today. The goal of our discussion is to help begin identifying the ethical dimensions of these dilemmas—and help PTs as they search for solutions.

Davis: The #1 ethical dilemma in America today is that we want to provide universal health care but we cannot afford it. The distribution and availability of services, and the primary relationship between PT and patient, are at stake. Is there even enough *time* to deliver services to all the people who want them?

Snyder: Even *before* the implementation of health care reform in the United States, we are beginning to deal with the cost-containment imperatives of managed care. Of course, the Canadians have been dealing with cost-containment for a long time.

"Living in a Kind of Disneyland"
Purtilo: It may be argued that what we traditionally have taught our students to do—help patients reach their maximum rehabilitation potential—PTs can no longer do under the constraints of managed care and health care reform. Can PTs retain the goal of maximum rehabilitation potential under cost-containment? If not, what are the ethical implications?

Davis: In defining "maximum rehabilitation potential," the patient's condition and age and other factors must be considered. Many of our new graduates don't have the experience to determine maximum potential or to know how far they should go with each patient to reach that potential... We need to help new professionals understand the parameters of "maximum potential"—regardless of cost-containment issues.

Snyder: Historically, we've been able to treat patients for extended periods of time, and that treatment has included passive therapies. We've believed that patients need to be "under our wing" to reach their maximum rehabilitation potential. That has been the approach of the entire medical community, and that approach needs to change.... Although we still may see patients achieving high levels of function under our direct care in the future, we increasingly will need to teach them to deal with their own back pain and resolve their own weaknesses, *giving them the skills to help themselves.* That's our ethical duty under the principle of beneficence. Ironi-

cally, we are being *forced* into this approach by insurers who may limit us, for example, to six visits to rehabilitate a patient who's had reconstructive knee surgery.

Purtilo: Is it the PT's job today to put responsibility back on the patient, saying, "We can empower you, but we can't continue to treat you"?

Snyder: No. But the PT who has had the opportunity to see a patient with low back pain for as many as 30 or 40 treatments, for example, needs to understand the link between that practice pattern and why cost-containment measures are being instituted in

the first place. Is there something we can do to reduce costs in our own practices in terms of how we treat and educate patients? This relates to the second level of ethical consideration—those actions and behaviors that may not be "ethically ideal" but that may be morally permissible ["What is 'Morally Required' of PTs?", page 46]. How much can or will we accommodate? In this case, how much will we "squeeze down" our care? We don't want to *withdraw* care, we want to provide care more *efficiently.*

Purtilo: In the United States, we may have been living in a kind of Disneyland. We've always said to our patients, "Just keep com-

The Participants

Marion Briggs, PT, is Administrative Facilitator, Patient Care Design Project, University of Alberta Hospitals, and Clinical Associate Professor, Faculty of Rehabilitation Medicine, University of Alberta, Edmonton.

Kenneth Davis, PT, is Assistant Administrator, Mid-America Rehabilitation Hospital, Overland Park, Kan. As former APTA Director of Practice , he served as liaison to the Joint Commission on Accreditation of Healthcare Organizations, the Commission on Accreditation of Rehabilitation Facilities, and the National Athletic Trainers' Association/APTA Task Force. Davis is a member of PT's Editorial Advisory Group.

Ruth Purtilo, PhD, PT, FAPTA, is Professor of Clinical Ethics, Center for Health Policy and Ethics and Department of Physical Therapy, Creighton University, Omaha, Neb, and Immediate Past President, American Society of Law, Medicine, and Ethics. She previously was Henry Knox Sherrill Professor of Medical Ethics and Ethicist-in-Residence, Massachusetts General Hospital, Boston, Mass.

Judy Sebring, PT, is Director of Physical Therapy, San Jose Medical Center, San Jose, Calif. She formerly was President and currently is Chief Delegate, APTA California Chapter.

Jayne Snyder, MA, PT, is President, Knortz & Snyder Physical Therapy, Lincoln, Neb. She served on APTA's Task Force on Health Care Reform and as President of the Nebraska Chapter and currently is a member of the Nebraska Chapter's Legislative Committee.

Jenneth Swinamer, PT, is Manager, Rehabilitation Services, and Chair, Steering Committee, Patient Focused Care Project, Royal Alexandra Hospital, and Clinical Associate Professor, Faculty of Rehabilitation Medicine, University of Alberta, Edmonton. Swinamer also is President, Physiotherapy Foundation of Canada, and Chair, Practice Review Board, College of Physical Therapists of Alberta.

Bob Sydenham, PT, COMP, is Director, RW Sydenham Associates Physical Therapy Services, and Clinical Assistant Professor, Faculty of Rehabilitation Medicine, University of Alberta, Edmonton. He serves on the Disciplinary Committee of the Alberta Physical Therapy Licensing Board and is President, International Federation of Manipulative Therapists (IFOMT).

What is "Morally Required" of PTs?

Purtilo: As we discuss some of the ethical issues facing physical therapy practice today, we first must ask ourselves, "Is something morally required of us, and, if so, why?"

Davis: But how do we define what is "moral"?

Purtilo: "Morality" is a community enterprise. We use it as a guide for preserving the very fabric of the human community and for helping people live together in peace and harmony. Our understanding of what is moral comes from many sources—religious and philosophical beliefs, family, and society, for example. Sometimes writers talk about a "professional morality" to designate that some duties, rights, and virtues are appropriate for a given context or community.... The type of moral relationship *physical therapists* have with patients and clients is partly determined by the societal expectation that therapists, as professionals, will behave in certain ways. Society expects, for example, that we will not harm patients. Society expects that we will not only *do something* for patients but that we will do what is best for them, according to the principle of beneficence. And society expects that certain types of physical therapy activities will be performed only with the patient's informed consent. The very context in which we operate, then, puts constraints on what we do.... We also have professional association codes of ethics, the public statements by which others measure our actions and by which we measure our own actions.

Davis: So we have subsets of community expectations—those of society at large, those of the medical society, those of our own professional society, those of our own clinics or departments, and those of the individual.

Briggs: The context in which we practice has many layers and influences both patient and care provider. There are "third parties"—and not just insurers!—lining up behind the patient and provider in the primary partnership. Behind the values and morals of the patient, there are those of the family, spouse, and surrogate decision maker. Then there are the community's interests, which can take two forms: the interests of the patient's ethnocentric community—which may be a minority in the general community—and the individual legal interests protected by state law. Lining up behind the values and morals of the *care provider* are the professional ethical code, hospital or facility policies, government funding policies, and legal interests of the community. There also are the values of the international community in terms of the "mega-allocation" of resources. The agenda for morality changes to some extent in each of these dimensions.

Purtilo: And the agendas may come into conflict... My personal definition of an ethical dilemma is that there may be two "right" things to do, but doing one thing compromises the other. Those are the times when we wake up in the middle of the night, unable to sleep.... One example of an ethical dilemma is that we teach our students to help patients reach maximum rehabilitation potential, but we practice under the constraints of cost-containment. How do we reconcile these two imperatives? This becomes a *moral* problem because we profess to society in our codes and our practice standards that *we will do what's best for the patient.*

ing—it's all here." Well, it's not all here anymore!

Who Determines Maximum Rehabilitation Potential?

Briggs: An underlying value among PTs—perhaps more so among Americans than among Canadians at this point—seems to be that we as professionals are the best ones to determine a patient's maximum rehabilitation potential and that somehow our determination becomes more accurate with experience. But does this respect the ethical imperative of patient autonomy in decision making? After all, what matters is not so much the maximum rehabilitation potential given the x, y, and z of a set of physiological factors. What matters is care that is *meaningful to the patient*. If we approach practice with that in mind, the economic imperatives may recede to play a more manageable role, instead of driving care as they now threaten to do. We won't be constricted—or, more importantly, our patients won't be constricted—by the belief that we as professionals know what needs to be done and we've got to be the ones who do it.... Unless we change our approach, we'll fail in our ethical duty to do what's best for the patient.

Swinamer: The major question, then, is who determines what the patient needs.

Davis: But the other part of that question *must* be, "What can the PT deliver to work effectively toward meeting the patient's needs, given the patient's prognosis and the PT's intervention skills?" The new graduate has a blank-slate expectation about working toward maximum rehabilitation potential.

Purtilo: Let's say that experience can serve as a guide in reaching realistic goals, and

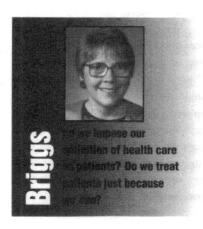

Briggs

"If we impose our definition of health care on patients? Do we treat patients just because we can?"

that, with experience, the PT's assessment begins to be informed. What if a therapist who has treated x number of patients with back pain encounters a new patient who says, "It's my back pain, and I need 50 treatments"? Many would conclude that the therapist's experience should govern—though, of course, the patient should be dealt with respectfully.

Snyder: We just can't give patients 50 treatments today! Under health care reform in the United States, we will have a "gate-keeper," or primary-care provider, who will decide how much care a patient will receive to achieve a certain level of quality of life. This means that PTs need to determine functional outcomes in each clinic, region, and specialty area... The fact is, we haven't defined maximum rehabilitation potential for certain diagnoses. There are many different types of strokes and stroke-related damage, for example. The long-term goal for the patient with stroke may be to ambulate x number of feet in the home setting. But what if 90% of patients with stroke in a clinic in one state reach this goal with 15 treatments over 2 months, and in a clinic in another state it takes 40 treatments? We need to scrutinize these differences.

Davis: We also presuppose that what we *do* results in the rehabilitation outcomes we *document*. Can we really differentiate between a natural recovery process and that which the PT effects through treatment?

Purtilo: I think we know—and are moving in the direction of more fully documenting—how the patient is improved through our interventions. But we aren't completely "there" yet.

Sebring: Even when we *do* know the maximum potential for a particular condition, we still need to determine *which route* is best for reaching that potential. Is it through teaching the patient in a home program with frequent monitoring? Or is it through a group setting rather than on a one-to-one basis? Ethically and otherwise, we must help the patient reach maximum

potential—but we can't burden the patient with treatment the insurer won't cover. Again, we need to educate the patient and family to supplement what we do.

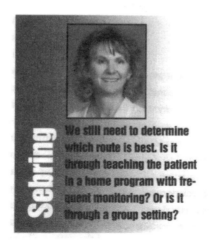

Sebring

We still need to determine which route is best. Is it through teaching the patient in a home program with frequent monitoring? Or is it through a group setting?

Swinamer: PTs still can provide hands-on care, but the emphasis needs to shift so that PTs serve as "consultants" to patient, family, and nursing staff. PTs need to look for *opportunities to be flexible* both in serving as consultants and in providing hands-on care. This is already happening in many settings across Canada.

Sydenham: Believing that you are going to help the patient reach *maximum* rehabilitation potential is not being in touch with reality! Maximum potential is not equivalent to *optimal* rehabilitation in these times of fiscal restraint. If you, the PT, were *paying* for the services instead of *being paid* to deliver them, how many times—and over how many weeks—would *you* have the patient come back for treatment?

Purtilo: Once again we are confronted with today's bottom line of cost-containment.... We therapists may be tempted to say that government, facility, or society is keeping us from what we know we "ethically" need to do, such as working toward maximum rehabilitation potential. But this group seems to be saying that there may be other ways for PTs to meet that goal: through the generation of outcomes data; through greater respect for patient autonomy; and through consultation with patients, families, and caregivers.

What *is* Health Care?

Sydenham: In Canada, physical therapy is defined as a "nonessential medical service." It's held that physical therapy improves quality of life but that it's not a matter of life or death.... The *level* of quality depends on who's paying. It's like buying a car. How much money you have determines the quality. In Alberta and other parts of Canada in which the state is the payer, the state is determining the bare-bones minimum of treatment that can be delivered to provide essential medical services. The Cadillac type of treatment that's been reimbursed on a fee-for-service basis is a thing of the past—unless it's allowed through a private insurance plan [ie, a non-Provincial health plan, such as that provided through an employer].

Briggs: When we talk about quality, it's important to realize that some patients may overstate their need for care—and that others may not *want* as much care as we give them.

Sebring: I agree. How many of us have heard patients finally say, "I'm weary of coming in for physical therapy"?

Briggs: Again, what is meaningful to *us*—walking 50 feet, for example, or dressing independently—may not be so for the patient. Especially in tertiary and quaternary facilities that use a great deal of high-tech medical procedures, many patients are vastly overtreated medically and, on a moral and social level, are treated more frequently than and differently from what would be meaningful for them. Do we impose our definition of health care on patients? *Do we treat patients just because we can?* As genetic engineering projects unfold, there will be even more fundamental ethical questions. As health professionals, we must ask ourselves not what *can* we do, but what *ought* we to do, for the individual patient.

Davis: In talking with Kansas legislators about health care reform initiatives, it's become clear to me that one of the basic dilemmas is how to define health care. Traditionally, health care has been defined

from a World Health Organization perspective—that is, in part, in terms of pathology, impairments related to pathology, and medical and surgical intervention. But our *society* has never really defined what health care should or should not include. One of the dominant costs to society is not the medical services themselves, but the social support systems that help patients return to their roles within society or, when patients cannot return to their roles, the systems that absorb the burden of their care.

Purtilo: And PTs often work at the boundary between medical and social services. What, then, is our ethical responsibility in regard to the amount and type of care that patients have a right to expect from us?

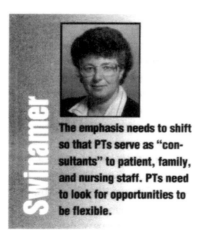

The emphasis needs to shift so that PTs serve as "consultants" to patient, family, and nursing staff. PTs need to look for opportunities to be flexible.

Snyder: On the first visit, I ask the patient about his or her goals and timeframes. My expertise should be used to modify the patient's goals so they're realistic and involve the family.... The third-party payer will write physical therapy goals if we don't establish realistic ones.

Sebring: And we need to continually reevaluate goals. After all, patients change their expectations.

Sydenham: But how *often* do you monitor the patient over a period of time? Does the *family* monitor the patient? As Ken [Davis] alluded to earlier, we don't know how much progress patients would achieve on their own.

Snyder: We also may see different recovery rates depending on who pays the bill. In my experience, cash-paying patients who have a large deductible tend to reach their goals more quickly than those whose physical therapy is being covered.

Sydenham: In Canada, Workers' Comp pays 90% of wages, tax-free; in Sweden, it pays 110%. When a patient can stay at home and receive 90% of his or her wages through Workers' Comp, the agenda for rehabilitation may be very different from what it would be if the patient were not receiving wages.

A Moral Imperative to Change Policy?

Purtilo: Should PTs take reimbursement policy as *the* governing authority? Is it the therapist's job, for example, to advocate for a system that is more similar to that of Canada or Sweden?

Sydenham: Alberta, for example, is changing the acceptable parameters of operation, cutting down on long-term care, implementing managed care, reviewing cases that involve multiple-year treatment, and moving patients from facilities that have been giving multiple-year treatment. PTs *definitely* should be involved in those types of decisions.

Purtilo: Let's look at the bigger picture, too. As we've discussed, what we used to do as therapists—and what we teach our students to do—we may no longer be able to do under health care reform. Do we, at our level of professionalism in Canada and the United States, have a moral imperative to become involved in *policy* changes?

Briggs: Yes—when we're talking about *micro-allocation*, or care for one patient, and *meso-allocation*, or hospital and clinic policies that determine patient care. However, in *macro-allocation*, which involves policymaking at the government and third-party level, the appropriateness of our influence becomes less clear. The PT *may* have a moral imperative to act as a clinical expert

"Patient Clusters"

"If we were going to create a brand new world for our patients," asks *Marion Briggs*, "What would it look like?"

That's the question the Patient Care Design Project—headed by Briggs at the University of Alberta Hospitals (UAH), Edmonton—hopes to answer by September of this year. As the primary teaching hospital and medical center for northern Alberta and parts of the Northwest Territories, UAH has more than 6,000 staff—all of whom will be affected by the project. Formerly Director of Rehabilitation Services, Briggs says the complexities of this project are preparing her for a second career—in corporate ethics.

"Through redesign and reengineering, UAH plans to reduce its $240 million budget by $40 million over the next 3 years," explains Briggs. Consultant to the project is APM, an American management consulting firm.

Fourteen multidisciplinary teams of 20 to 30 professionals and managers are clustering patients based on the services those patients need. The goal is to make *fundamental* changes—changes in how, when, and by whom services will be provided.

A team may decide, for example, that a particular cluster of patients needs physical therapy immediately postsurgery, an immediate turnaround of laboratory tests, some occupational therapy, and a particular type of relationship with the referring physician. It is then the task of the "supplier design teams" to determine how to meet those needs in the most cost-effective way possible.

Other project teams include the patient support team (eg, personnel who provide pastoral care, nutrition, laundry services); the corporate support team (eg, personnel concerned with human resources, finance, and administration); and the information management team, which supports all

teams with computer and other technology. Briggs estimates that, in all, as many as 300 staff will be involved in the team process. "Nothing is excluded from review," she adds, "whether it's how many VPs we need or what types of tests and interventions a patient needs or how to fold the bed linen."

Briggs believes that this project is the only one of its kind worldwide. "Many academic health centers in the United States, for example, have reengineered themselves; however, none has simultaneously undertaken operational restructuring [*how* things should get done] and clinical resource management redesign [*what* things should get done, based on DRGs or case mix groupings, or CMGs]." One of UAH's advantages is that it already underwent "decentralization" last year, replacing the traditional physical therapy, occupational therapy, respiratory, speech-language, nursing, and medical departments with patient service teams. Total quality improvement staff training implemented 4 years ago also helped pave the way for the project.

"We've been moving steadily toward an ever greater focus on patient need," says Briggs, who believes all health care facilities, regardless of size, should and must move in that direction.

Briggs cites care maps, which are designed to reduce variation in treatment, as part of the movement. "The usage of some treatments, such as radical mastectomy and colostomy, varies widely from region to region," she says. "Care maps aim to reduce that variation." Critics suggest that care maps remove the "right and obligation to make decisions outside the parameters of the maps" and will create "technicians" who apply cookbook procedures, she explains, whereas proponents claim that care maps require the practitioner to examine clinical decisions

critically. "Is the health outcome for hospitalized patients different with daily versus weekly chest radiographs, for example?" asks Briggs. "The goal is not to take away clinical judgment. The goal is to enhance it. Do physicians need to order screening tests that have multiple results when they have to wade through information they *don't* want to get the information they *do* want?"

In Briggs's view, health care *must* change. "The world is different from the way it was when many of us entered physical therapy practice. There are so many ways to keep people alive.... The global economy cannot continue to support the large percentages of gross national product spent on health care." For Briggs, the key is to decide what constitutes "defensible practice."

"The truth is, we don't know the impact of 80% of what *any* health professional does for patients." The data, says Briggs, show health is more influenced by education, diet, and environment than it is by "sick intervention," but a greater proportion of resources is spent to manage illness than is spent to promote health.

Quality of life, asserts Briggs, will gain increasing importance over the next few years, and "alternative" therapies will become standard, "which has implications for the overall use of health dollars to promote health rather than treat sickness." If massage can be used in conjunction with physical therapy to prevent deterioration or complications, she says, it's an investment—an investment that may be less expensive than traditional physician-driven services.

"Traditionally, we've thought of health care as a way to 'fool' death. But is *death* the real enemy?" *PT*

—*Jan Reynolds*

with a sound body of knowledge to recommend policy based on a population rather than on individuals.

Snyder: The moral imperative is clear-cut for me. PTs need to be very active in changing state and federal regulation on health care.

Purtilo: Would you generalize this as a responsibility that all your colleagues share?

Snyder: Yes—Association members and nonmembers alike. PTs also need to be active on utilization review boards. Because policy affects our patients, we need to be making changes at the level of policy.

Davis: It's not so much an imperative to make changes, it's an imperative to raise level of awareness... Society traditionally has defined health care as hospital-based and physician-delivered, but society has evolved to a point at which health care costs go beyond that definition to include the support of social roles. And it's in that realm that rehabilitation plays its major role. If rehabilitation is not included adequately in health care reform, society will eventually pay the price, *because the definition of health care will have been narrowed.* PTs should play a key role in helping the public understand that.

Sebring: I agree. Our moral role as professionals is not so much to change policy but to educate politicians and the public about choices. The public can't make informed choices right now about physical therapy, partly because we haven't given them the information they need about the benefits of physical therapy. If we give them the data, they may or may not decide to change the policies... Invite legislators into the clinic. Show them what you do and what results you achieve.

Snyder: It's never been more critical to educate the legislators. There will be a major lag time between the public's responses and our responses to the health care reform proposal.... Many legislators have no contact with rehabilitation. When I hear Bob [Sydenham] suggesting that reha-

bilitation could become optional or elective care in Canada, it scares me. In Nebraska, we fought hard to keep physical therapy as a standard benefit under Medicaid. We need to tell legislators about how physical therapy intervention can reduce costs.

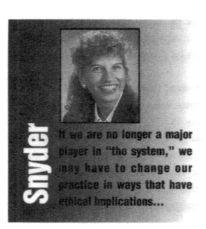

If we are no longer a major player in "the system," we may have to change our practice in ways that have ethical implications...

Gatekeepers, POPTS, and Ethics

Purtilo: Many PTs in the United States do not think of themselves as being skilled in the political process. Can our Canadian colleagues help guide us in these efforts?

Sydenham: We can offer our experience. For example, the Canadian physical therapy profession recently has had to respond in a formal way to the chiropractic profession, which has proposed to the governments of Alberta, Ontario, and Manitoba that chiropractors should serve as "gatekeepers" for patients with low back pain. They've used the "Manga Report"[1] to support their position, a report that, like so many others, equates physical therapy with modalities and chiropractic with manipulation.... It's likely that the same proposal will be made to US legislators.

Purtilo: Why are issues such as gatekeeper roles *ethical* issues?

Snyder: We've been trained to improve quality of function and quality of life. If we are no longer a major player in "the system," we may have to change our practice in ways that have ethical implications... For example: In 5 years there may be no other place for PTs to practice but physician-owned practices or joint ventures [physician-and-PT-owned practices] that comprise many of the health care alliances now being formed across the United States.

Purtilo: But why, specifically, is physician-owned physical therapy services [POPTS] an *ethical* issue?

Snyder: Because of the potential for abuse and unethical conduct when the physician profits from referral to his or her own physical therapy clinic. Data from the state of Florida, for example, have indicated that utilization and cost of care is higher in joint ventures.[2]

Sydenham: In Canada, POPTS are restricted by law; only Ontario allows POPTS. In Alberta, for example, 75% of a physical therapy service operation must be owned by a PT.

Briggs: Would the ethical dilemma in the United States include PTs owning more than one clinic and cross-referring to one of their own clinics?

Snyder: That's a good question, and it hasn't really been answered yet. People have asked—legitimately—"What is the difference between a physician owning the clinic and a PT owning the clinic?" In the United States, however, most insurers still require physician referral, so the abuse primarily is in physicians referring patients to their own physical therapy clinics.

Davis: This issue requires a much broader discussion about controlling referral, especially in terms of hospital systems that refer within themselves... I would argue, however, that the ethical issue is not the POPTS. The *real* ethical issue is whether a given service to patient or community is being provided by the health professionals who are best prepared to help patients achieve the best outcomes possible. Whether those professionals are PTs, OTs, or nursing staff is not necessarily the ethical issue at stake.

Snyder: But we haven't documented yet who can provide the best-possible care. We

haven't documented that PTs are more efficient in rehabilitating an ankle joint than are, for example, ATCs. That's why people outside the profession question us.

Purtilo: The underlying current here seems to be that there is a moral requirement to provide the best setting possible for optimal care, and that clinical judgment may be influenced or even blocked in some settings.

Swinamer: I don't believe PTs in the United States will ever be limited to practicing in only POPTS or joint ventures. But PTs *should* worry about the economic value that is attributed to their services. They should make sure the value supports them—whether it's through physician practice, hospital practice, or private practice.

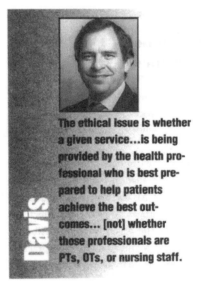

The ethical issue is whether a given service...is being provided by the health professional who is best prepared to help patients achieve the best outcomes... [not] whether those professionals are PTs, OTs, or nursing staff.

Davis

Snyder: The fact remains, however, that for years many PTs in the United States have felt there is a strong potential for abuse of both patient and PT in joint ventures and physician-owned clinics. As health care alliances become a fact of life, how can we be involved in those alliances *and* reconcile this long-standing ethical dilemma?

Purtilo: These are issues of professional identity involving what is required of any health professional. We are legitimately concerned about changes in the system that might mitigate our potential to be the best-prepared practitioners to deliver a given ser-

vice... The onus of responsibility is on us to prove that what we're doing for our patients is best. The companion ethical dimension is that, *if we are doing what's best for the patient, we ought to be able to continue doing it.*

Snyder: And if we are the best-prepared professionals to serve the patient in the rehabilitation arena, what are the ethical implications when we have a limited amount of money, such as under capitation or DRGs, and we have only $600 to rehabilitate an injured shoulder, and we begin to overutilize ancillary personnel to reach patient goals? What happens when—as part of the strategy to make ends meet—we utilize on-the-job-trained physical therapy aides with high school degrees to perform 90% of care?

Briggs: This again raises the fundamental ethical question: What does the professional, by virtue of his or her training, *need* to do? What is morally permissible, morally impermissible, and morally debatable? I would argue that there is very little that PTs could rightfully claim as an absolute moral imperative, as something that *only* the physical therapy professional must do.

Davis: We often say that issues are "ethical" issues when, in truth, they're not.

Briggs: *Why* do we utilize ancillary personnel and multiskilled practitioners? If the net effect is that a profession "downloads" undesirable or unpleasant tasks to personnel who are lower on the hierarchical ladder, that's an ethical problem based on a lack of respect for individuals. It wouldn't necessarily—but it could—have a negative impact on patient care. On the other hand, if using ancillary personnel enhances everyone's capacity to contribute, that's a positive. Professionals, by not doing tasks they don't *need* to do, can concentrate on the tasks they're especially skilled to do. In that scenario, nonprofessionals, who have skills and abilities they're currently not able to use because of professional territorial guarding, could contribute more fully. The ethical dilemma disappears. And everybody "wins."

"Patient-Focused Care"

As Manager of Rehabilitation Services and Chair of the Steering Committee of the Patient Focused Care Project at Royal Alexandra Hospital in Edmonton, Alberta, *Jenneth Swinamer* has encouraged her staff to "embark on a different style of practice, emphasizing consultation as well as hands-on care... Today, with discharge happening more and more rapidly, we need to learn how to do more with less." The consultant, explains Swinamer, teaches not only patients but family caregivers and other health care providers to ensure continuity and consistency of care and achievement of patient goals *throughout* the 24-hour day.

Swinamer and her staff assembled a "teaching package" containing information on adult learning styles—particularly on how learning styles may differ among patients and different types of health professionals. The package addresses behavioral issues (eg, how to be "assertive" versus "aggressive"), problem solving, and direct teaching (eg, of nursing staff). Staff also engaged in role-playing exercises to explore how their interactions would be different as "consultants." They asked themselves, "Am I the only person who can give the patient a particular type of care?"

"In the acute care setting, the patient may see the PT for only one half hour out of the 24 hours a day that the patient is in the hospital," says Swinamer. "How can the PT 'maximize' that half hour, making it meaningful for the remaining 23½ hours? One way is through teaching other health professionals."

Swinamer says she welcomes involvement by nursing and other professionals in specific tasks that previously may have been viewed as strictly physical therapy tasks, such as patient ambulation or chest physical therapy—"tasks that should belong to all caregivers."

The utilization of therapy assistants, or service aides (including the therapy aide, therapy technician, therapy attendant, and other on-the-job-trained support personnel) is one key to the transition toward a more consultative role for PTs. In Winnipeg, Manitoba, Swinamer headed a Physiotherapy Regulatory Board committee on supervision of therapy assistants. Two types of supervision were identified: administrative (eg, monitoring aspects such as dress code, punctuality, and general safety behaviors, especially important for the large traveling therapy teams that staff rural hospitals and whose members typically are hired by nursing staff) and clinical direction (eg, ensuring that therapy assistants do not assess, act on clinical judgment, or progress the treatment, but follow the program of care as defined by the therapist).

Swinamer served as clinical consultant for a subsequent multiprofessional study on "multiskilled second-level practitioners," supported by the Canadian Physiotherapy Association, the Canadian Association of Occupational Therapists, and the Canadian Association of Speech-Language Pathologists and Audiologists and funded by the National Health Research Development Program (NHRDP) through the University of Alberta. She hopes the results, released last year, will form the basis for training and supervision models across Canada.

"Each province has control over the education programs within its borders," says Swinamer. "Our fear is that these programs are too 'province-specific.' With 'national' training models, there would be generic training of support personnel in addition to some province-specific training.... We need to build in flexibility so we can keep up with the changes in health care." Adding to the fear is the fact that most university-based physical therapy education programs are not yet training PTs how to supervise.

How do Canadian PTs feel about moving from hands-on practitioner to consultant? "Many fear role erosion," Swinamer says. "They ask, 'Will I become obsolete?'" Over the past few years, the number of PTs at Royal Alexandra Hospital has dropped from 30 to 24; the number of support staff has increased from 3 or 4 to 7.

Swinamer predicts that as acute care settings move into patient-focused care, fewer PTs will be employed on a salaried basis and more will be employed on a contract basis as independent practitioners working in a number of hospitals. What impact would this have on the patient-therapist relationship?

"There should be no 'lessening' of care; however, services may be rendered on an ongoing basis by support personnel, with the therapist seeing the patient only three times per week. This would place an even greater emphasis on PT interview, problem-solving, and goal-setting skills... What the PT may lose in traditional patient contact and collective professional identity, however, the PT may gain in the building of more consultative, and collegial, relationships with physicians. There will be loss—but there also will be opportunity." *PT*

—*Jan Reynolds*

Cross-Training: Ethical Issue or Matter of Self-Protection?

Sebring: I believe PTs are the best-qualified personnel to provide physical therapy; I also believe we can utilize PTAs and aides under our direction and supervision to achieve maximum rehabilitation potential. But if we delegate tasks to an aide who takes three times as long as the PT to achieve results, that would be neither ethical nor effective. As we know, the term "ancillary" today also can refer to patient-focused care programs, in which there is cross-training of nursing staff to provide the services of more than one profession.

Snyder: In the Midwest, patient-focused care has become a role model for extended care and nursing home settings.

Purtilo: Can the cross-trained person be viewed as a care extender, or, in a richer sense, can cross-training be viewed as a collaboration that helps patients receive the care they need?

Sebring: The cross-trained aide can assist in the delivery of physical therapy under the direction of the PT in the morning, for example, and deliver x-ray services under the direction of an x-ray technician in the afternoon. That makes sense for patient and professional. But if a patient is not receiving needed physical therapy services under the direction of a PT because a gatekeeper has determined that a nurse or a nursing aide can provide those services and no physical therapy needs to be ordered—that *doesn't* make sense.

Purtilo: Self-interest, then, can exist within certain ethical constraints; however, "ethics" should not be used as an excuse to "dump" tasks you don't want to do yourself.

Davis: Marion [Briggs] brought up professional territorial guarding. Protection of our own interests is not necessarily in the best interests of the patient and community. We sometimes carry turf battles into state legislatures when in fact a principal

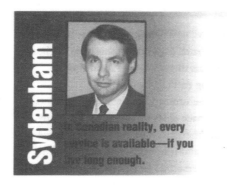

Sydenham

In Canadian reality, every service is available—if you live long enough.

purpose of licensure is to protect the public from harm and to identify credentials to perform services. We need to ask ourselves to what degree cross-training is an ethical issue or a self-protection issue.

Is it Rationing or Triage?

Snyder: If we involve support personnel 50% of the time in providing some of the rehabilitation techniques that PTs traditionally have provided, and if those personnel earn 50% of what the PT professional traditionally has earned, should we be reducing our charges to reflect the decrease in the cost of providing that service?

Davis: Yes.

Snyder: But are we? Or are we overcharging for the level of care the consumer is receiving?.... Likewise, if I have a patient who receives treatment three times a week, but that patient would recover just as quickly receiving therapy once a week, that's overutilization—another ethical issue.

Davis: If the PT facility reduces quality by overutilizing aides, for example, to reduce cost and then uses that reduced cost in a competitive fashion, that also would be ethically inappropriate.

Briggs: In Alberta, under the provincial government health care system, services provided by the physical therapy attendant or aide cannot be billed at all in private practice. The private practitioner must absorb the cost.

Sydenham: Workers' Comp and third-party insurance, however, *will* pay for those services.

Swinamer: Which underscores a double standard. In the publicly funded system in Canadian hospitals, attendants or aides are part of global funding and may be used at the discretion of the department or the PT.

Sydenham: Our Provincial insurance fund pays us approximately $20 [Canadian] per treatment; in American money, that's about $15. Does that mean American PTs are *over*charging for treatments—or that we are *under*charging?

Purtilo: This discussion of cost is important. The implication is that the costs of our services will lead policymakers to make decisions about *which* of the available services will in fact be covered. Among PTs and other health professionals—and health care consumers—there is general concern about "rationing" in universal health care. When one "rations," one has made a conscious choice about the criteria for allocation of scarce resources, a choice that has ethical dimensions.

Davis: We have not yet reached a consensus about the criteria to be used. But I would ask whether the process is "rationing" or "triaging." In triaging, it is agreed that care must be given, but the process is based on prioritization, and the decision making is distributed to the levels at which care can be appropriately delivered. In the emergency department, for example, decisions are made about the priority of the patient's condition and how quickly services need to be rendered. Because services are delivered to all who come to the emergency department, it's not so much a matter of rationing as it is a matter of allocating resources, or assigning service delivery, to the appropriate level, using a priority system.

Briggs: The two principles of the Canadian Health Act are universality and accessibility. Those principles...suggest that the concept of rationing cannot be on the health care agenda. That's the official view.

Sydenham: In Canadian reality, every service is available—if you live long enough.

Purtilo: In talking about long-term care, a high-level Swedish official once told me that if the care is needed, "you find a way to pay for it...end of discussion." In the United States, however, the focus today is on *getting rid of care that cannot be provided because it costs too much*. Under the principles of universality and accessibility—or, as the United States calls it, "universal access," which is a linchpin of the Clinton health care reform plan—rationing is precluded much as it is in Canada.

Briggs: It could be said, however, that triage is the Canadian version of rationing. Waiting lists are managed by degrees of acuity and urgency and by time-economics.

Sydenham: It was reported in *Back Letter* [1993;8(7)] that a particular health care organization in Canada was going to gross approximately $25 million in 1993 by providing "rationed" treatments, that is, x number of treatments for x number of dollars per treatment for x condition—with the expectation that the patient would return to work at the end of the treatment course. As it turns out, a great number of these patients were *not* able to go back to work; however, regardless of patient outcomes, the third-party insurer was billed the x number of dollars.

Davis: In the United States, there are multiple sources of payment and multiple levels of coverage provided by third-party payers. Determination of patient need is based on availability of funds and coverage, and the PT is placed in the situation of making an internal value judgment on whether the coverage is consistent with the clinical needs that need to be met. There's one level of coverage for Medicare, one for Workers' Comp—and yet the clinician is being asked to make treatment decisions about "how long" and "when."

Snyder: We have an even greater discrepancy when the insurer is Blue Cross/Blue Shield. Is it a regular policy, an HMO policy, or a PPO policy? The amount of care allowed differs under each one of those policies, but all are administered under the same company.

Davis: Harkening back to Ruth's [Purtilo] question about whether reimbursement policy is the governing authority, we need to determine, once and for all, whether "patient need" is a universal clinical measure—or a matter of what coverage provides.

To Meet the Demands of Patient, Society, and Profession

Purtilo: We've asked a number of provocative questions today. What do you feel is the most *pressing* ethical issue?

Briggs: To raise ethics as an agenda item for discussion among all PTs—period.

Davis: To search for an answer about who our profession is serving: itself, its community, or its individual patients. The profession demands one thing of us, the patient demands another, and society demands yet another. How do we find the commonality among those demands?

Sebring: To balance the need to achieve patient goals with the need to contain costs, appropriately using patient education and home programs, group treatments, and support personnel—without overutilizing or underutilizing any of them—and making certain that we are driven not by our own economic concerns but by society's needs.

Snyder: To realize that we have new ethical issues and that we need to look at previous ethical issues in a new light. All PTs need to bring issues to the forefront as we evolve in our new role in the health care system.

Swinamer: To distribute and allocate physical therapy services among the hospital patient population, among the professionals and the ancillary personnel, and between the private sector and the public sector.

Sydenham: To confront the inappropriate treatment, diagnosis, and omission of factors in patient management that are causing credibility problems regarding the necessity for physical therapy services—problems that are resulting in PTs being left out of managed care in Canada.

Purtilo: Canadian and American PTs will have the opportunity to continue discussing these issues at Joint Congress in Toronto in June—formally, during the Health Care Systems panel on "The Paradigm Shift in Service Delivery" [June 5] and informally, among colleagues and friends. In addition, *PT* will continue to provide a forum for the discussion of ethics in physical therapy, and I encourage readers to participate in this ongoing dialogue. *PT*

Postscript: Participant Judy Sebring acted on Marion Briggs' challenge to raise ethics as an agenda item for discussion among PTs, suggesting and chairing a discussion on ethical issues in managed care at the Tri-County District meeting of APTA's California Chapter in Santa Barbara in March.

References

1   Manga P, Angus D, Papadopoulos C, Swan W. *The Effectiveness and Cost-Effectiveness of Chiropractic Management of Low Back Pain.* Report presented in 1993 to the Ontario Ministry of Health. Copies can be obtained from the Ministry.

2   *Joint Ventures Among Health Care Providers in Florida.* Tallahassee, Fla: Health Cost Containment Board of the State of Florida; 1991.

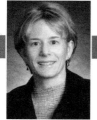

board perspective

By Janet Bezner, PT, PhD

Getting to the Core of Professionalism

A list of core values for physical therapists seeks to define what others should expect of you—and what you should expect of yourself.

As a kid I attended many Little League Baseball games—my mom was president of the local league for a time, so we spent many a Saturday at the ballpark. Being a very active child, my tolerance for sitting in the stands and watching was limited, so, after convincing my mom that I wouldn't go too far, I'd wander off to find some other kids to hang out with.

Once when I was bored and looking for something to amuse me, I was kicking the dirt under the bleachers and found a $5 bill! Looking around furtively and not sure what to do, I wondered whose it was and what I should do. I can remember standing there with my foot covering the money, feeling torn between picking it up, running to the snack bar, and spending every penny on candy and popcorn, or giving it to my mom, who would pat me on the head in a "good girl" kind of way and try to return it to its rightful owner.

After thinking through the two possible courses of action and considering the consequences, I determined that the best decision would be to turn in the money. The consequences of eating all of that candy *and* trying to explain where I got the funds seemed too great. Besides, I reasoned, if nobody claimed the money maybe my mom would let me keep it.

Maybe you had a similar experience as a child: an early lesson in values in which you sacrificed a desire or prize in order to "do the right thing." Although the stakes weren't that high in my experience at the ballpark, I learned a valuable lesson about honesty that I still reflect on today in situations in which

the stakes are much higher. Dishonesty or lack of integrity today could cost me my license, a business deal, my membership in APTA, and my reputation—stakes that are very significant and important to me and to my future as a professional.

Of Vision and Values

Whatever values you adopt as an adult and as a professional, they guide your decision-making and thus are important to consider and develop. Stephen Covey talks about this process in his book *The 7 Habits of Highly Effective People*.[1] One's beliefs and ideas are based on one's values, which generate one's behaviors, which in turn determine the outcomes one experiences. In the case of young Janet and the $5 bill, because I *valued* honesty (and feared a good talking-to!), my *behavior* was to hand over the money to my mom. The *outcome* I experienced was praise and reinforcement for my behavior and my beliefs. (And the fact that I can't even remember whether I got to keep the money says something, I think, about the power of praise and reinforcement.)

Until recently, APTA hadn't spent a great deal of time or resources on the development of professional values. Although many "value" words can be found in the *Guide to Physical Therapist Practice*,[2] *A Normative Model of Physical Therapist Professional Education*,[3] and various APTA core documents,[4] the Association had not created a core set of values it could use to communicate to others the ideals we believe are most important, or to guide the individual member seeking to develop further professionally.

With the adoption of the APTA *Vision Statement for Physical Therapy 2020* (see box on page 27) by the House of Delegates in 1999, the importance of professionalism was identified as critical to the future of physical therapy and specifically to the movement of physical therapy toward a doctoring profession. It is tempting to argue that we are all professionals simply because we graduated from accredited physical therapy programs and obtained licensure—and that we thus need not pay further attention to the subject. On the contrary, however, professionalism is so critical a part of realizing Vision 2020 that it was of great import to the Association to further define this quality and to identify the attributes relative to professionalism that a graduate of a physical therapist (PT) program ought to demonstrate and that individual practitioners should display on a daily basis.

Toward this end, APTA held a consensus conference in July 2002 at which 18 members with expertise in physical therapy education, practice, and research discussed and agreed upon the core values of the profession and the indicators (judgments, decisions, attitudes, and behaviors) consistent with those values. I was fortunate to be able to participate as Board liaison to this group, which was led by Joe Black, PhD, MDiv, and Jody Gandy, PT, PhD, of APTA's Education Department.

Everyday Indicators

During the 3-day conference, the participants generated an impressive list of values that all PTs should possess. The group pared that list down to seven core values that represent the critical or essential elements of professionalism in PTs. These core values and their definitions appear in alphabetical order in the table on this page. Conference participants also created a list of indicators for each core value to describe what one would see if the PT were demonstrating that core value in his or her daily practice. While space limitations prohibit publication here of the entire list of indicators (for that, go to www.apta.org, click on "Education," then click on "Professionalism in Physical Therapy: Core Values"), what follows are brief descriptions of some of the indicators associated with each core value.

Accountability. A PT demonstrates accountability by acknowledging and accepting the consequences of his or her actions, by responding to the patient's or client's goals and needs, and by maintaining membership in APTA and other organizations.

Altruism. A PT demonstrates altruism by placing the patient's or client's needs above those of the PT, by providing *pro bono* services, and by providing services to the patient or client that go beyond expected standards of practice.

Compassion and caring. A PT demonstrates compassion and caring by being an advocate for patients' or clients' needs, understanding an individual's perspective and the various influences on that person's life in his or her environment, and demonstrating respect for others and considering them as unique and of value.

Excellence. A PT demonstrates excellence by internalizing the importance of using multiple sources of evidence to support professional practice and decisions, seeking out and acquiring new knowledge throughout his or her professional career, and by demonstrating high levels of knowledge and skill in all aspects of the profession.

Integrity. A PT demonstrates integrity by abiding by the rules, regulations, and laws applicable to the profession, adhering to profession's highest standards (in practice, ethics, reimbursement, and other areas), confronting harassment and bias in oneself and others, being trustworthy, and choosing employment situations that are congruent with practice values and professional ethical standards.

Professional duty. A PT demon-

Professionalism in Physical Therapy: Core Values

Core Value	Definition
Accountability	Active acceptance of the responsibility for the diverse roles, obligations, and actions of the physical therapist, including self-regulation and other behaviors that positively influence patient/client outcomes, the profession, and the health needs of society.
Altruism	Primary regard for or devotion to the interests of patients/clients, thus assuming the fiduciary responsibility of placing the needs of the patient/client ahead of the physical therapist's self interest.
Compassion/Caring	Compassion is the desire to identify with or sense something of another's experience; a precursor of caring. Caring is the concern, empathy, and consideration for the needs and values of others.
Excellence	Physical therapy practice that consistently uses current knowledge and theory while understanding personal limits, integrates judgment and the patient/client perspective, embraces advancement, challenges mediocrity, and works toward development of new knowledge.
Integrity	The possession of and steadfast adherence to high moral principles or professional standards.
Professional Duty	The commitment to meeting one's obligations to provide effective physical therapy services to patients/clients, serve the profession, and positively influence the health of society.
Social Responsibility	The promotion of a mutual trust between the profession and the larger public that necessitates responding to societal needs for health and wellness.

APTA Vision Statement for Physical Therapy 2020

(HOD 06-00-24-35)

Physical therapy, by 2020, will be provided by physical therapists who are doctors of physical therapy and who may be board-certified specialists. Consumers will have direct access to physical therapists in all environments for patient/client management, prevention, and wellness services. Physical therapists will be practitioners of choice in clients' health networks and will hold all privileges of autonomous practice. Physical therapists may be assisted by physical therapist assistants who are educated and licensed to provide physical therapist-directed and -supervised components of interventions. Guided by integrity, life-long learning, and a commitment to comprehensive and accessible health programs for all people, physical therapists and physical therapist assistants will render evidence-based service throughout the continuum of care and improve quality of life for society. They will provide culturally sensitive care distinguished by trust, respect, and an appreciation for individual differences.

While fully availing themselves of new technologies, as well as basic and clinical research, physical therapists will continue to provide direct care. They will maintain active responsibility for the growth of the physical therapy profession and the health of the people it serves.

strates professional duty by facilitating the achievement of each patient's or client's goals for function, health, and wellness; promoting the profession; mentoring others; and getting involved in professional activities beyond the practice setting.

Social responsibility. A PT demonstrates social responsibility by promoting cultural competence within the profession and the larger public; promoting social policy that affects the function, health, and wellness needs of patients and clients; promoting community volunteerism; and working to ensure the blending of social justice and economic efficiency of service delivery.

Matters of Communication

The achievement and demonstration of these core values, the Board believes, is essential if our profession is to realize Vision 2020. They are the values that society and the profession itself expect from a doctor of physical therapy (DPT) who practices autonomously. They also are the beliefs and behaviors we want the greater public to associate with physical therapy and PTs. Because of their primary importance and their relationship to our major goals (direct access, evidence-based practice, the DPT, being seen as practitioner of choice, and autonomous practice), the Board is carefully considering how best to communicate and use them.

The core values will be integrated into the next revision of *A Normative Model of Physical Therapist Professional Education*—Version 2004—and thus will influence future physical therapist students. Their application to the practitioner is equally important and is being discussed by the Board at this writing (in late October). If you have thoughts or ideas about how these core

values can be most useful to the membership and best applied, please contact me or any Board member.

In the interim, I would encourage each of you to review these core values and reflect on the extent to which your daily actions and decisions are consistent with them and the greater good they represent. Identify areas in which you can improve. Seek out all the indicators of each core value, observe others who exemplify them, and select activities and situations that challenge you to demonstrate each value. The next time you find yourself faced with a difficult decision, use the opportunity to reflect on the values upon which you rely to make decisions.

Perhaps you can recall a childhood encounter that offered you a choice that led you to integrity. Or, you might reflect on a more-recent situation in which you've seen someone choose the less value-driven path and experience the consequences; unfortunately, the media is full of stories such as these. Whatever your current situation, remind yourself that candy and popcorn may be great in the moment, but they won't get you as far in the long run as will giving back that $5 bill! **PT**

Janet Bezner, PT, PhD, is vice president of APTA and senior vice president of PeakCare Inc. She can be reached at janetbezner@apta.org.

References

1. Covey SR. *The 7 Habits of Highly Effective People.* New York: Simon & Schuster; 1990.
2. Guide to Physical Therapist Practice. 2nd ed. *Phys Ther.* 2001;81:9-744.
3. *A Normative Model of Physical Therapist Professional Education.* Alexandria, Va: American Physical Therapy Association: Version 2000; 2000.
4. APTA core documents. Available at www.apta.org/About/core_documents.

Research Report

Using Clinical Outcomes to Explore the Theory of Expert Practice in Physical Therapy

Background and Purpose. Theoretical models of physical therapist expertise have been developed through research on physical therapists sampled solely on the basis of years of experience or reputation. Expert clinicians, selected on the basis of their patients' outcomes, have not been previously studied, nor have the patient outcomes of peer-nominated experts been analyzed. The purpose of our study was to describe characteristics of therapists who were classified as expert or average therapists based on the outcomes of their patients. Subjects. Subjects were 6 therapists classified as expert and 6 therapists classified as average through retrospective analysis of an outcomes database. Methods. The study was guided by grounded theory method, using a multiple case study design. Analysis integrated data from quantitative and qualitative sources and developed a grounded theory. Results. All therapists expressed a commitment to professional growth and an ethic of caring. Therapists classified as expert were not distinguished by years of experience, but they differed in academic and work experience, utilization of colleagues, use of reflection, view of primary role, and pattern of delegation of care to support staff. Therapists classified as expert had a patient-centered approach to care, characterized by collaborative clinical reasoning and promotion of patient empowerment. Discussion and Conclusion. These findings add to the understanding of factors related to patient outcomes and build upon grounded theory for elucidating expert practice in physical therapy. [Resnik L, Jensen GM. Using clinical outcomes to explore the theory of expert practice in physical therapy. *Phys Ther.* 2003;83:1090–1106.]

Key Words: *Clinical competence, Grounded theory, Low back pain, Physical therapy profession, Qualitative methods.*

Linda Resnik, Gail M Jensen

Expert practitioners are thought to "do something better," because they know how to do the "right thing at the right time," and thereby "provide better care."[1] In their pivotal work, Jensen et al[2] have articulated the need to understand and enhance expertise and to apply the lessons learned through the study of expert therapists to improve physical therapy education and patient care. Rothstein[1] and Purtilo[3] have agreed that if the knowledge, skills, and decision-making capabilities of the expert therapist can be identified, nurtured, and taught, the result will hold important ramifications for physical therapist practice and patient care.

The work of Jensen and colleagues[2,4–6] has shaped the current understanding of expertise in the field. The first in a series of studies conducted by these researchers focused on the differences between novice and experienced physical therapy practitioners.[4] Eight physical therapists practicing in outpatient orthopedic settings who had varying levels of experience were studied through nonparticipant observation of intervention sessions. Using a grounded theory method, the authors identified a number of themes that distinguished novice therapists from experienced therapists. They reported that experienced therapists spent more time with patients than did novice therapists in providing hands-on care, seeking information, and evaluating and educating the patient. Experienced therapists appeared able to handle interruptions of direct intervention more efficiently than did novice therapists. The experienced therapists also spent more time in social interchange with patients, and with patient education, than did the novice therapists.[4]

In a subsequent study,[5] Jensen et al investigated attributes of master and novice physical therapists. Subjects of this study were clinicians, identified as either master or novice clinicians, working in orthopedic outpatient settings, nominated by a panel of academic coordinators of clinical education. Each of the researchers collected data through on-site observation of 1 novice clinician and 1 master clinician with at least 3 patients. The researchers reported that master clinicians' knowledge was more extensive and that master clinicians were more comfortable with their knowledge base than were novice clinicians. They also found that master clinicians individualized their evaluation and teaching for each patient, were more responsive in their therapeutic interaction with patients, and integrated more verbal encouragement and tactile cues with intervention than did the novice clinicians.[5]

Finally, Jensen and colleagues[6] studied 12 experts nominated by officers of the American Physical Therapy

L Resnik, PT, PhD, OCS, is Postdoctoral Fellow, Center for Gerontology and Health Care Research, Brown University, 2 Stimson Ave, Providence, RI 02912 (USA) (linda_resnik@brown.edu). Address all correspondence to Dr Resnik.

GM Jensen, PT, PhD, FAPTA, is Associate Dean for Faculty Development and Assessment and Professor of Physical Therapy, School of Pharmacy and Health Professions, and Faculty Associate, Center for Health Policy and Ethics, Creighton University Medical Center, Omaha, Neb.

Both authors provided concept/idea/research design and data analysis. Dr Resnik provided writing, data collection, and project management. Dr Jensen provided consultation (including review of manuscript before submission). The authors acknowledge Leah Nof, PT, PhD, Melissa Tovin, PT, PhD, and Dennis Hart, PT, PhD, for their dissertation committee work and Susan Allen, PhD, for her constructive critique of the manuscript.

This study was approved by the Institutional Review Board for the Protection of Human Subjects, Nova Southeastern University, Fort Lauderdale, Fla.

This article was received November 14, 2002, and was accepted June 27, 2003.

Association's (APTA) specialty sections for geriatrics, neurology, orthopedics, and pediatrics. The researchers selected subjects based on frequency of nomination and geographical convenience. Three experts were chosen in each of 4 practice arenas: geriatrics, neurology, orthopedics, and pediatrics. Data were collected throughout the episode of care for at least 2 patients of each clinician. The researchers reported that the expert clinicians had an inner drive for lifelong learning and a broad knowledge base consisting of formal knowledge and knowledge of movement, of patients, and of their clinical specialty. Expert clinicians shared a focus on patient education and an understanding about working within the health care system to maximize resources. Experts understood their own limitations and appreciated what they did know as well as what they needed to learn. The expert clinicians' clinical reasoning focused on patient-specific functional outcomes and was based on collaborative problem solving and decision making. Experts shared a belief in patients' responsibility for their own health. The experts studied demonstrated a well-developed ability for self-reflection, with continual reassessment of their own practice. The experts intertwined intervention and evaluation to fine-tune the patients' programs.

Theories of physical therapist expertise, disseminated in the literature and through programming at national and regional conferences, have the potential to improve physical therapy education, administration, and practice. A central limitation of the research on physical therapist expertise, however, is that the theoretical models of expertise have been developed through research on therapists sampled solely on the basis of years of experience or reputation.[4–12] The methods of subject selection in prior studies ensured a pool of subjects who were actively involved with APTA, known to APTA section leadership, and active in educational activities. Although this type of reputation is an important facet of being recognized as an expert, it is not clear how it affects patient outcomes. Although experts are assumed to be those who achieve the best clinical outcomes,[1] prior research has not documented this relationship. Expert clinicians, selected on the basis of their patients' outcomes have not been previously studied, nor have the patient outcomes of peer-nominated experts been analyzed.

We believed, therefore, that there was a need to identify therapists whose patients have the best outcomes in order to understand the characteristics of these therapists and to compare their qualities with those of peer-nominated experts reported in the literature. Thus, the purposes of our study were to describe the characteristics of clinicians whose patients with lumbar syndromes had excellent outcomes and to build upon the prior theoretical framework of physical therapist expertise.[13]

Method

Subjects

Our research was guided by the grounded theory approach. The intent of grounded theory is the generation of a theory relating to a particular situation.[14] In accordance with this method, subjects are chosen by a form of theoretical sampling defined as data gathering, driven by concepts derived from the data analysis process. The purpose of theoretical sampling is to gather data that will maximize opportunities to discover variations among concepts and deepen the understanding of the relationships between the concepts under study. Although the researcher must make some initial sampling decisions regarding the group to be studied and the number of observations or interviews, theoretical sampling requires flexibility in determining the precise number of subjects and the number and types of follow-up. In grounded theory, the researcher continues sampling until the participants say nothing new about the concepts under exploration and the collected data have reached a saturation point.[15] Saturation, the stopping point in data collection and analysis, is the point in research where collecting additional data does not add to the explanation of the concepts.[15]

Our initial sampling decisions resulted from retrospective analysis of the data from the Focus On Therapeutic Outcomes Inc (FOTO) database (Knoxville, Tenn).[16] For our study, we operationally defined therapist expertise on the basis of collective patient outcomes. We used health-related quality-of-life (HRQL) outcomes data contained in the FOTO database for patients with lumbar spine syndromes (24,276 patients seen by 930 therapists) to calculate mean patient outcomes for each therapist participating in the database.

Health-related quality-of-life measurements have been widely recommended as reliable, valid, and sensitive for determination of outcomes for patients with low back pain.[17–19] The FOTO database contains an HRQL measure called the overall health status measure (OHS) that measures both mental and physical dimensions of health. Internal consistency of items in the OHS constructs with 2 or more items has been reported (α=.57–.91).[20,21] Internal consistency reliability statistics of the items of the OHS constructs[20,21] are comparable to the internal consistency reliability statistics calculated from the same items embedded in the 36-Item Short-Form Health Survey (SF-36) questionnaire[22] and the 12-Item Short-Form Health Survey (SF-12) questionnaire.[23] Test-retest reliability of data obtained with the OHS was good (intraclass correlation coefficient [ICC(2,1)]=.92).[20] Validity of data obtained with the OHS has not been examined, but there is evidence that an overall HRQL measure with similar items is responsive for patients receiving outpatient therapy.[24]

Overall health status scores are calculated by averaging scores from the 8 embedded HRQL constructs: general health (1 item from the SF-12),[25] physical functioning (10 items from the physical functioning scale [PF-10] of the SF-36),[22] role physical (2 items from the SF-12),[23] bodily pain (2 items from the SF-36),[22] vitality (1 item from the SF-12),[23] mental health (2 items from the SF-12),[23] role emotional (2 items from the SF-12),[23] and social functioning (1 item from the SF-12).[23] The OHS physical functioning construct also includes 3 new questions pertinent to clients with upper-extremity impairments.[26] Scoring of item responses followed published algorithms.[22,23] Raw ordinal scores were transformed to interval scores varying from 0 to 100 for each question.[22,23] Transformed item scores were grouped by construct and averaged to obtain the score for each of the 8 OHS functional scales.

To control for the effect of patient factors that influence HRQL outcomes, we calculated predicted discharge OHS scores by developing a general linear model that included patient age, severity of condition, sex, onset of condition, number of surgeries for condition, reimbursement, exercise history, and employment status. Patient age (in years) was entered into the model as a continuous variable. Severity of the condition was also entered as a continuous variable, measured by the intake score of the OHS scale. The variable called "onset of condition" represented the number of days from the onset of the condition until the beginning of intervention. In the FOTO dataset, onset of condition was classified as: 0 to 7 days, 8 to 14 days, 15 to 21 days, 22 to 90 days, 91 days to 6 months, and over 6 months. Number of surgeries for the low back was categorized as: none, 1, 2, 3, and 4 or more. Reimbursement was the primary source of the payment for the patient's physical therapy. Reimbursement was classified as: indemnity, litigation, Medicaid, Medicare, patient, health maintenance organization or preferred provider organization, workers' compensation, or other. Exercise history was a measurement of the patient's self-reported exercise prior to the episode of physical therapy. Exercise history was classified as: at least 3 times a week, 1 to 2 times a week, or seldom/never. The variable called "employment status" measured the patient's employment at the time of intake for physical therapy. The categories of employment status were: full-time, modified work, employed but not working, previously employed and receiving disability, unemployed, retired, or student.

The residual scores for the OHS discharge measure were calculated for each patient after general linear modeling and saved. Residual scores were defined as the difference in actual scale points between the patient's actual discharge scores and the predicted discharge scores after modeling. Patient data were aggregated by therapist, and mean residual discharge scores for each therapist's patients were calculated. We then selected for inclusion in the expert group the 10% of therapists whose patients had the highest mean residual scores (n=94) and for inclusion in the average group the 10% of therapists whose patients had average mean residual scores (45th-55th percentiles) (n=94).

We used SPSS software* to randomly select 30 therapists from each of the theoretical sample groups (expert and average). We anticipated that this sample would yield between 4 and 10 potential participants for each group. Clinician code numbers were used by FOTO representatives to identify the employment site of each selected therapist. The work sites of all 60 therapists were contacted by FOTO representatives to inform them about the study and to obtain the clinicians' names and contact information. After receipt of employer authorization, FOTO representatives mailed each clinician a letter that described the study and contained an informed consent form. Those who agreed to participate in the study returned their consent forms to the first author.

In accordance with grounded theory methods, the number of participants in the qualitative study was not determined a priori, but was guided by the data analysis process. Four therapists from the group classified as average and 12 therapists from the group classified as expert responded to the initial request by returning their signed informed consent forms. A follow-up request that was sent to members of the group classified as average yielded 2 additional respondents. Therapists from each group were contacted in the general order in which their responses were received. Therapists were not told about the study's classification scheme and did not know if they were categorized as expert or average. Participants were asked to provide a copy of their curriculum vitae, to submit a written statement of philosophy explaining their approach to the clinical management of patients with low back pain, and to schedule an appointment for a telephone interview. Participant interviews and subsequent case analyses proceeded until no new or contradictory findings were discovered and resulted in 12 participants—6 from each of the 2 groups (expert and average).

The professional profiles of participants from the group classified as expert are summarized in Table 1. During the process of data analysis, we sorted participants from this group into experienced and novice subcategories based on their years of clinical experience, as there

---

* SPSS Inc, 233 S Wacker Dr, Chicago, IL 60606.

Table 1.
Professional Profiles of Therapists Classified as Expert[a]

Clinician	Age (y)	Years of Clinical Experience	Education	Advanced Certification	Practice Settings	Professional Membership
Liz	59	39.0	BS PT/OT	McKenzie diploma	Spine specialist Outpatient Home care Pediatrics Mental health	APTA
Pam	44	21.0	BS in PT	Certified Manual Therapist 2001	Acute care Outpatient	No
Kathy	45	13.5	MS PT BS in biology/psychology	No	Outpatient Acute care Geriatrics	APTA
Sarah	31	2.5	BS PT BS ATC/health education	No	Outpatient	APTA NATA
James	32	4.5	MS PT BS in exercise science	No	Acute care Outpatient	No
Dawn	32	6.0	MS PT BS in exercise science/ physiology	No	Outpatient	No

[a] Pseudonyms are used instead of clinicians' actual names. ATC=Certified Athletic Trainer, BS=bachelor of science, MS=master of science, PT=physical therapy, OT=occupational therapy, APTA=American Physical Therapy Association, NATA=National Athletic Trainers Association.

seemed to be 2 distinct subgroups of therapists in this category. The 3 participants in the experienced subcategory were aged 44 to 59 years. Two of these participants had been practicing for more than 20 years, and 1 participant had been practicing for 13.5 years. The 3 participants from the novice subcategory were aged 31 to 32 years and had 6 years or less of clinical experience. All novice therapists from the expert group had undergraduate degrees in exercise science and an employment history as a physical therapy aide or athletic trainer prior to becoming a physical therapist.

Participants from the group classified as average were aged 28 to 48 years and had a wide range of experience and training. Their professional profiles are summarized in Table 2. The majority of their clinical experience had been in outpatient orthopedic settings. Two of these therapists divided their time between administration and clinical practice. All 6 therapists in this group held professional (entry-level) bachelor's degrees in physical therapy. One therapist also had a master's degree in business administration. Four of the 6 therapists in the group classified as average had between 7 and 12 years of experience, 1 therapist had less than 5 years of experience, and 1 therapist had 19 years of experience. Because this range of experience among participants was more uniformly distributed, no subgrouping by experience was needed in the group classified as average.

Data Collection

A semiguided interview process (Appendix) was conducted by the principal investigator (LR), who was aware of each participant's classification group. The semiguided format allowed flexibility in sequencing and wording of interview questions and allowed for additional probing to clarify specific participant responses. Each initial interview lasted approximately 45 minutes. All interviews were tape recorded and transcribed. Follow-up interviews, telephone calls, letters, or e-mails were used as needed to gather more data, test emerging hypotheses, and seek negative case examples (ie, instances of therapists whose characteristics varied from those of others in their group).

Data Analysis

Data analysis began with open coding by the principal investigator of initial interviews, philosophy statements, and résumés. Open coding is a means of reducing the data to a set of important themes or categories. Coding continued until no new information was obtained and no new categories were formed. Our design involved 3 phases of data analysis: within-case, cross-case, and cross-group analysis.[27–29]

The within-case analysis was performed by synthesizing data for each therapist into a report consisting of a summary of all information provided by the participant and relevant information contained in the FOTO database and subsequently by analyzing that information.

Table 2.
Professional Profiles of Therapists Classified as Average[a]

Clinician	Age (y)	Years of Clinical Experience	Education	Advanced Certification	Practice Settings	Professional Membership
Beverly	48	19.0	BS PT	No	Outpatient Acute care Outpatient rehabilitation Skilled nursing facility	No
Tim	37	10.0	BS PT	No	Outpatient Sports Home care	APTA
Sharon	33	10.0	BS PT	No	Pediatrics Inpatient Outpatient	No
Crystal	28	4.5	BS PT	OCS 2000	Outpatient Acute care	APTA
Mike	30	7.5	BS PT/ATC	MS administration	Outpatient	NATA
Ann	33	12.0	BS PT	No	Outpatient Acute care	APTA

[a] Pseudonyms are used instead of clinicians' actual names. ATC=Certified Athletic Trainer, BS=bachelor of science, MS=master of science, PT=physical therapy, OT=occupational therapy, OCS=Occupational Certified Specialist, APTA=American Physical Therapy Association, NATA=National Athletic Trainers Association.

The within-case analysis involved the evaluation of main themes, impressions, and summary statements and the generation of explanations, speculations, and hypotheses, as well as alternative interpretations, explanations, and disagreements.[30] The next steps for data collection in each case also were identified, and implications for revision and updating of the coding scheme were noted.[2,30]

Cross-case analysis began when the main points, explanations, and summaries for the within-case analyses were organized by category and compiled. During this analysis, the coding categories were continually refined and organized into 4 overall key categories: knowledge base, clinical reasoning, values, and virtues. Comparison matrices[30] were constructed to compare properties and dimensions among therapists in each of the groups. Comparison matrices are an analytic tool used to visually display data in a systematic way.[30] The matrices we developed took the form of spreadsheets displaying rows of data for each therapist and columns denoting key attributes. Follow-up interviews, telephone calls, letters, or e-mails were used to gather the additional data needed to complete the matrices, follow up on the analyses, and enable comparisons. These later stages of data collection and sampling were guided by the data analysis process, consistent with the tenets of the grounded theory approach.[31]

Cross-case analysis resulted in the development of 2 composite case studies (expert and average) that merged common elements of cases within each group. Cross-case analysis also was used to focus axial coding, or the identification of the subcategories, properties, and dimensions of each category.[32] The next step in data analysis was the cross-group analysis, which summarized the findings from composite case studies and elucidated the similarities and distinctions between groups. The data analysis process is summarized in Figure 1.

At each stage of data collection and analysis, the literature was consulted to determine how findings and interpretations compared with other research and theories. The key concepts and emerging theories that were uncovered were checked against the literature and discussed among the authors. Data collection and analysis continued until no new categories were discovered in the last 2 therapists' interviews. The cross-group comparison facilitated the development of an initial theoretical framework and identified a central phenomenon using criteria advocated by Strauss and Corbin.[32] The *central phenomenon* is defined as the main theme of the research. Memos of the researcher's analytical thought process, integrative diagrams, and review of the literature were used in conjunction with further analysis of the composite.[32] Memos, frequently used in qualitative analysis, are notes of the investigator's thought and decision-making processes recorded throughout the data collection and analysis. Integrative diagrams are schematic drawings showing the relationships among the concepts.

Accuracy of the analysis was enhanced by using the following verification strategies: source triangulation, examination of researcher bias, member checks, use of thick description, peer reviewing and debriefing, and an audit trail of methodological and analytic decisions.[33] In our study, triangulation was performed by considering

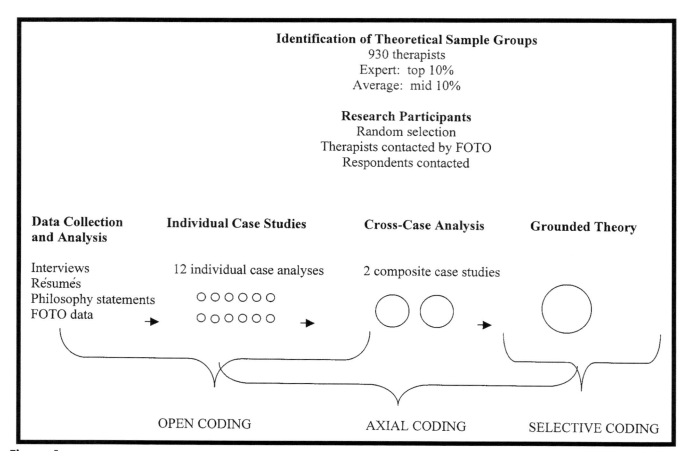

Figure 1.
Summary of analytical process. FOTO=Focus On Therapeutic Outcomes Inc.

multiple sources of data in the analysis. Multiple data sources included information contained in the outcomes database on each therapist's patients, written statements of philosophy, each therapist's curriculum vitae, and interviews. Participant checks were conducted by asking several of the research participants to review transcripts and case studies to verify the researcher's interpretation. "Thick description" is the inclusion of meaningful quotations to represent important themes and categories when reporting data analysis. The second author and an external auditor reviewed the case studies and discussed and commented on emerging themes and coding categories after case construction.

Findings

We have chosen to organize our findings around 3 core topics: (1) the central phenomenon and grounded theory resulting from the study, (2) unique attributes of practitioners classified as expert, and (3) commonalities across groups of therapists classified as expert or average. The central phenomenon in our study was expert practice within the context of excellent outcomes for patients with low back pain. We first present the primary attributes and relationships identified in our theory and

then explain the derivation of the theory by describing the unique attributes of practitioners classified as expert and the commonalities across the 2 groups of therapists. In support of our theory, we have chosen representative statements from study participants as short exemplars of the themes. The sections on unique attributes of practitioners classified as expert and on commonalities across groups of therapists classified as expert or average follow the order of themes outlined in Table 3.

Theory of Expert Practice

Therapists classified as expert in our study were distinguished by a patient-centered approach to care. In this approach, patients are viewed as active participants in therapy, and a primary goal of care is the empowerment of patients—which is achieved through a collaboration between therapist and patient, clinical reasoning, patient education, and establishment of a good patient-therapist relationship. The patient-centered approach results from the interplay of clinical reasoning, values, virtues, and therapist knowledge and permeates and guides the clinician's style of practice.

Table 3.
Summary of Coding Themes From Cross-Group Analysis

Themes	Expert Group	Average Group
Clinical reasoning		
Patient empowerment a primary goal of therapy	√	
Collaborative problem solving	√	
Context of clinical practice: identity of teacher/coach	√	
Knowledge base		
Eclectic academic backgrounds	√	
Undergraduate degrees in exercise science	√	
Field experience prior to physical therapy school	√	
Frequent utilization of collegial knowledge	√	
Greater use of movement observation	√	
Reflection on practice	√	
Amount of clinical experience	√	√
Specialty knowledge from continuing education	√	√
Knowledge from patients	√	√
History as a patient receiving physical therapy	√	√
Athletic	√	√
Values and virtues		
Love of clinical care	√	
Humility	√	
Inquisitiveness	√	
Caring	√	√
Commitment to professional growth	√	√
Clinical practice style		
Patient education central to practice	√	
Individualizing intervention	√	
Limited delegation of care to support personnel	√	
Growth opportunities in the workplace	√	√

Excellence in patient-centered care involves clinical reasoning that is centered around the individual patient, enhanced by a strong knowledge base, skills in differential diagnosis, and self-reflection. The primary goals of empowering patients, increasing self-efficacy beliefs, and involving patients in the care process are facilitated by patient-therapist collaborative problem solving. This approach alters the therapeutic relationship and emphasizes the professional's primary role in supporting and enhancing patients' abilities to make autonomous choices.[34]

In our theory, the foundation for the expert clinician's approach to care is an ethic of caring and a respect for individuality. Clinicians who value and appreciate patient individuality garner more information from and about patients. This knowledge is gained through attentive listening, trust building, and observation. Our findings suggest that therapists' passion for clinical care—and their desire to continually learn and improve their skills coupled with the qualities of humility and inquisitiveness—drive their use of reflection, or thinking about practice. This combination of factors helps accelerate the acquisition and integration of knowledge.

The patient-centered approach is exemplified by the therapist's emphasis on patient education and by strong beliefs about the power of education. In this study, therapists classified as expert emphasized the patient-practitioner relationship and carefully regulated their delegation of care to support personnel. It is our theory that these efforts promoted patient empowerment and self-efficacy, better continuity of services, more skillful care, and more individualized plans of care.

The therapists classified as expert in our study possessed a broad, multidimensional knowledge base. Multidimensional knowledge is a mixture of knowledge gained from professional education, clinical experience, specialty work, colleagues, patients, continuing education, personal experience with movement and rehabilitation, and teaching experience. It is our theory that specific types of knowledge such as years of clinical experience are not as critical as the sum total of the knowledge base. Knowledge acquisition appears to be facilitated by work experience prior to attending physical therapy school. A synopsis of our theoretical model is presented in Figure 2.

Clinical Reasoning

Patient empowerment. The goal of empowering patients and increasing patient self-efficacy was central to the group classified as expert. Liz, for example, spoke of helping the patient realize that "he is in control" and can "become independent from PT [physical therapy]," and she described their efforts to discourage helplessness and dependency. [Editor's note: pseudonyms are used instead of the clinicians' actual names.] Patient empowerment was accomplished through patient education, avoiding passive modalities, minimizing unnecessary visits, and helping patients to develop self-management strategies for preventing exacerbations of their conditions.

> I think that it's really important from day 1 to put the responsibility for a lot of things back on the patient. I think it gives them more of a feeling of control, which a lot of people lose in our health care system, and that leads to a lot of stress and sometimes makes them worse. I think if you can empower a patient to some degree and give them a sense of control back and the feeling like they are doing something, that, in a large part, has to do with your success. (Kathy)

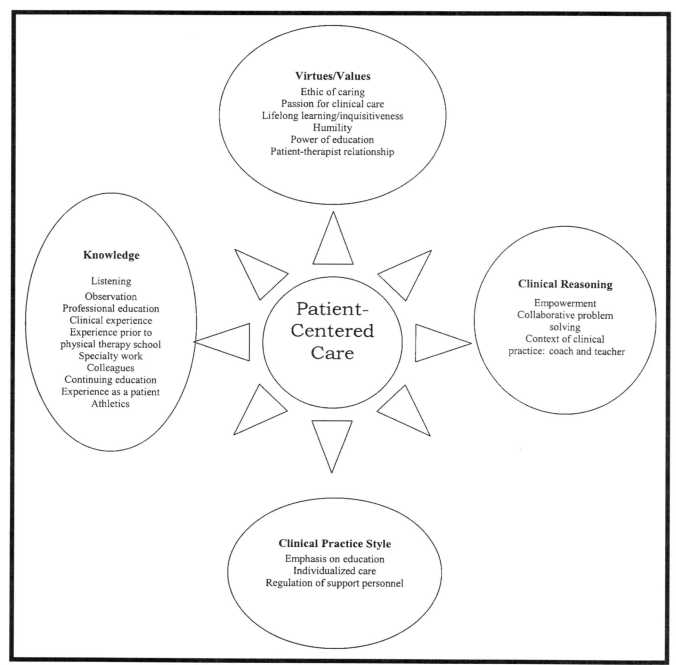

Figure 2.
Theory of expert practice.

"Engaging people in their own care" and patient empowerment also were mentioned by some therapists in the group of therapists classified as average. However, none spoke with the conviction or knowledge of self-efficacy issues that were demonstrated by the clinicians classified as expert. Beverly's comments were representative of the group of therapists classified as average:

I try to teach them something to do to make them feel a little bit better. So, what I might teach them is some body mechanics, about their posture, and about their activities, that

right off the bat they didn't know or they didn't realize they were doing wrong. And I try to, right away, teach them a couple of exercises that may, if you're in spasm, try to reduce the spasm and gently start increasing some flexibility. (Beverly)

Collaborative problem solving. Expert therapists used collaborative problem solving with their patients to help patients learn how to resolve problems on their own, discover solutions to everyday challenges, and take responsibility for their own care.

I'm a firm believer in educating back patients. [I] do lots of dos and don'ts, lots of body mechanics, lots of joint protection, lots of problem solving. You know, "How would you do this if . . . ? What would you do if . . . ?" You know, lots of, "Okay, you're going to have a bad day, we all have good days and bad days, what do you do on a bad day? How would you modify your behavior, or what can you do to make yourself more comfortable when you have a bad day?" (Kathy)

Problem solving in the group of therapists classified as average revolved primarily around the process of mechanical assessment—finding "the position of comfort and proper posture to relieve stress/pain on the injured tissue."

I try to identify structures that are causing the problem—muscle tightness, joint tightness, pain—and then I try to correct that or improve it, or have them recognize it and change it themselves. (Ann)

Context of clinical practice.

The clinical practice theme represents the context of care and, therefore, is complex in nature. The clinical practice theme incorporates the therapist's philosophy of practice and types and sources of knowledge, as well as clinical reasoning.[2] Its central components are therapists' beliefs and values about their roles as therapist.[5] Many similarities in clinical practice themes existed among clinicians in the group classified as expert. Four of the 6 therapists classified as expert (Liz, Kathy, James, and Pam) identified their primary role as educators who fostered patient self-efficacy. Two others (Sarah and Dawn) viewed their primary role as diagnosticians and movement analysts.

I've never been one of those practitioners who believe you [the patient] come in, and I do something to you, and that gets you better. I guess because of the background that I've had, my emphasis tends to be: we're coaches, we're teachers, we're educators. I feel sometimes that's not done enough. (Kathy)

A wider variety of clinical practice themes existed among members of the group classified as average. Three therapists (Sharon, Tim, and Crystal) identified their primary roles as manual therapists and healers, 2 therapists (Ann and Mike) identified their roles as educators and coaches, and 1 therapist (Beverly) expressed her primary role as a reassuring comforter. These themes contrast with those of expert group members, which were more consistent in their focus on patient education and empowerment.

I'm not certified as a manual therapist, but I would consider myself a manual therapist, I'd probably say maybe 40% to 50% of the time. The rest of the time is getting the patient to exercise and to stretch, and stuff like that. So, if they have a joint problem that needs to be mobilized, my hands are on them. If it's purely a flexibility issue in the spine, I'm stretching it, then I'm teaching them how to stretch. (Crystal)

You know, right away, when a patient comes in, I just want to reassure them when they are a little bit nervous and they are already in pain. Backs are very, very painful, [so] that I want them to understand that we are not going to try to increase their pain level. [I] to try to be very reassuring. (Beverly)

Multidimensional Knowledge Base

Academic and field experience prior to attending physical therapy school.

Our analysis revealed that there were differences in group professional preparation that extended beyond the professional degree. Participants in the group classified as expert were distinguished by 1 of 2 patterns of preprofessional preparation: diverse academic backgrounds or, for the novice therapists classified as expert, an undergraduate degree in exercise science coupled with work experience (Tab. 1). Examples of eclectic academic and career backgrounds included those in veterinary science, professional dance, occupational therapy, and clinical experience in international settings. Liz, for example, had graduated with a combined physical therapy/occupational therapy degree and had worked in both fields. Earlier in her career, she specialized in pediatrics, earned a master's degree in developmental disabilities, and was certified in both neurodevelopmental treatment and sensory integration. None of the participants from the group classified as average possessed the varied academic backgrounds or the combination of exercise science and extensive work experience found in the group classified as expert (Tab. 2). The least experienced participant in our group classified as expert (Sarah) had the most pre–physical therapy clinical experience (8 years).

Frequent use of collegial knowledge.

Expert therapists used the rich knowledge base of colleagues who, they explained, were "all very willing to answer questions" and described how they used their peers for consultation and examination of patients. Therapists sought out knowledgeable mentors to assist them in challenging cases. Most described a work environment that offered numerous opportunities for professional growth. Regardless of the actual amount of money reimbursed for continuing education, working in a supportive atmosphere with "knowledgeable staff" apparently provided opportunities for growth.

Everyone is really up on the research and up on what's going on. It really keeps you on your toes. It's a nice reinforcement of some of the things you do know, and a very rude awakening, of, "Oh my God, no matter how much I think I know, there's always more to learn!" What's neat with this health care system and the other therapists here, too, [is that] there's always someone where, if I go into an [evaluation] and start seeing some things, then I can come out and go to one of the other therapists and say, "I need you to take a look at something. Give me your impression, just go in take a look and see what you think." I think that helps tremendously. It's important sometimes to have another pair of eyes, another pair of hands, even after you've been seeing somebody for a while. It's nice to have a fresh approach, bring somebody else in that maybe is seeing something that you are not. It keeps you from getting biased, also. (Kathy)

In contrast, 5 out of 6 therapists in the group classified as average did not report consulting specifically on each other's patients in this way. Instead, they described how they learned from observing colleagues in action, discussed problems, and handed over a patient to another therapist for specialized care.

We throw ideas back and forth, we share, especially when we come to a road block. You know, "I've tried this and this, what do you think?" (Mike)

Whether it's therapists in my office, or other therapists that I meet at courses or therapists that I meet out, I talk to them about things. You learn ideas from them, and it really comes from just trying things, whether it's established or not. (Tim)

Use of movement observation. Members of the group classified as expert spoke frequently about observing movement. One therapist described how she observed her patients, "when they are in the clinic, how they get in and out of the chairs in the clinic," and outdoors. Observation of patients during normal, everyday activities helped therapists gain knowledge of patient function that augmented the information gained through observation of static postures and structured exercises. This strong emphasis on functional movement observation was not noted in the group classified as average.

We have a lot of windows, so I watch them getting in and out of their cars. Some of the things I've been observing just from when we're sitting in there talking: how are they sitting, how did they walk in, how are they standing, how are they holding themselves, how did they put their purse down on the floor, how did they take their shoes off? (Pam)

Reflection on practice. The process of reflecting on practice helped the therapists defined as expert to refine and improve their approach to practice. Most participants described the way that they thought about and analyzed their practice, and they spoke of "figuring out how things help," "practicing and changing your approach," and "changing the way that you instruct." Dawn described her strategy for integrating new material through purposeful practice as "choosing a new patient each day" to apply what she had learned in continuing education. This way, she was able to "use each little thing that I'd learn" and become more confident in her abilities. Pam stated:

I think it's just years of figuring out how things help, and just practicing and changing the way that you approach things, or changing the way that you instruct, to get more compliance.

The majority of participants from the group classified as average did not discuss reflecting on their practice, and several noted difficulties in thinking about practice.

It's very difficult for me to think about my whole career and how I practice, which I don't know if that's a good thing. I should have a better idea of how I treat back patients, but I don't. (Ann)

Values and Virtues

Love of clinical care. Therapists in the group classified as expert expressed a passion for clinical care and described the satisfaction they experienced from "helping other people." One therapist commented that it was really "fun to work" and said that she planned "to work at least until I am 70." These comments are consistent with this group's view of physical therapy as a vocation or "a calling."

In general, I love what I do. I love getting up and going to work, because you are there to help people. There are always challenges in every day in some shape or form, but it keeps you interested, and, plus, you are involved with people all day long, and I enjoy working with people. So, I think that being a therapist is a good job to see good outcomes, plus have fun at the same time at what you're doing. (Liz)

Although many of the professionals in the group classified as average also expressed an enjoyment of work and caring for patients, the same level of passion and enthusiasm was not evident, and one expressed his desire to shift his responsibilities away from patient care.

My goal at this point is to be completely involved in administration and out of patient care unless I can be very selective. If I can work with a cycling team or see only cyclists, I'd be happy. If I could work at a college and student athletes for half day and teach for half day, I would do that as well, but those jobs are few and far between. (Mike)

Humility. All therapists in the group classified as expert valued their continued professional growth and learning. Excitement about learning was obvious as they spoke about colleagues, their "responsibility to keep up-to-date with the literature," and opportunities for growth. Coupled with this drive to learn was a sense of humility that was not evidenced in the therapists from the group classified as average. The therapists classified as expert were quick to recognize their own limitations.

It is our responsibility to keep up-to-date with the literature and our responsibility to realize that it is a very large profession, and we can't know and do everything, and not be afraid to admit that you don't know something. I think that's what makes a good therapist, or a good physician. This field is too broad, you can't know it all. . . . You've got to be able to do a little bit of everything, and you've got to realize you can't do everything. (Kathy)

Inquisitiveness. Another quality that distinguished therapists classified as expert was inquisitiveness. This quality was evident from initial contact, throughout the interviews. Liz, for example, asked extensive questions while setting up the first interview appointment: "Why was I selected? What kind of degree are you getting? Where are you in school? What do you hope to do with your degree?" Dawn posed numerous questions about this research, trying to discern what kind of information would be most helpful. James described how he was "constantly asking questions" and how he had "bugged everyone around here about as much as I can." We believe that this quality contributes to lifelong learning; it was not noted in interviews with the therapists classified as average.

Patient Clinical Style

Patient education central to practice. Expert participants emphasized patient education and had a good understanding of teaching methods and their relationship to patient empowerment. One participant classified as expert, Liz, explained her belief that patients' home programs should be "as simple as possible" and "originate from collaborative discoveries made during the treatment session. . . . This helps so that the patient can remember them [the exercises] and incorporate them during the day."

> I try to keep everything really simple. I don't hand out huge lists of things to do. I try to teach the patient the whole sense of treatment. . . . So I really try to teach what the care is, so that they know, they don't inadvertently hurt themselves. I try to take away their fear of moving, so that they know that as long as they are not harmed by something that you know, they can continue to do things. Teach them how to test themselves to see if they are actually able to do something, then they'll know they are helping. (Liz)

Teaching philosophies of the group classified as average focused on teaching patients content, such as "what they need to know about their back," "what the diagnosis is," "showing them on the skeleton," and "the mechanics of how moving will affect your low back." No therapist in the group classified as average articulated a collaborative problem-solving approach.

> In terms of posture, I'll instruct just about everybody in proper positioning in the chair, good support using a towel roll or a pillow if they need it. If they are an office worker, I will talk to them about how their desk is set up, can they adjust the chair, can they adjust the computer, etc. But, just about everybody will be given or shown how to make a towel roll for lumbar support, just to get in that nice lordosis. I teach them how to go from supine to standing, sitting to standing, vice versa, bed mobility, etc. (Mike)

Individualizing of intervention. Therapists classified as expert put their patients first, and adapted intervention to address the needs and concerns of each patient. They described their efforts to "treat people individually" and develop "rapport with just about anybody." Participants classified as expert also spoke about individualizing the examination process, adapting the sequence and content to the patient. Half of the participants classified as average spoke about individualizing intervention for each patient, while the other half described their use of standardized examination and protocols for a variety of patient problems. Mike, for instance, discussed his treatment protocol, saying it "always includes hamstring flexibility" and "an abdominal bracing/core strengthening program which includes concentrated partial sit-ups and lower abdominal strengthening."

Limited delegation of care to support personnel. The pattern of care delegation was quite different between the participants classified as expert and those classified as average. In general, the group classified as expert provided more of their own direct intervention, limited the nature of delegated tasks more stringently, and supervised their support staff more closely than members of the group classified as average. In addition, they tended to work in teams, with only a single support person. This enabled the participants classified as expert to control the episode of care and may have provided greater continuity of care to the patient.

Two participants classified as expert worked without any support personnel. One participant did not have the option to work with an aide or assistant because there were none on staff, while the other participant chose not to use support personnel because her patient management philosophy did not include a role for them, "because my patients are always so different." This therapist was reluctant to use physical therapist assistants (PTAs) for exercise supervision, saying that if the patients did not require her skills, then they "would probably be independent enough to come in and do the gym work without help anyway."

The others in the group classified as expert did delegate care to a PTA or athletic trainer, but most believed in close supervision of the process. They worked with a single PTA "in a team" and conferred about patients "several times per week," "sitting, talking, hashing things out" with PTAs on a daily basis. "We do not bounce patients around," one participant commented. Therapists described their ability to control each intervention session, deciding on that day which aspects of care would be delegated.

> Every patient is different, and [when] they come in, I have to re-evaluate every time. You know there are exceptions to that, and once they are stable, I discharge them, or get them on their own. (Liz)

In contrast, all therapists in the group classified as average routinely delegated portions of patient care to PTAs or aides. Some told of delegating portions of manual therapy to their assistants, and half indicated that they often shared patients among multiple therapists and had 2 or more assistants helping them. One therapist commented that the hospital department was flexible in allowing patients to arrive late and "be seen by whichever therapist was available at the time."

> Well, we work in teams. So, you have a therapist who is teamed with an assistant or the athletic trainer. So, with any therapist, you may have 2 assistants helping them out, depending on how the patient schedules. If they want a particular time, sometimes they get bumped around, and that happens. We try to keep them with 2 to 3 therapists at a max. But, you know, we have technicians, also. (Tim)

Commonalities Across Groups of Therapists

For the purposes of this study the commonalities between therapists classified as expert and those classified as average (Tab. 3) were considered core dimensions of physical therapist practice, whereas the distinguishing characteristics described above were considered unique attributes of expert practitioners.

Knowledge Base

Amount of clinical experience and specialty knowledge.
Overall, the participants classified as expert were not distinguished from participants classified as average by years of experience, continuing education, or specialty training. Four out of 6 members of each group possessed advanced clinical training and specialty knowledge gained from continuing education course work. One expert therapist received McKenzie diplomate certification prior to data collection for this study. Another had become a certified manual therapist after the FOTO data collection period and was enrolled in a manual therapy residency. In the group classified as average, 1 participant had completed a year-long manual therapy course, 1 was in the process of becoming manual therapy certified, and 1 passed her orthopedic certified specialist examination after the data collection period.

History as a patient receiving physical therapy and as an athlete.
All members of the group classified as expert had previously received physical therapy, most having been managed for athletic injuries unrelated to back pain. At least half of the group classified as average also had experienced an injury that required physical therapy. Some participants reported that injury and rehabilitation had sensitized them to the patient's experience. This sensitization helped them to develop empathy, because, as Mike explained, he knew "when it is hurting and what is hurting, and how it feels, and whether that's

good or not for pushing patients, particularly those who are not able to push themselves."

All members of the group classified as expert, and most members of the group classified as average, had been, or were currently, involved in sports. At least half were drawn into the profession of physical therapy because of their personal interest in sports. Many therapists had taught or coached within their sport. This background provided personal knowledge of exercise and was a resource for relating to patients.

> I know how much time and how much work it takes to get to where you want [to be] physically. And I think that I pass that on to my patients, too, in their rehab. (Sharon)

Values and Virtues

Caring.
Caring for and about people was a fundamental ethic in both groups of physical therapists. They articulated a strong desire to help others and an enjoyment of "working with people," and they described themselves as "believers in helping others." It was also common for the therapists to describe themselves as "a people person" and speak proudly of "making a difference in somebody's life." The majority of therapists portrayed themselves as good listeners who learned from their patients. As one therapist in the group classified as average explained, "I listen to what patients are telling me is wrong with them. I have a whole hour with them. I write down their concerns, what they are telling me."

Commitment to professional growth.
Virtually all participants expressed a high regard for continued professional growth and lifelong learning. This was demonstrated by their pursuit of continuing education and advanced credentialing and by their enthusiastic remarks about learning.

> Continuing education, continuous learning, is a vital part of my professional existence. (Ann)

Clinical Practice Style

Utilization of opportunities in the workplace.
Most participants described a work environment that offered opportunities for professional growth. For some participants, such as Kathy, this included a "wonderful education program," with ample reimbursement for professional conferences and numerous opportunities to attend weekly in-services and study groups. For others, such as James, money for continuing education was minimal. "They won't reimburse you for anything," he said.

Most therapists described regular (usually monthly) in-services provided by colleagues. As Beverly explained, "When anyone, any therapist, does go to a conference, then they usually come back and give us an in-service." This enabled therapists to be exposed to a new idea or technique and to "incorporate it into our clinic."

Discussion

Implications of the Theoretical Model

Our findings provide one explanation of the characteristics and work environments of the therapists we classified as expert in the management of lumbar syndromes. Our work builds upon previous theoretical models of expertise and describes attributes of therapists whose patients who had excellent clinical outcomes. Our findings challenge a basic assumption that extensive experience as a physical therapist is essential for the development of physical therapist expertise.[5,35] The assumption that expert therapists have many years of experience has guided the sampling of subjects in prior studies of expertise.[4–6,8–10,35,36]

Our method of selecting subjects according to the outcomes of their patients differed from methods used in previous studies on expertise in physical therapy. Our selection method did not limit participation to experienced clinicians or to those with widespread collegial recognition. Our selection method had the potential to include subjects with diverse professional profiles, "ordinary" clinicians who were extraordinary in their level of patient outcomes. In prior expertise studies, subject selection was based on years of experience or peer nomination from APTA specialty section leadership. The methods used in these studies provided a subject pool of therapists who were actively involved with APTA, known to section leadership, and active in educational activities. The 12 subjects in the study by Jensen et al,[6] for example, had practiced in a minimum of 3 different practice settings and had 10 to 31 years of experience. Most had master's degrees, 11 out of 12 were APTA members, and all were teaching in some capacity.

The participants classified as expert in our study were different from those studied by prior researchers.[4–12,37] In reviewing the professional profiles of the participants in our group classified as expert, it is doubtful that all of them would be recognized as "experts" by their colleagues and communities. Some participants had not practiced in multiple settings, but had worked in the same practice environment since graduation. Their experience varied from 1.5 to 40 years; half were APTA members, and the minority had formal teaching experience. We believe that several therapists within this group may have been considered experts by their peers. Participants from the novice subcategory, however, were the unlikely "experts," because they were not at an advanced point in their career development. In all likelihood, they had not yet been labeled as experts by their peers, and

their caseloads may not have reflected the level of challenge or difficulty often reported by the experts in the prior studies.[2]

While the professional profiles of our participants were more diverse than those found among participants in previous studies, the theoretical model that emerged bears strong resemblance to other models of expertise.[2,4–6] Our theory supports and expands the understanding of a multidimensional knowledge base previously identified as a dimension of expertise in physical therapy.[2] Jensen et al[2] identified this dimension as a dynamic, multidimensional knowledge base that is centered on the patient and evolves through reflection. Our model of multidimensional knowledge includes professional education, continuing education, personal knowledge, clinical experience, and pooled collegial knowledge. It is our theory that all of these components of knowledge are facilitated by the use of reflection and a work environment that allows therapists to consult with and learn from colleagues.

A patient-centered approach was also identified by Jensen et al and called "collaborative, problem-solving clinical reasoning."[2] Jensen et al[2] reported that expert therapists shared a belief in patients' responsibility for their own health. Although few studies have tested the outcomes of a patient-centered approach, the benefits are discussed in the literature.[34,35,38,39] The findings of studies of clinical decision making in expert nurses[40] and physical therapists[2] have suggested that experienced clinicians are more likely than average clinicians to reflect a patient-centered approach. A client-centered approach to care has been endorsed by the Canadian Association of Occupational Therapists, with the assumption that this approach will lead to improved satisfaction and effectiveness of care.[34]

Patient-centered care describes a process of care guided by a philosophy of practice. This approach is characterized by the practitioner's beliefs, values, and attitudes about the rights of patients and patients potential to help themselves with.[38] In this model, patients are viewed as active participants in therapy and as partners in the therapeutic process who are responsible for making their own informed choices.[34] A patient-centered approach contrasts with a traditional medical model of care, or a practitioner-centered approach, which places the responsibility for health decisions chiefly in the hands of the clinician.[39] Thus, patient-centered care has implications for the patient-practitioner relationship.

Underpinning the patient-centered model is an ethic of caring and a respect for individuality. This is a similar finding to the dimension that Jensen and colleagues[6] called "caring and commitment" to patients. Patient-practitioner relationships influence the degree of involvement that patients have in their own care. Patient education is considered one of the most important strategies for empowering patients to become involved in their own care.[38] In our opinion, therefore, those therapists who place more emphasis on education, and have better communication skills, would be more effective at enhancing patient empowerment.

Continuity of care is recognized as a strategy for improving patient-practitioner communication. We theorize that delegation of care to multiple support personnel has implications for the therapeutic relationship and can interfere with patient-practitioner communication. Expert therapists' emphasis on the patient-practitioner relationship shapes the way that they regulate delegation of care to support personnel. This regulation may affect outcomes of care by promoting better continuity, more skillful care, and more individualized interventions.

We maintain that the practitioner's values and virtues are instrumental in using and gaining knowledge. This attribute is also consistent with prior grounded theory on expert practitioners.[5,6] In prior studies, expert practitioners also were found to have an inner drive for lifelong learning, understand their own limitations, appreciate what they did know as well as what they needed to learn, and demonstrate a well-developed ability for self-reflection and reassessment of their own practice.[6]

Limitations

Because this was a qualitative study of a specific group of therapists, the findings cannot be generalized to a broader population. The selection of therapists for sampling, based on retrospective analysis of a clinical database containing HRQL data, has limitations due to problems with missing observations, data control, patient selection bias,[41–43] and assumptions of construct validity. The construct validity of the data in our study is predicated on the use of HRQL measurements as outcomes of physical therapy. Another, related limitation is the manner in which therapists were classified as expert (90th percentile) and average (45th–55th percentiles) and the restriction of the sample to only those 2 groups. Perhaps most important, there are limitations in the exclusive use of intake and discharge HRQL measurements to measure the benefits of intervention. These measurements may not include all areas of significance to the clinician and the patient.[2] As Jensen et al[2] have noted, it is possible that aspects of physical therapy intervention, such as patient education, have lifelong health effects, which cannot be captured with HRQL measurements or assessed at the time of discharge. In our study, there was no method for tracking long-term HRQL outcomes within the existing FOTO database. Although these measurements may not reflect the actual

long-term effect of physical therapy, other research[44] has shown that SF-36 scores obtained at discharge are good indicators of long-term outcomes for patients with low back pain. We also did not examine the characteristics of therapists with poor patient outcomes. Although both groups of therapists in our study demonstrated similarities in caring about patients and commitment to the profession, it is possible that therapists with poor patient outcomes do not share these qualities.

Our interpretation of the therapists' style of clinical reasoning was limited by the research method and data collection. The method did not allow an analysis of clinical reasoning in actual intervention sessions or in regard to specific clinical examples. Interpretation of therapists' clinical reasoning was based on the comments made during interviews and the written philosophy of practice. Our data sources captured only the therapists' attitudes and beliefs about their professional lives. To limit the scope of this project, we did not seek input from patients, families of patients, colleagues, or administrators to obtain their viewpoints. Subtleties of communication, nonverbal behavior, and clinical reasoning could not be appreciated without observation of clinical encounters. Future research is recommended to address other aspects of clinical expertise and to add to improving this theory.

Although our study design did not include observation of therapists during management of patients, there is good reason to believe that beliefs and values that were expressed during our interviews are an accurate reflection of the therapists' emphasis on teaching. Sluijs et al[45] examined the beliefs and attitudes toward patients to see if there were correlations between the amount and type of education and the therapists' attitudes. Therapists who believed that education would lead to better adherence (where patients are more interested in intervention and thus have a quicker recovery) were found to pay more attention to this element of care, provide more and better education, and spend more time with their patients than those who did not believe in its effectiveness.[45]

Further research is recommended to test the hypotheses developed through this research and to address its limitations of method and design. Additional research on the effect of physical therapist use of support personnel is recommended. Although APTA has general guidelines on supervision and delegation,[46] individual state practice acts regulate this aspect of care in varying ways. Some states have general requirements for supervision of PTAs, some states have periodic on-site requirements, and the most stringent states require on-site supervision.[47] We found no published research that has evaluated the effect of supervisory patterns on outcomes of care.

Our findings have implications for physical therapy education, practice, and administration. Therapist effectiveness might be facilitated through the adoption of a treatment philosophy similar to the one espoused by the therapists who were classified as expert in our study and through the efforts of supervisors and managers who promote a collegial climate of continuous learning and reflection. The hypotheses generated from this study can be used to develop and test a "best practice model" for the management of patients with lumbar syndromes.

Educators can use this information to help new therapists achieve better patient outcomes, and to stimulate mid-career therapists to better performance. Practitioners can increase attention to psychosocial aspects of rehabilitation and behavioral change strategies. Clinical educators can help students to develop effective methods of patient education and coaching, and promote the development of reflective practitioners with patient-centered values.

Conclusions

Practitioners classified as expert in our study were distinguished by a patient-centered approach to care, which is characterized by collaborative problem solving, patient empowerment through education, and cultivation of the patient-practitioner relationship. We believe that this philosophy of care contributed to the style of delegation to support personnel, maximized continuity of care, and promoted individualized intervention. These findings both confirm and build upon the prior theoretical framework of expertise. In contrast to widespread assumptions about experience and expertise, we did not note a relationship between years of experience and patient outcomes. Other components of knowledge, including the use of pooled collegial knowledge, reflection on practice, and experience prior to physical therapy school, facilitated the acquisition of knowledge.

References

1 Rothstein JM. Foreword II. In: Jensen GM, Gwyer J, Hack LM, Shepard KF. *Expertise in Physical Therapy Practice*. Boston, Mass: Butterworth-Heinemann; 1999:xviii.

2 Jensen GM, Gwyer J, Hack LM, Shepard KF. *Expertise in Physical Therapy Practice*. Boston, Mass: Butterworth-Heinemann; 1999.

3 Purtilo RB. Foreword I. In: Jensen GM, Gwyer J, Hack LM, Shepard KF. *Expertise in Physical Therapy Practice*. Boston, Mass: Butterworth-Heinemann; 1999.

4 Jensen GM, Shepard KF, Hack LM. The novice versus the experienced clinician: insights into the work of the physical therapist. *Phys Ther*. 1990;70:314–323.

5 Jensen GM, Shepard KF, Gwyer J, Hack LM. Attribute dimensions that distinguish master and novice physical therapy clinicians in orthopedic settings. *Phys Ther*. 1992;72:711–722.

6 Jensen GM, Gwyer J, Shepard KF, Hack LM. Expert practice in physical therapy. *Phys Ther*. 2000;80:28–52.

7 Embrey DG, Yates L, Nirider B, et al. Recommendations for pediatric physical therapists: making clinical decisions for children with cerebral palsy. *Pediatric Physical Therapy*. 1996;8(4):165–170.

8 Embrey DG, Yates L. Clinical applications of self-monitoring by experienced and novice pediatric physical therapists. *Pediatric Physical Therapy*. 1996;8(4):156–164.

9 Embrey DG, Hylton N. Clinical applications of movement scripts by experienced and novice pediatric physical therapists. *Pediatric Physical Therapy*. 1996;8(1):3–14.

10 Embrey DG, Guthrie MR, White OR, Dietz J. Clinical decision making by experienced and inexperienced pediatric physical therapists for children with diplegic cerebral palsy. *Phys Ther*. 1996;76:20–33.

11 Embrey DG, Adams LS. Clinical applications of procedural changes by experienced and novice pediatric physical therapists. *Pediatric Physical Therapy*. 1996;8(3):122–132.

12 Embrey DG. Clinical applications of decision making in pediatric physical therapy: overview. *Pediatric Physical Therapy*. 1996;8(1):2.

13 Morse JM. Theory innocent or theory smart? *Qual Health Res*. 2002;12:295–296.

14 Strauss AL, Corbin J. Grounded theory methodology: an overview. In: Denzin NK, Lincoln YS, eds. *Handbook of Qualitative Research*. Thousand Oaks, Calif: Sage Publications Inc; 1994:273–285.

15 Cutcliffe JR. Methodological issues in grounded theory. *J Adv Nurs*. 2000;31:1476–1484.

16 Dobrzykowski EA, Nance T. The Focus On Therapeutic Outcomes (FOTO) Outpatient Orthopedic Rehabilitation Database: results of 1994–1996. *Journal of Rehabilitation Outcomes Measurement*. 1997;1(1):56–60.

17 Jette AM. Outcomes research: shifting the dominant research paradigm in physical therapy. *Phys Ther*. 1995;75:965–970.

18 Delitto A. Are measures of function and disability important in low back care? *Phys Ther*. 1994;74:452–462.

19 Enebo BA. Outcome measures for low back pain: pain inventories and functional disability questionnaires. *Chiropractic Technique*. 1998;10(1):27–33.

20 Hart DL. Test-retest reliability of an abbreviated self-report overall health status measure. *J Orthop Sports Phys Ther*. In press.

21 Hart DL. The power of outcomes: FOTO Industrial Outcomes Tool—initial assessment. *Work*. 2001;16:39–51.

22 Ware JE Jr, Snow KK, Kosinksi M, Gandek B. *SF-36 Health Survey: Manual and Interpretation Guide*. Boston, Mass: The Health Institute, New England Medical Center; 1993.

23 Ware JE Jr. *How to Score the SF-12 Physical and Mental Heatlh Summary Scales*. Boston, Mass: The Health Institute, New England Medical Center; 1995.

24 Hart DL, Dobrzykowski EA. Impact of exercise history on health status outcomes in patients with musculoskeletal impairments. *Orthopaedic Physical Therapy Clinics of North America*. 2000;9(1):1–16.

25 Ware JE Jr, Kosinski M, Keller SD. A 12-Item Short-Form Health Survey: construction of scales and preliminary tests of reliability and validity. *Med Care*. 1996;34:220–233.

26 Hart DL. Assessment of unidimensionality of physical functioning in patients receiving therapy in acute, orthopedic outpatient centers. *J Outcome Meas*. 2000;4:413–430.

27 Muzzin LJ, Norman GR, Feightner JW, et al. Expertise in recall of clinical protocols in two specialty areas. *Proc Annu Conf Res Med Educ*. 1983;22:122–127.

28 Merriam SB. *Qualitative Research and Case Study Applications in Education.* 2nd ed. San Francisco, Calif: Jossey-Bass Inc Publishers; 1998.

29 Winegardner K. The Case Study Method of Scholarly Research. The Graduate School of America. Available at: http://www.tgsa.edu/online/cybrary/case1.html. Accessed November 27, 2001.

30 Miles M, Huberman AM. *Qualitative Data Analysis: An Expanded Sourcebook.* 2nd ed. Thousand Oaks, Calif: Sage Publications Inc; 1994.

31 Glaser BG, Strauss AL, Corbin JM. *The Discovery of Grounded Theory: Strategies for Qualitative Research.* Chicago, Ill: Aldine; 1967.

32 Strauss AL, Corbin JM. *Basics of Qualitative Research: Techniques and Procedures for Developing Grounded Theory.* 2nd ed. Thousand Oaks, Calif: Sage Publications Inc; 1998.

33 Lincoln S, Guba EG. *Naturalistic Inquiry.* Beverly Hills, Calif: Sage Publications Inc; 1985.

34 Law M, Baptiste S, Mills J. Client-centred practice: what does it mean and does it make a difference? *Can J Occup Ther.* 1995;62:250–257.

35 Noll E, Key A, Jensen GM. Clinical reasoning of an experienced physiotherapist: insight into clinician decision-making regarding low back pain. *Physiotherapy Research International.* 2001;6(1):40–51.

36 Jensen MP, Turner JA, Romano JM, Lawler BK. Relationship of pain-specific beliefs to chronic pain adjustment. *Pain.* 1994;57:301–309.

37 Shepard KF, Hack LM, Gwyer J, Jensen GM. Describing expert practice in physical therapy. *Qual Health Res.* 1999;9:746–758.

38 Ersser S, Atkins S. Clinical reasoning and patient-centred care. In: Higgs J, Jones ME, eds. *Clinical Reasoning in the Health Professions.* London, England: Butterworth-Heinemann; 1995.

39 Ellis S. The patient-centred care model: holistic/multiprofessional/reflective. *Br J Nurs.* 1999;8:296–301.

40 Benner PE, Tanner CA, Chesla CA, et al. *Expertise in Nursing Practice: Caring, Clinical Judgment, and Ethics.* New York, NY: Springer Publishing; 1996.

41 Jette DU, Jette AM. Physical therapy and health outcomes in patients with spinal impairments. *Phys Ther.* 1996;76:930–945.

42 Jette DU, Jette AM. Physical therapy and health outcomes in patients with knee impairments. *Phys Ther.* 1996;76:1178–1187.

43 Pryor DB, Lee KL. Methods for the analysis and assessment of clinical databases: the clinician's perspective. *Stat Med.* 1991;10:617–628.

44 Gatchel RJ, Mayer T, Dersh J, et al. The association of the SF-36 health status survey with 1-year socioeconomic outcomes in a chronically disabled spinal disorder population. *Spine.* 1999;24:2162–2170.

45 Sluijs EM, van der Zee J, Kok GJ. Differences between physical therapists in attention paid to patient education. *Physiother Theory Prac.* 1993;9(2):103–117.

46 Direction and Supervision of the Physical Therapist Assistant. In: HOD 06–00–16–27 [amended HOD 06–99–07–11; HOD 06–96–30–42; HOD 06–95–11–06; HOD 06–93–08–09; HOD 06–85–20–41; initial HOD 06–84–16–72/HOD 06–78–22–61/HOD 06–77–19–37]. Alexandria, Va: American Physical Therapy Association.

47 Summary of Physical Therapy Practice Acts and Rules on PTA Supervision. Available at: https://www.apta.org/Advocacy/state/PTA_supervision_summary. Accessed December, 20, 2001.

Appendix.
Examples of Questions for Guided Telephone Interview

1. Please provide your name, age, years of experience, year of graduation, and type of practice setting.

2. What is the size of your current practice? The number of colleagues within the practice?

3. Do you work with any support personnel? If so, how do you delegate to them?

4. What are your job responsibilities?

5. Approximately how many patients with low back pain do you see per week? Per month? Per year?

6. What is the percentage of patients who fill out intake FOTO[a] forms?

7. How long have you participated in FOTO?

8. Why do you participate in FOTO?

9. Approximately how many patients do you see per week?
   Number of patients per day
   Time spent with each patient
   Time spent on evaluation

10. Talk about experiences that have affected how you think about physical therapy.

11. Talk about experiences that have affected how you practice with patients with low back pain.

12. Do you think that your knowledge of physical therapy for patients with low back pain has changed over time? If so, how? To what do you attribute these changes?

13. What are the sources for your knowledge base? (Your knowledge base includes your knowledge of facts and theories and of how to perform professional activities [procedural knowledge] and your appreciation of the meaning and relationships of facts and theories for each patient.)

14. What do you consider to be the milestones in your learning that have led to your becoming the clinician you are today?

15. Talk about the most memorable patient you had with low back pain.

16. What does being a professional mean to you?

17. What is your view of yourself as a professional? What are you most proud of in your professional life?

18. What are you least proud of? What would you like to change or do differently in your physical therapy practice?

19. Talk about your practice environment, including your caseload, the type of facility in which you work, your colleagues, and the support staff. What are the strengths and limitations?

20. What does it mean to you to grow as a professional? In what ways does your work environment support your professional growth?

21. Do you subscribe to any specific practice philosophy (beliefs or tenets) in your approach to patients with low back pain? For example, would you describe yourself as a manual therapist? A McKenzie therapist? Do you follow any specific guidelines in your care of patients with low back pain?

[a] FOTO=Focus On Therapeutic Outcomes Inc.

HABITS OF THOUGHT

by Ruth B Purtilo, PhD, PT, FAPTA

Revisiting the Basics of Professional Life

*"The way in which my profession is being perceived
...no longer represents what I studied long and hard to achieve." (Letter to the editor)*

Sometimes I'm asked, "How did you go from being a physical therapist to being a 'philosopher'?" I usually reply, "I *didn't*. It's just that the questions that were raised for me during my years of clinical practice turned out to be important philosophical questions, and what I learned from my study of philosophy turned out to be relevant to my practice."

All physical therapists raise important philosophical questions—that is, all therapists who accept that the study of philosophy is the search for that which is "real," or "essential," or "basic."

Are you searching for what is "real" in your professional identity? If so, you are not alone. Many therapists today feel that the very core of their professional identity is being shaken by profound changes in health care delivery. Managed care, capitation, cross-training, reengineering, outcomes management, the new language of customer satisfaction—any or all may seem to be an earth tremor to persons who went through rigorous formal preparation for professional service, who signed a social contract with society through professional licensure, and who agreed to abide by the American Physical Therapy Association's *Code of Ethics.*

As you search for the essential elements of your professional identity, you need to reflect on the concepts, ideals, values, practices, and commitments that have been identified with professionalism throughout the ages. Ethics is one important area of philosophical inquiry

> The therapist who wishes to maintain his or her professional identity... must be mindful of policies or practices that undermine the principle of beneficence—and reject them.

that gets right to the point.

In the first Habits of Thought in January 1993, I named some criteria (principles) so basic to the idea of a profession that I think of them as the "ABCs" of health care ethics. I revisit them below.

Autonomy

During a recent discussion about health care, a therapist turned to me to say, "Well, what do you think? Does a managed care approach protect, enhance, or threaten the therapist's professional autonomy?" This therapist wanted clarity about a very basic dimension of her professional identity.

Autonomy includes freedom from impingement on a profession's judgments and activities. But the larger challenge is to combine this ideal of freedom with a clear understanding of what the freedom is *for*. Professional autonomy does not mean

simply "following your bliss." It means being responsive to patients' needs and focusing on patients' satisfaction. It also means being attuned to societal needs and resources and applying independent but informed judgments about how the health care needs of patients should be addressed when resources are limited.

Is professional autonomy protected, enhanced, or threatened by managed care? In the context of the two imperatives listed above, each of you may have a somewhat different answer.

Beneficence

The principle of beneficence requires therapists (and other health professionals) to act always in their patients' best interests. The *ideal* of service, which has characterized professional ethics, is duty-driven. It is not the prerogative of the physical therapist to engage in policies and practices that have as their goal some other end. A key element of professional identity, then, is adherence to the duty to serve (act as an advocate for) the patient or client.

If cross-training, the movement of professionals into groups, capitated payment systems, or any other aspect of the evolving health care system begins to impinge on the professional's ability to be beneficent, the identity, then, of the professional who accepts this impingement will be transformed into something other than that of a professional. And that acceptance will become complicity in transforming the identity, of the profession itself into something else.

"In trying to determine what is 'real' or 'essential' about our professional identity, I am reminded about how we study anatomy. Our 'real' quest in anatomy class is not to identify, for example, the superior vena cava in the cadaver before us on the lab table. The superior vena cava is only one small aspect of a larger system—human circulation. The instructors, whose job it is to distinguish fundamentals from nonfundamentals, may subtract one point if we miss the examination question about where the superior vena cava is located, but, more importantly, they will not allow into professional practice the student who fails to grasp the underlying basic concept of human circulation.... That's the way it is with professional identity. If we know what professional autonomy is—but we fail to know what it is for—we cannot hang on to the essentials of our professional identity."

—Ruth B Purtilo

The therapist who wishes to maintain his or her professional identity, and the identity of professionalism per se, must be mindful of policies or practices that undermine the principle of beneficence—and reject them.

Considered Constraint

When physicians were the only health professionals, the definition of "the professional" was "one who exercises not only the science but the art of medicine." This ancient definition is useful and relevant in assessing the identity of all health professions as they are perceived today.

A key component of health care is to act with considered, thoughtful restraint: to act skillfully, to not make decisions rashly, to not use privileges to exercise autonomy for ends other than the good of patient and society.

Today the idea of constraint or containment often is applied to the constraint or containment of costs only. This distorts professional identity because it ignores the well-being of the patient as the organizing focus for determining the conditions under which it is morally justifiable to apply constraint based on limited funds or other resources.

The principle of justice is designed to help professionals (and society) deal with the distribution of any scarce but valuable resource. This principle holds that similarly situated persons will be treated similarly; arbitrary decisions about who will receive the desired goods (eg, health care) are not allowed. Criteria such as the relative degree of need for the resources and the likelihood of benefit from them help establish initial priorities. As the resources become more scarce, however, these criteria become more compelling, and the decisions about who will receive the resources, more tragic.

Under the guidance of the principle of justice, the emphasis always is on fairness, even when it is not possible to provide persons with everything they need or everything that would benefit them. This disposition to fairness is essential to professional identity, and any necessary constraint should be tempered by the desire to treat everyone fairly.

In her letter to the editor (page 14), Patricia Lemcke writes, "The way in which my profession is being perceived...no longer represents what I studied hard and long to achieve." As *you* consider your professional identity, take time to reflect on the basic, unchanging tenets of professional life. They can act as critical markers for you during this time of change.

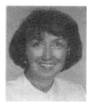

Ruth B Purtilo, PhD, PT, FAPTA, is Professor of Clinical Ethics, Creighton University Center for Health Policy and Ethics, Omaha, Neb, and is Past President, American Society of Law, Medicine, and Ethics. She is coordinator Habits of Thought.

HABITS OF THOUGHT

By Ernest Nalette, EdD, PT

Truth-Telling and Deception In Practice

Your colleague has justified her actions as being in the best interest of not only Mr Doe but all similar patients, current and future. But is she lying to achieve her purposes?

*H*abits of thought predispose us not only to *think* in a certain way but to *act* in a certain way. "Good" thoughts are prerequisite to "good" actions. We learn what is "good" from our families, friends, communities, and religious leaders. But our beliefs about the "good" continually are challenged in our personal and professional lives. The following case example raises questions about one component of the "good"—truth-telling in professional practice.

You are sitting with a colleague and friend who is telling you about a current patient, Mr Doe, and her success in helping him improve his level of function. She mentions that Mr Doe's insurance plan does not reimburse physical therapists for the type of services she is providing him. She says it is irritating to have to "play the game" with the insurance company in order to be reimbursed for services that she believes are necessary to the patient's health and well-being. The "game," she explains, involves choosing words to enter into the medical record, words that will ensure reimbursement for her services—even when those words do not accurately reflect the patient's status.

You are surprised. "But aren't you lying when you intentionally misrepresent the patient's status?" you ask. Your colleague does not answer you directly; instead, she replies that she is acting *in the patient's best interest.* "The insurance company's policies are unreasonable," she says. When you ask whether she has done anything to try to change those policies,

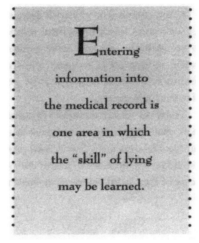

*E*ntering information into the medical record is one area in which the "skill" of lying may be learned.

she responds that she does not have the time to treat patients *and* work to change policy. "Besides," she adds, "It's *useless* to try to change policy. You know we're powerless to influence the insurance industry." Your colleague explains further that if reimbursement for this patient and all patients with similar conditions is denied, the practice at which she works will be forced—by financial necessity—to stop providing services to this patient population.

Your colleague has justified her actions as being in the best interest of not only Mr Doe but all similar patients, current and future. You understand her reasoning, but the question remains: Is she *lying* to achieve her purposes?

Bok[1] defines *lying* as "an intentionally deceptive message in the form of a statement." According to this definition, your colleague is lying, because she intentionally is recording a deceptive picture of Mr Doe's status. *But is your colleague telling a "justifiable lie"?*

After further discussion with your colleague, you decide a lie is called for to protect Mr Doe's interests. Your decision may be influenced by a number of factors:

- The patient referral had been accepted with good intentions.
- The services being provided are beneficial to the patient, who has shown improved function as documented through tests and measures.
- The insurance company's past pattern of nonreimbursement in this type of case is clear.
- Mr Doe lacks private funds to pay for the services.
- Mr Doe trusts that the therapist will help him recover his function, and maintaining this trust—by whatever means necessary—is critical to ensuring that the services continue to be beneficial to him.
- To offer pro bono services to all patients with conditions such as that of Mr Doe would result in the financial failure of the practice at which your colleague works.

As children we are taught that we should tell the truth and avoid lying; however, almost all of us can imagine a situation in which telling a lie—that is, being intentionally deceptive—may serve the best interest of a patient. Such a lie might not seem "right"; however, it might seem "justifiable." No discussion of lying can be limited, however, to the idea that the therapist will treat a particular lie as a tragic exception to a more general moral guideline. In practical terms, lying becomes easier to do each time it is done.

Entering information into the medical record is one area in which the "skill" of lying may be learned. In fact, some health professionals become experts at writing medical records that are just vague enough to create a picture of the patient's status that is inaccurate. If we lie about patient status frequently, the result is to practice lying and to become skillful at lying, and as we practice lying, we inevitably create a predisposition to lying—and form a habit of thought. We begin to slide down that slippery slope, lying not only when we believe lying serves the best interest of the patient but when lying serves our own self-interests—such as enhanced reimbursement.

The vast majority of physical therapists and other health professionals do not enter their professions or their particular practice environments intending to lie. It is more likely that a set of circumstances within the practice environment subtly shapes our behaviors—including the way we write in the medical record—to result in deception. By default, we may become game players, and playing the game may mean that we allow ourselves to become liars.

When lying becomes a habit, we forget what we used to know—that lying is wrong. The habit of lying also allows us to avoid making the extra effort to change the circumstances that lead us to believe a lie is required in order to do our professional duty.

To practice truth-telling, we may need to take specific actions:

- Decide when and why to act differently than those with whom we practice.
- Work with peers and others to change policies that support lying and create ethical dilemmas for therapists.
- Join with patients to foster necessary policy changes.
- Practice trustworthiness, that is, be a person who keeps a confidence and is "thoughtful about the impact of ... decisions on others, sensitive to their needs and claims ...."[2]

Lying *is* wrong. But if we *do* choose to lie, we should do so with the understanding that we are taking the risk of *becoming a liar* and a less-virtuous person, no matter what other ends are being achieved in the short term. That is, if we choose to lie, we should lie in the hope that, next time, we will choose *not* to lie. Truthfulness is a virtue worthy of our continual practice to improve ourselves as persons and professionals through good habits of thought. *PT*

Ernest Nalette, EdD, PT, *is Manager, Physical Therapy Department, Medical Center Hospital of Vermont, and Clinical Associate Professor, Department of Physical Therapy, University of Vermont, Burlington, Vt.*

References
1 Bok S. Lying: *Moral Choice in Public and Private Life.* New York, NY: Vintage Books; 1979.
2 Lebacqz K. *Professional Ethics: Power and Paradox.* Nashville, Tenn: Abingdon Press; 1985;79.

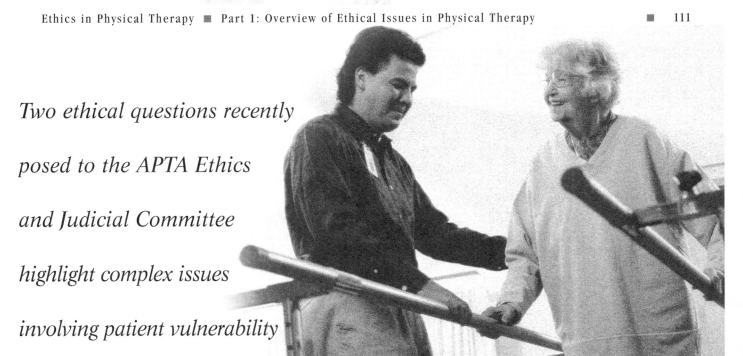

Two ethical questions recently posed to the APTA Ethics and Judicial Committee highlight complex issues involving patient vulnerability in the physical therapist– patient/client relationship.

By Susan W Sisola PT, PhD

Patient Vulnerability:

Ethical Considerations for Physical Therapists

Physical therapists established the foundation for their ethical obligations to patients in the earliest days of the profession.[1] Today, physical therapists' acceptance of their professional status as autonomous practitioners requires continuing in-depth and diligent consideration of these ethical responsibilities.[2,3] The privilege and influence that accompany professional practice obligate physical therapists to look beyond literal or superficial interpretations of their ethical code, and to consider the complexities of the ethical issues evident in the current practice environment. Thoughtful deliberation of ethical issues followed by a commitment to action is a sign that the trust of patients and society is warranted.

Two ethical questions recently posed to the APTA Ethics and Judicial Committee (EJC) reflect physical therapists' recognition of this obligation. This article highlights two seemingly straightforward, yet complex, issues. One involves romantic and sexual relationships with former patients; the other involves physical therapists recommending or selling products to patients. (See Ethics and Judicial Committee Opinions at www.apta.org/PT-Practice/ethics_pt/ejc_opinions for full opinions.)

Although the situations giving rise to these questions are quite different, both questions involve considerations of patients' vulnerability in the physical therapist/patient relationship.

Romantic or Sexual Relationships With Former Patients

"Is it ethical for a physical therapist to engage in a sexual relationship with a patient after care for that patient has been transferred to another therapist?"

On the surface, this question appears to be readily addressed by the APTA Code of Ethics (Code) and Guide for Professional Conduct (GPC).[4] Principle 2.1.C. of the GPC states, "A physical therapist shall not engage in any sexual relationship or activity, whether consensual or nonconsensual, with any patient while a physical therapist/patient relationship exists." Further review, however, underscores the complexities of the question and the level of consideration required for a thoughtful and ethical response.

Scott[5] describes the relationship between a physical therapist (PT) and patient/client as one of the most intense among health care disciplines, given the length of time the PT may be in close physical contact with patients. Patients must be considered vulnerable within this relationship due to their level of trust in the PT and the inherent power differential between the patient and PT. The losses a patient may face due to illness or injury, coupled with the power of expertise, skill, and information held by the PT, create a significant disparity of power within the relationship.[6] Furthermore, during the process of examination and evaluation, the physical therapist may elicit significant personal information from patients, including the sharing of private and perhaps intimate aspects of their lives.

These circumstances may at times lead some patients to develop a degree of affection for the PT. Principles 1 and 2 of the APTA Code of Conduct, and related EJC interpretations of the Guide (1.1.B, 1.1.C.),[4] address the physical therapist's position of trust, obligating him or her to act not only in the best interests of patients, but also as a fiduciary—one who places the patient's interests above all others, including any self-interest on the part of the PT. Act-

ing as a fiduciary, the physical therapist has ethical and legal obligations to avoid any exploitation or abuse of the patient. Thus, the PT must ensure that the therapeutic relationship does not become a personal one, and, as Scott has suggested, "any natural reciprocal feelings that may arise for the therapist must be sublimated to prevent sexual abuse of a patient."[7(p78)]

Recognizing that an attraction between a PT and a patient occasionally may occur, the APTA Code of Conduct and Interpretative Guide (2.1.E.)[4] states, "In the event the physical therapist or patient terminates the physical therapist/patient relationship while the patient continues to require physical therapy services, the physical therapist should take steps to transfer the care of the patient to another provider."

Active involvement of the PT in transferring the care of a patient is required to avoid any potential abandonment of the patient. But the question now becomes whether the ethical obligations inherent in the patient–therapist relationship are lifted for the PT at the time that care of the patient is transferred to another PT. Literal interpretation of this question would suggest that

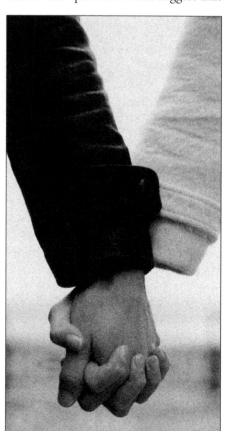

the ethical obligations for the physical therapist in question (therapist A) cease when he or she has assisted in transferring the care of the patient to another provider (therapist B) prior to initiating a sexual relationship. In an obvious sense, the patient–physical therapist relationship could be said to end once the PT stops treating the patient. A broader and more comprehensive interpretation, however, suggests several conditions that could affect the PT's ethical obligations.

Does a patient deemed to be too vulnerable on Monday somehow cease to be too vulnerable on Tuesday simply because his or her last treatment with the PT in question occurred on Monday? The basic rationale for the GPC restriction against sexual relationships between a physical therapist and patient is that the patient has (or is likely to have) such a special vulnerability in relation to his or her physical therapist that the risk of exploitation inherent in a romantic or sexual relationship is too great. While the patient's vulnerability is not something that can be assumed to dissipate immediately at the end of the final treatment session, it is difficult to suggest any defined timeframe for when, if ever, initiation of a romantic/sexual relationship with a former patient would be ethically permissible.

This concern for vulnerability of the patient is consistent with the reasoning of the Council on Ethical and Judicial Affairs (CEJA) of the American Medical Association (AMA), which has stated with regard to physicians that having a sexual or romantic relationship with a former patient is unethical "if the physician uses or exploits trust, knowledge, emotions, or influence derived from the previous professional relationship."[8] Similarly, the Oregon Physical Therapist Licensing Board condemns as unprofessional conduct any sexual contact with a patient, which it views as including "entering into a sexual or romantic relationship with a former patient, if facilitated by the former patient's trust or attraction rising out of the therapeutic relationship."[9(p19)]

Patient Vulnerability: *Ethical Considerations for Physical Therapists*

Some professions have advocated a waiting period of 6 months to several years following the termination of a professional/patient relationship before beginning a sexual relationship.[5,9] It is felt that a significant waiting period minimizes the potential for exploitation of patients, and signals acceptance by the provider of her or his ethical obligations. The EJC does not believe that any arbitrary period of time (eg 3 months or 2 years) can answer whether initiation of a romantic or sexual relationship with a former patient would be ethical. Determining whether the PT would be exploiting a patient's trust depends on circumstances unique to the particular case, and thus calls for the PT to exercise extra diligence in considering his or her conduct.

The passage of time, by itself, cannot provide assurance against the possibility of exploitation of a former patient. Key factors in determining the potential for exploitation relate to the patient and the character of the patient's relationship with the PT. It is possible to imagine that in some cases a romantic or sexual relationship would not be considered unethical if initiated with a former patient soon after the termination of treatment. In other cases, a romantic or sexual relationship with a former patient could never be considered ethically permissible.

The determination as to whether initiating a romantic or sexual relationship with a former patient would be ethically permissible depends not on a quantitative measure of time since the last treatment session but rather on a host of qualitative circumstances relating to the patient, the physical therapist, and the relationship between them. Any significant disparity between the power, status, and emotional vulnerability of the former patient and that of his or her PT strongly suggests the potential for an exploitive relationship. Consider the following questions in assessing the risk of exploitation:

❖ Does the patient seem vulnerable?
❖ Is the age difference between the PT and the former patient substantial?
❖ Is the patient considerably poorer or less educated than the physical therapist?
❖ Does the patient have significant psychiatric or psychological problems?
❖ Does the patient have problems with substance abuse?
❖ Has the patient been the victim of abuse, especially sexual abuse?
❖ Is the patient particularly lonely or extremely shy?
❖ Is the patient suffering from a recent separation or divorce, death of a loved one, or economic difficulty?
❖ Is the patient undergoing psychological adjustment to a significant illness or injury?

The physical therapist's own circumstances also are potentially relevant to a determination of ethical obligation. For example, if the PT is in the midst of a personal crisis, the risk of exploitation of a former patient might be greater. Consultation by the PT with a trusted colleague before initiating a romantic or sexual relationship with a former patient could be helpful in weighing the risks.

When the decision to transfer a patient's care is precipitated by a romantic or sexual attraction to the patient, this decision requires special considerations. Determining where a patient should be referred, under these circumstances, is a practical one that the PT must consider, with attention to the particular circumstances of the situation and the patient's best interests. If the patient's condition required particular skills or expertise not held by other PTs at the facility, the referring PT ethically would be obligated to refer the patient to another clinic, where the necessary skills or expertise would be available, in

---

Relevant principles from the APTA Code of Ethics (Code) and Guide for Professional Conduct (GPC)[4]

Principle 1. A physical therapist shall respect the rights and dignity of all individuals and shall provide compassionate care.

GPC 1.1.B. A physical therapist shall be guided by concern for the physical, psychological, and socioeconomic welfare of patients/clients,

GPC 1.1.C. A physical therapist shall not harass, abuse, or discriminate against others.

GPC 2.1.A. To act in a trustworthy manner the physical therapist shall act in the patient/client's best interest. Working in the patient/client's best interest requires knowledge of the patient/client's needs from the patient/client's perspective. Patients/clients often come to the physical therapist in a vulnerable state and normally will rely on the physical therapist's advice, which they perceive to be based on superior knowledge, skill, and experience. The trustworthy physical therapist acts to ameliorate the patient's/client's vulnerability, not to exploit it.

GPC 2.1. B. A physical therapist shall not exploit any aspect of the physical therapist/patient relationship.

GPC 2.1.E. In the event the physical therapist or patient terminates the physical therapist/patient relationship while the patient continues to require physical therapy services, the physical therapist should take steps to transfer the care of the patient to another provider.

order to act in the best interests of the patient.

Merely transferring a patient's care to another physical therapist in order to initiate a romantic or sexual relationship with that patient does not, in and of itself, relieve the PT of his or her ethical obligations. At no time should a romantic or sexual relationship take precedence over the physical therapist's recognition of the vulnerability of patients in her or his care, and full acceptance of the therapist's ethical obligation to act first and foremost in the patient's best interest. Failure to do so signals a failure to fully accept the ethical obligations required of autonomous professionals and could result in unethical conduct by a physical therapist.

Recommending and Providing Clinical Products for Patients

Physical therapists in all practice settings frequently are in a position to recommend, and perhaps sell, clinical equipment to their patients. Because of their expertise in movement dysfunction, PTs are uniquely qualified and positioned to recommend to patients/clients the "best" equipment to prevent further injury and enhance patient function and recovery. Failure to provide this valuable service certainly could be argued as not acting in the best interest of patients. The myriad business arrangements surrounding the practice of providing or selling equipment, however, can lead to many ethical questions. A physical therapist recently posed the following scenario:

A physical therapist working in the area of ergonomics recommended certain products for improving work sites for patients. While he recommended products from various vendors from time to time, he tended to suggest products from one particular vendor, as this company had the most complete line of products and seemed to meet the needs of his patients/clients. The physical therapist had not received

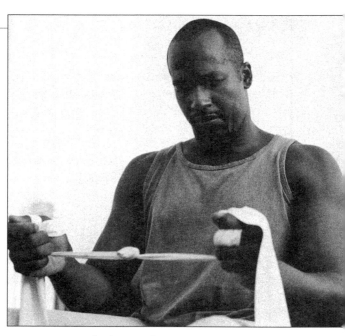

compensation of any sort from any of the vendors. The vendor of the product line the physical therapist recommended most frequently then contacted him, suggesting the possibility of paying him a financial "reward" that would be tied to the number of orders placed by patients/clients. The physical therapist asked, "Is it unethical to accept incentives from this company for suggesting that my patients utilize this particular company's products? Could this arrangement be considered "good business" for all the parties involved?"

Recommending products for patients requires a physical therapist to attend to the patient's "physical, psychological, and socioeconomic welfare" (GPC 1.1.B.).[4] A physical therapist's recommendation of any device or product always must be based on the PT's sound professional judgment that use of this product will be beneficial to the health of the patient. Thus, PTs must assess the efficacy and effectiveness of a new product before incorporating it in their practice. In addition, PTs must promote only those products that they consider to be a good value (promoting socioeconomic welfare of patients). A physical therapist would not be acting in the patient's interests when recommending a clinically useful product that was extremely overpriced (eg, in comparison with competitive products).

Physical therapists frequently find that the most efficient and effective way to ensure that patients/clients have access to devices that will be beneficial to their health and function is to actively assist them in selecting and purchasing the equipment. It certainly could be argued that a physical therapist satisfies an ethical duty to act in the best interests of patients when he or she recommends an appropriate product and then

facilitates the patient/client's access to that device. Making necessary equipment readily available to patients with impaired mobility or limited access to transportation is an important component of service offered by physical therapists.

When the physical therapist has a financial interest in the product he or she recommends, however, additional ethical obligations arise. The Code and GPC clearly caution against any financial exploitation of the patient/client–physical therapist relationship. Although recommending or selling products offered by a third party is not unethical for the physical therapist, receiving compensation or other forms of incentive raises serious questions regarding the professional's ethical obligations, given the vulnerability of patients/clients. First, when a physical therapist recommends a product, the decision behind the recommendation must be based on the therapist's professional judgment that the product will be in the patient's best interest—not that it is in the physical therapist's financial self-interest.

In addition, a physical therapist who recommends a product must disclose to the patient any financial interest in having the patient follow his or her recommendation and purchase the product. Further, a PT who makes a recommendation for which he or she is compensated must respect and promote the patient's freedom of choice with respect to that product.

Patient Vulnerability: *Ethical Considerations for Physical Therapists*

Despite what must be assumed to be reasonable intentions of the PT when recommending or selling products to patients, the presence of a financial interest must be considered a potential influential factor in the decision-making of any physical therapist, even if only at the subconscious level. Therefore, the PT's behavior in the absence of a financial interest cannot be a sure guide to how he or she might behave under a compensated arrangement. For this reason, physical therapists promoting products for patient/client use must be particularly attentive to the possibility that the financial interest might distort their professional judgment.

The disclosure obligation for a PT who recommends or sells products to patients also incorporates the ethical obligation of trustworthiness, because a financially interested physical therapist who fails to reveal her or his interest might mislead the patient into believing that the recommendation was purely disinterested. An informed, competent patient may well choose to follow a physical therapist's recommendation while fully understanding that doing so would benefit the PT financially, and that patient would have no reason to feel that he was deceived about the PT's financial benefit. On the other hand, a patient who was unaware of the physical therapist's financial interest well might feel that she had been misled by the PT's failure to disclose that arrangement. Gaining and maintaining the patient's trust is at the heart of the physical therapist–patient/client relationship. Actions that undermine that trust threaten not only that particular interaction, but also societal perceptions of the trustworthiness of physical therapists as a whole.[1]

Respecting a patient's freedom of choice also involves the degree of influence the PT actually holds with a particular patient. As noted previously, patients must be considered to be vulnerable within the relationship due to their level of trust in the PT and the power differential inherent in such relationships.[5-7] Under certain circumstances, a physical therapist might have such influence over a patient that his or her recommendation of a particular product would have the effect of negating the patient's freedom to choose another product. This reality requires that the PT be particularly zealous in making sure that the recommendation of a product in which he or she has a financial interest is motivated primarily by concern for the patient's best interests. Although disclosure of a financial interest must be considered mandatory, the vulnerability of particular patients could render that disclosure to be, in fact, meaningless. Thoughtfully considering the level of vulnerability of patients receiving care at a particular physical therapy clinic is an important step in determining an ethical process for recommending or providing clinical products for patients at that site.

The privileges inherent with professional stature require a heightened level of diligence and insight for all physical therapists. The potential for knowledge and expertise to strongly influence and create or exploit vulnerability in patients must be balanced by full acceptance of our ethical obligations to patients and clients, and to society. **PT**

Susan W Sisola, PT, PhD, is associate professor, Doctor of Physical Therapy Program, College of St Catherine, Minneapolis, Minnesota. She is a member of the APTA Ethics and Judicial Committee. Also on the committee are Chair Gail Wheatley, PT, Linda E Arslanian, PT, MS, Carol M Davis, PT, PhD, and Laura "Dolly" Swisher, PT, PhD. To contact Committee members, please call John J Bennett, APTA General Counsel, at 800/999-2782, ext 3107, or via e-mail at johnbennett@apta.org.

Sections 7.2.A and 7.2.B of the Guide for Professional Conduct[4] provide a basis for considerations of a physical therapist's ethical obligations when endorsing products.

❖ 7.2.Endorsement of Products or Services

A. A physical therapist shall not exert influence on individuals under his/her care or their families to use products or services based on the direct or indirect financial interest of the physical therapist in such products or services. Realizing that these individuals will normally rely on the physical therapist's advice, their best interests must always be maintained, as must their right of free choice relating to the use of any product or service. Although it cannot be considered unethical for physical therapists to own or have a financial interest in production, sale or distribution of products/services, they must act in accordance with law and make full disclosure of their interest whenever individuals under their care use such products/services.

B. A physical therapist may receive remuneration for endorsement or advertisement of products or services to the public, physical therapists, or other health professionals provided he/she discloses any financial interest in the production, sale, or distribution of said products or services.

REFERENCES

1. Purtilo RB. Thirty-First Mary McMillan Lecture: A time to harvest, a time to sow: ethics for a shifting landscape. *Phys Ther.* 2000;80:1112-1119.
2. Magistro CM. Clinical decision-making in physical therapy: a practitioner's perspective. *Phys Ther.* 1989;69:525-534.
3. Swisher LL. A retrospective analysis of ethics knowledge in physical therapy (1970 2000). *Phys Ther.* 2002;82:692-706.
4. American Physical Therapy Association. *Code of Ethics and Guide to Professional Practice.* Adopted by APTA House of Delegates, June 1991; amended June 1999.
5. Scott R. *Professional Ethics: A Guide for Rehabilitation Professionals.* St. Louis, MO: Mosby; 1998.
6. Purtillo R, Haddad A. *Health Professional and Patient Interaction,* 5th ed. Philadelphia PA: WB Saunders; 1996.
7. Scott R. Habits of thought: sexual misconduct. *PT—Magazine of Physical Therapy.* 1993;1(10):78-79.
8. Council of Ethical and Judicial Affairs, American Medical Association. Sexual misconduct in the practice of medicine. *JAMA.* 1991;266:2741-2745.
9. Oregon Physical Therapist Licensing Board. Available at http://www.ptboard.state.or.us/pdf/bdpres.pdf. Accessed April 17, 2003.

Professional Perspective

Gift-giving or Influence Peddling: Can You Tell the Difference?

Physical therapists are faced with an ever-increasing array of advertising ventures, "free" gifts, and enticing offers from equipment and supply companies and various health care agencies. Concerns are raised about the ethical implications of gift exchange in professional activities. Basic motives governing gift exchange are examined from a sociological standpoint. The obligation of the professional to act in the best interest of the patient and to guard against the impression of impropriety to the public is paramount in decisions concerning gifts. Opinions from the medical and pharmaceutical professions are explored to glean criteria that have applicability to physical therapy. These criteria are presented in the form of questions that may be helpful for physical therapists. [Finley C. Gift-giving or influence peddling: Can you tell the difference? Phys Ther. 1994;74:143–148.]

Key Words: *Ethics; Physical therapy profession, professional issues; Professional-patient relations.*

Claudette Finley

Is it unethical to accept gifts of minimum value distributed freely by equipment vendors and other business enterprises advertising at state and national American Physical Therapy Association (APTA) meetings? Is it ethically sound to send flowers or other gifts to a referral source in recognition of the opening of a practice or a significant anniversary? Are there differences in ethical implications between situations in which physical therapists are presented small gifts from grateful patients and situations in which equipment, drug, or supply companies present substantial gifts to facilities? Should companies subsidize the cost of physical therapists attending continuing educa-tion meetings and professional conferences? Is it unethical for equipment companies to seek substantiation of their product by subsidizing research? If a company requests to furnish equipment for a classroom with the company's name clearly marked on the materials, is this acceptable? These situations arise frequently in physical therapy practice, education, and research, yet they hold the potential for compromising professional ethical standards. The purposes of this article are to discuss ethical implications in gift exchange in physical therapy and to convey information from other professions that may be helpful in establishing criteria to assist in the decision-making process.

With the increase in the number of equipment and supply vendors and the "mushrooming" of new agencies for home health, rehabilitation, and hospitals, a physical therapist walking through an exhibit area at a conference is bombarded with small gifts, raffles, free trips, scholarships, and numerous other methods of advertising to entice the initiating of a business venture. In addition, representatives from these companies pay frequent visits to clinics and educational facilities for the purpose of selling their products. Advertising is a necessary part of economic survival for these companies.

At what point in this "economic" process do we begin to feel concern about whether an activity has ethical implications? Concern arises when gifts or other considerations, whether accepted or offered, foster obligatory

C Finley, PT, is Associate Professor, Department of Physical Therapy, Health Science Center, University of Florida, PO Box 100154, Gainesville, FL 32610 (USA). She is a former member of the American Physical Therapy Association Judicial Committee.

The views expressed in this article are those of the author and do not reflect official opinions of the American Physical Therapy Association Judicial Committee.

This article was submitted October 22, 1992, and was accepted August 10, 1993.

conditions. There is concern when the gift holds the potential for affecting the objectivity of professional judgment. There is concern with the appearance of impropriety to the public. There is concern with who carries the responsibility for control over the content, faculty, educational methods, and materials when business enterprises subsidize the expenses of a physical therapy conference. These concerns point to the necessity for physical therapists to weigh carefully these situations to determine what is the basic motive behind the gift (ie, to express appreciation for services, to advertise, to obligate, to promote the self-interest of the physical therapist, or to influence professional judgment).

Do Gifts Convey Messages?

To understand the principles behind this necessary form of goods exchange, we need to be aware of the role of gift exchange in "early" societies. Marcel Mauss, a French social anthropologist, in his classic essay *The Gift: Forms and Functions of Exchange in Archaic Societies*, asks, "In primitive or archaic types of society, what is the principle whereby the gift received has to be repaid? What force is there in the thing given which compels the recipient to make a return?"[1(p1)] Gift exchange between clan and clan, in which individuals and groups exchanged everything, constitutes the oldest economic system we know and is the basis from which gift exchange arose. Mauss studied the social significance of gift exchange as a means of initiating and sustaining relationships. He explained

> The gift itself constitutes an irrevocable link especially when it is the gift of food . . . . For it is not only the person who gives it that is bound but also the one who receives it . . . . Gifts carried a certain danger, for the receiver must always give back in return more than he received . . . . The danger represented by the thing given or transmitted is possibly nowhere better expressed than in very ancient Germanic language . . . the double meaning of the word "gift" as gift and poison . . . . In addition, gifts established the hierarchy. To

give is to show superiority . . . . To accept without returning or repaying more is to face subordination.[1(pp61–72)]

Thus, we see at work some of the fundamental motives of human activities that have implications for professionals who face situations involving gift exchanges daily.

The role of "reciprocity" in a number of societies was studied by Becker.[2] He states that the point of reciprocity is to create and sustain balanced social relationships. He explains that the return gift must be perceived by the receiver as good and must also be "in kind" and "fitting." A personal exchange requires a personal response. If the benefit, instead, is aimed at sustaining a social structure that provides benefits to many people rather than just one person, then the return would be "fitting" if it also benefits many people. The social transaction generated an "obligation," which carries the sense of a requirement. This author warns

> An obligation to reciprocate for the goods we receive puts too much power in the hands of others. Enterprising people can shower us with unasked-for benefits . . . simply to get benefits in return . . . . Do we really want a principle that puts the extent of our obligations so thoroughly in the hands of others? . . . The problem is the control others have over the extent of our obligations.[2(p135)]

Thus, Becker asks the same questions as Mauss,[1] but adds

> How can a benefit, unasked for by the recipients, obligate them to make a return? The justification for such non-contractual obligations is obscure, yet it is the crux of the matter . . . . If it (reciprocity) is to have a useful place in moral theory at all, it will be for an account of nonvoluntary obligations— the kind we acquire whether we ask for them or not. Ethnographers, social anthropologists, historians and sociologists report in unison that people everywhere do "feel" such obligations . . . it is a pervasive feature of human social life. It will not go away.[2(pp73–74)]

Then, can a gift be "free"? Does pure benevolence exist? "[T]here are some

acts of benevolence . . . which would be undermined by the attempt, on the part of a recipient, to force them into the pattern of a reciprocal transaction," argues Becker.[2(p94)] The gift of blood or charitable donations would be examples of pure impersonal benevolence. According to this author, the appropriate response to pure benevolence would be a simple gracious acceptance and gratitude. We have read the donor's intentions and have responded with gratitude, which completes the reciprocal response.

Professional Responsibility and Gift Exchange

If we accept that gift exchange does introduce the possibility of an "obligation," then should certain restrictions be imposed on professionals to govern ethical behavior in their practice? Many professions have recognized the inherent dangers that gifts pose for objective decision making.[3] A distinction must be made, however, between those professions with the primary motive of making a profit (ie, of promoting the self-interest of the company) and those professions that bear the obligation of putting the interests of their clients or patients over self-interest. For example, Levy and Mishkin[4] point out that if a car salesperson says, "This is the car for you," the buyer knows that the sale is in the self-interest of the salesperson and his or her company. On the other hand, if an audiologist says, "This is the hearing aid for you," one would expect the decision to be in the patient's best interest.

Do certain professions have higher moral obligations? Pellegrino[5] explores this question and asks

> Do we really wish the special human predicaments with which medicine, law, and the ministry deal to be conducted like our relationships with auto mechanics, merchants, or bankers? . . . Is there something intrinsic to the activities of the professions that distinguishes them from business and the trades? . . . I submit that there is such justification and that it can be found in the nature of the human needs the

professions address and the human relationships peculiar to them.[5(p169)]

Why do we need to make this distinction between certain professions? Thomasma and Pellegrino derived an axiom of vulnerability that reads

> In human relations generally, if there are inequalities of power, knowledge, or material means, the obligation is upon the stronger to respect and protect the vulnerability of the other and not exploit the less advantaged party.[6(p41)]

Veatch reminds us of the commitment in the Declaration of Geneva that states, "The health of my patient will be my first consideration."[7(p25)] A further definition of the difference between professions is pointed out by Pellegrino[5] in that the needs the professions address are of the most personal kind. He writes

> [T]he patient or client must open up the most confidential aspects of his or her life . . . and must trust that [the professional] has the knowledge he or she claims to have and will use it in the best interest of the client . . . . Trust, therefore, is mandatory . . . . [There is] the promise of help, in the face of human vulnerability. This promise gives a special moral quality to the professional relationship . . . that one will use that knowledge to advance the best interests of the one who needs help and not one's own interest . . . . They [the nature of the relationships] impose moral obligations that must transcend standards of moral behavior in society at large.[5(pp173–175)]

The medical community has also reacted in numerous publications to the expressed concerns of its members on this issue. Chren et al[8] warn that physicians are not seasoned business people and miss the subtle, but compelling, sales pitch. We often overlook the vulnerability of conscientious practitioners to the obligation that comes with a gift.

Reports of research studies on the influence of gifts are mostly found in medical and pharmaceutical literature. There are no reports of research studies on this issue to date in the physical therapy literature. The impact

of drug company funding on the content of continuing medical education was explored by Bowman.[9] After a content analysis of audiotapes from two educational courses on calcium channel blockers, Bowman reported a bias. The two courses were presented by different drug companies. Each drug company was found to make more positive and more frequent statements about its own product.

Bowman and Pearle[10] studied changes in drug prescribing patterns related to commercial company funding of continuing medical education and reported that overall the sponsoring drug company's products were favored.

Avorn et al[11] studied scientific versus commercial sources of influence on the prescribing behavior of physicians. Their findings showed that physicians are not always able to recognize the commercial messages and inputs that ultimately bear on therapeutic decisions. The physicians were strongly influenced by nonscientific sources.

Chren et al[8] point out that gifts that affect prescribing practices can threaten the fiduciary relationship between physician and patient. Gifts cost patients money, and the use of patients' money to pay for gifts can be unjust. The cost is ultimately passed on to patients without their explicit knowledge and consent. These authors explain

> [P]hysicians' acceptance of gifts may contribute to the further erosion of the common perception that the medical profession serves the best interests of patients . . . . We believe it is unjust to have a system in which patients pay for gifts that benefit doctors or drug companies. The burdens (payment) are the patient's (or patient's insurers'), but the benefits (beach bag or trip) accrue to the physician, who controls the patient's choice of medication, and to the company, which enjoys the profits . . . . [T]he injustice to the patient is heightened by lack of disclosure . . . .[8(pp3449–3450)]

Although these authors are directing their remarks to physicians, the ideas expressed are applicable to physical therapy practitioners and our relationships with equipment and supply companies.

Several examples of the problems gifts impose when outside pressures come to bear upon this fiduciary relationship are described by Levy and Mishkin.[4] With the outright cash gift or the all-expenses-paid trip, the authors point out that ethical problems arise when the giveaway is targeted to individuals, in contrast to a random giveaway at a conference. They explain

> The trip helps expand the influence of a vendor on a professional's judgment in the context of an ongoing commercial relationship . . . . The dynamic human relationship helps to create subtle feelings of obligation on the part of the professional.[4(p49)]

Volume discounts are also examined, and the authors ask whether the professional's judgment in choosing a product will be affected by the discount. The 1987 resolution of the American Surgical Association denounces the active participation of physicians in promotional exercises for which they receive compensation:

> Giving papers at the behest of a health care industry for the primary purpose of promoting a pharmaceutical, an appliance or any other health care supply item is not an acceptable professional service warranting remuneration.[12(p1690)]

Levy and Mishkin[4] remind us that we need to protect the public impression of the appearance of impropriety. They state

> [T]he public image of the profession is tarnished by the impression that clinicians gather information upon which they base independent judgments for patients at junkets paid for by the very vendors soliciting their business . . . that a professional's judgment somehow is intertwined with the promotional activities of vendors . . . . [P]rofit incentives tend to influence the professional by creating a motivation to follow self-interest rather than the interest of those served professionally . . . .

Where substantial likelihood exists that professionals will be influenced to prefer their self-interest over the client's and where the consumer has no way of knowing about or evaluating the effect of that influence, the practice is unacceptable.[4(pp49–50)]

Making Decisions About Gifts

A number of professional associations have incorporated into their codes of professional responsibility specific statements addressing the issue of gift exchange.[3] In the APTA Code of Ethics and Guide for Professional Conduct,[13] the ethical principle of concern for the interest of the patient over the self-interest of the physical therapist is paramount. In January 1993, the following statements addressing the issue of gifts were added to the Guide for Professional Conduct:

5.4 Gifts and Other Considerations

A. Physical therapists shall not accept nor offer gifts or other considerations with obligatory conditions attached.

B. Physical therapists shall not accept nor offer gifts or other considerations that affect or give an objective appearance of affecting their professional judgment.

The focus of these statements is on whether an obligation is established and professional judgment is impaired. The exercise of sound professional judgment is basic to decisions involving gifts.

Physical therapists may find it helpful to study how the medical profession has addressed some of the controversial issues between individual physicians and industry. In 1990, the American College of Physicians issued guidelines in a position paper published in *Annals of Internal Medicine*.[14] Position 1 reads

Gifts, hospitality, or subsidies offered to physicians by the pharmaceutical industry ought not to be accepted if acceptance might influence or appear to others to influence the objectivity of clinical judgment. A useful criterion in determining acceptable activities and relationships is: Would you be willing to have these arrangements generally known?[14(p624)]

Shortly thereafter, the American Medical Association's House of Delegates adopted guidelines recommended by their Council on Ethical and Judicial Affairs.[15] These guidelines state that it is considered unethical for physicians to accept the following from pharmaceutical companies: subsidies to pay for the costs of travel, lodging, or other personal expenses incurred by physicians while attending meetings; any gifts that are of substantial value and do not primarily entail a benefit to patients; any gift that entails an obligation; and cash payments of any kind.

The need to distinguish between personal and institutional gifts is discussed by Chren et al.[8] They explain

[O]bligations are minimized when gifts are institutional rather than personal. Therefore, we argue that it is ethically acceptable for drug companies to give money to institutions for books, educational activities, journals . . . in exchange for only an explicit acknowledgement; this situation poses less of a danger because no personal relationship and no obligation to respond in any way are established between the individual physician and the drug company's representative . . . . [F]ull disclosure, avoidance of extravagance and waste, and the primary goal of improving patient care by physician education make these activities ethically acceptable.[8(p3450)]

The recipient's use of the gift is emphasized as a guideline by Camenish[16] in his essay "On Being a Professional, Morally Speaking." Will the gift benefit those in need of our professional services, or does the professional receive the primary benefits?

Goldfinger warns that the monetary value that would render a gift unacceptable cannot be set with precision:

Few would consider the acceptance of a notepad or a ballpoint pen an improper act. But those who espouse overall restraint might balk at a more expensive amenity, such as a dinner or a country club outing.[14(p625)]

As Chren et al explain, "The key here is not the monetary value of a gift but whether it is instrumental in fostering a personal relationship."[8(p3451)]

Physical therapists face an array of situations involving gift exchange, from the patient who wants to express gratitude with a small gift to the large equipment company donating products to the clinic for consideration. The assumption that one can accept the deluge of gifts from industry without any risk of being compromised is incredibly naive.[17] Decisions about gifts are not easy to make; the motives of the giver must be recognized. Throughout this article, various criteria for making decisions about gifts have been discussed. These criteria are summarized below in the form of a list of basic questions that may be helpful to physical therapists in situations involving gift exchange:

1. Is the gift-giving occurring in an effort to express gratitude for services rendered? Is the gift of minimal value?

2. Is the gift-giving an attempt to obligate or control a portion of a physical therapist's practice or research? Are there "strings" attached to receiving the gift?

3. Is the substance or quantity of the gift(s) large enough to be raised as an issue of "kickback"?

4. Is the gift to an institution or organization rather than personal?

5. Does the gift foster a personal relationship between the professional and the vendor?

6. Will the gift benefit those in need of our services, or does the professional receive the primary benefit?

7. Is the cost of the gift ultimately passed on to patients without their knowledge?

8. Would you be willing to have the gift generally known or disclosed to the patient, the public, or to one's colleagues?

9. Is the gift of financial support from companies to physical therapists to attend continuing education meetings, for the purpose of furthering the physical therapy education of the practitioner? Is there reimbursement for essential expenses such as travel, registration, and lodging, rather than personal expenses? Is it a personal pleasure trip with a token educational experience?

Summary

This article presents an overview of concerns related to the issue of gift exchange in physical therapy. Basic motives governing the giving or receiving of gifts are examined from the sociological aspect. The responsibility of the health professional to place the interest of the patient foremost in decisions is discussed. Criteria gleaned from the experience of other professions are posed as questions that may help the physical therapist in making decisions concerning gifts.

References

1 Mauss M; Cunnison I, trans. *The Gift: Forms and Function of Exchange in Archaic Societies.* Glencoe, Ill: The Free Press; 1954.

2 Becker LC. *Reciprocity.* London, England: Routledge & Kegan Paul Ltd; 1986.

3 Gorlin R, ed. *Codes of Professional Responsibility.* 2nd ed. Washington, DC: Bureau of National Affairs Inc; 1990.

4 Levy NI, Mishkin DB. In whose best interest is it, anyway? Solutions to ethical problems caused by influences outside the professional relationship. In: *Reflections on Ethics: A Compilation of Articles Inspired by the May 1990 ASHA Ethics Colloquium.* Rockville, Md: American Speech-Language-Hearing Association; 1990:47–51.

5 Pellegrino ED. What is a profession? *J Allied Health.* 1983;12:168–176.

6 Thomasma DC. The ethics of caring for vulnerable individuals. In: *Reflections on Ethics: A Compilation of Articles Inspired by the May 1990 ASHA Ethics Colloquium.* Rockville, Md: American Speech-Language-Hearing Association; 1990:39–45.

7 Veatch RM. *A Theory of Medical Ethics.* New York, NY: Basic Books; 1981.

8 Chren MM, Landefeld CS, Murray TH. Doctors, drug companies, and gifts. *JAMA.* 1989; 262:3448–3451.

9 Bowman MA. The impact of drug company funding on the content of continuing medical education. *Mobius.* 1986;6:66–69.

10 Bowman MA, Pearle DL. Changes in drug prescribing patterns related to commercial company funding of continuing medical education. *J Contin Educ Health Prof.* 1988;8:13–20.

11 Avorn J, Chen M, Hartley R. Scientific versus commercial sources of influence on the prescribing behavior of physicians. *Am J Med.* 1982;72:4–8.

12 Bricker EM. Industrial marketing and medical ethics. *N Engl J Med.* 1989;320:1690–1692.

13 *Code of Ethics and Guide for Professional Conduct.* Alexandria, Va: American Physical Therapy Association; 1993.

14 Goldfinger SE. Physicians and the pharmaceutical industry: American College of Physicians. *Ann Intern Med.* 1990;112:624–626.

15 American Medical Association, Council on Ethical and Judicial Affairs. Gifts to physicians from industry. *JAMA.* 1991;265:501.

16 Camenish PF. On being a professional, morally speaking. In: Flores A. *Professional Ideals.* Belmont, Calif: Wadsworth Inc; 1988: 14–26.

17 Goldfinger SE. A matter of influence. *N Engl J Med.* 1987;316:1408–1409.

Invited Commentary

The author has given an important ethical issue a level of visibility that is long overdue. As the author indicates, prior dialogue on this issue within our profession has essentially been nonexistent.

It is indeed difficult in certain situations to make the differentiation between gift-giving and influence peddling, and the level of difficulty ranges on a continuum dependent on the situation. For example, I have no ethical dilemma if a recipient of my professional services gives me a jar of homemade jelly; however, if that client offers me a season theater ticket worth several hundred dollars or a year's membership in the local country club, my ethical alarm is activated. In the examples given, the gifts were intended merely as an appreciative gesture without obligatory connotation. But the theater ticket and the country club membership have professional impropriety overtones that strongly conflict with my value system.

Decisions relating to gift-giving and sponsorships from vendors and referral networks are far more complex than are those pertaining to gifts from service recipients. My personal level of concern with this aspect of gift-giving has increased concomitantly with the expansion of our technology and the increased numbers of vendors who promulgate the sales of that technology. Also, with the ever-increasing numbers of health care alliances, organizational mergers, and provider networks—all trying to recruit and retain physical therapists—the enticements, special incentives, and sponsorships pose numerous dilemmas.

Perusing the exhibit halls at our various conferences is all too frequently an observational exercise in the art of sales seduction. In such scenarios, we are the object of influence peddling as we fill our shopping bags with plastic goniometers, samples of ultrasound gel, and a variety of other goodies. In addition, some colleagues have expressed concern regarding conference and meeting social events sponsored by vendors. Many of these events have become part of the tradition of such conferences at local, state, and national levels. Is there an obligatory aspect wherein the sponsor of the event is expecting some future consideration that other vendors are less likely to receive? One would be naive to miss the rhetorical nature of that question.

Referral networks present a very special problem. The reality is that we have to maintain and build on these networks for the viability and survival of our professional practices. But where do we draw the line in our own gift-giving and influence peddling?

We have colleagues, well-known within our profession, who serve as "consultants" and receive annual retainer fees. In effect, they allow their names to be listed as "consultants" and receive retainer fees. Is this influence peddling complicity of a differing type?

I would not presume to try to provide answers to all of these questions. This article, however, engenders many questions, all of which need exploration and dialogue. Hopefully, the publication of this provocative article will elicit more interest in the need to confront the gray areas of our ethical value systems.

Jane Mathews-Gentry, PT
Rehabilitation Team Leader
Visiting Nurse Association
*   of North Shore Inc*
8 Angle St
Gloucester, MA 01930

Author Response

I am pleased that Jane Mathews-Gentry was asked to write a commentary on this article concerning the issue of "gift-giving" versus "influence peddling." I appreciate her review of the manuscript and her supportive statements concerning the serious nature of this problem and its infiltration into our profession. As a physical therapy leader with an extensive clinical perspective in a variety of settings and a breadth of knowledge concerning issues facing our profession, she gives credence to the need to recognize and explore the potential problems involved with gift-giving.

In her commentary, Ms Mathews-Gentry raises the question of the conflict physical therapists face in needing to build referral networks without becoming caught in the problem of gift-giving and influence peddling. This conflict was only alluded to in my article, and more discussion and direction are needed. In addition, she raises the issue of "consultants" and annual retainer fees, which I did not address in my article. This area also needs further study.

The primary purposes of this article were to ask questions concerning the problems of gift-giving and to share information on how other professions have approached this issue. I hope that this article will provoke discussion and lead to better understanding of the complexities involved in the problems of gift-giving.

Claudette Finley, PT

Physical Therapy & ADVERTISING

As a health professional, you may use advertising to both obtain and communicate information about products and services. What issues should you be aware of?

By Carol Schunk, PsyD, PT, and Ron Hruska, MPA, PT

Advertising is part of today's global culture, a way of communicating information and ideas to large numbers of people. No matter what the medium, the amount of advertising can seem overwhelming, and we may feel *barraged* with advice on what to buy, what to eat, how to look, and what to believe. This holds true not only in our personal lives but in our professional lives as well.

Most publications depend on advertising dollars for survival; professional journals and magazines are no exception. Although the advertising-to-editorial ratio usually is lower in professional journals than it is in popular magazines, increasing the number of paid advertisements still is an ongoing financial goal for the managing editors of those professional journals that do accept advertising. Because physical therapists are consumers of physical therapy products and services, physical therapy's professional publications are an obvious medium-of-choice for companies that want to advertise their products.

Today most consumers are *informed* consumers who realize that the majority of individuals who appear in general advertisements are models and that many of the statements made in these advertisements may not be backed by empirical data. As advertisements for products and equipment used by health professionals begin to simulate advertisements for other types of goods and services, therapists should become informed *professional* consumers. That is, when therapists read advertising material in periodicals or product information distributed by companies at conventions or through direct mailings, they must keep in mind that although outlandish statements about the merits of a product may be commonplace in advertising for products such as breakfast cereal, advertisements for products and services related to the health professions should be following different guidelines.

Therapists should read brochures and advertisements objectively. If, for example, claims about treatment outcomes are made, the therapist should ask, "What is the evidence?" Many

companies do spend the time and money to conduct independent studies that provide potential buyers with specific, reliable data (see page 54). Each therapist knows the needs of his or her patients and the needs of his or her practice; each therapist is responsible for deriving relevant information from advertisements or seeking out more specific information from the advertiser.

"Testimonials"

In periodicals relevant to physical therapy, the number of advertisements using therapist testimonials has increased over the years. The format may range from photographs of individuals providing therapy-like services to actual therapist-written testimonials.

There are two types of apparent experts who may make "first-hand" claims about a product or service: the expert who is not identified, and the expert who *is* identified.

The unidentified expert. A product advertisement may include what apparently is a first-person statement next to a photograph of an unidentified person using the product. This person usually has an aura of professionalism—often complete with white jacket—that may imply the person is a physical therapist when in fact he or she is a model. The reader therefore may make the assumption that 1) the person in the photograph is a therapist and that 2) the "therapist" in the photograph is endorsing the equipment *as a therapist*. There is nothing illegal or unethical about an advertiser using a model; using an actual therapist can be complicated because of scheduling problems, for example, or because of a therapist's possible lack of ease before the camera. But the reader should be aware that the person in an advertisement may not be what he or she seems to be.

The identified expert. The endorsement of a product by a peer whose affiliations and credentials are identified provides the reader with a person to contact for more information or for verification of intent. It certainly is not illegal—or even necessarily negative—for therapists to be consultants for equipment or service companies. This growing trend is not inappropriate; after all, who is better qualified to determine whether a product is appropriate for clinical use or to advise therapists on a therapy-related product than a member of their own peer group? As a smart consumer, however, every therapist should realize that the individual who is endorsing a product may be in some way associated with the company itself.

Endorser Disclosure of Financial Interest

When it comes to general advertising, the consumer's assumption usually is that everyone who endorses a product is paid to do so. This assumption may be easier to make when the relationship between the product and the endorser is far-fetched—such as in the famous 1970s commercial in which football legend Joe Namath extolled the virtues of a particular brand of pantyhose.

In some cases, therapist-endorsers receive remuneration from product manufacturers for consultation services; in other cases, they merely provide the company with information on the product. In either case, in physical therapy product advertising, the endorser is—by virtue of being a physical therapist—knowledgeable about the appropriateness and applicability of the product. And this fact automatically adds credibility to the advertisement. The question is: Do we as professional consumers have the right to know whether the therapist endorsing a particular piece of equipment is a paid consultant?

Historically, the physical therapist's role in advertising and product endorsement has been minimal. The American Physical Therapy Association's (APTA) *Code of Ethics* provides the only professional guideline for therapists involved in product endorsement. Principle 5, Section 5.3B, Endorsement of Equipment or Services, states:

> Physical therapists may be remunerated for endorsement or advertisement of equipment or services to the lay public, physical therapists, or other health professionals, provided they disclose any financial interest in the production, sale, or distribution of said equipment or services.

Before 1990, this provision included advertisements for products only—not services. APTA's Judicial Committee revised Section 5.3 to include services in response to the increased number of advertisements for physical therapy management consulting services.

As noted in the *Code*, endorsements of equipment or services is within the ethical boundaries of physical therapy practice; however, the *disclosure of financial interest* is one part of the ethical obligation that may be overlooked.

In our informal review of current advertisements, minimal disclosure of financial interest was found. Was this because of a lack of financial interest or a lack of awareness? Therapists who are on company retainer or who receive remuneration from a company should identify that fact when providing written or verbal testimonial for or endorsement of that company's product because this type of disclosure provides additional information for the consumer who is making a decision to buy a product.

Advertisers and therapists alike must be made aware of the need to disclose—otherwise advertisements and endorsements may be viewed as misleading, and the therapists who appear in them may appear to be in violation of the *Code of Ethics*.

Deceptive Advertising

When determining whether an advertisement is outright deceptive, it is important to first ask, "Under what system of values is the issue of deception being considered?" Advertisements whose intent readers might misunderstand—and advertisements that most physical therapists' sense of taste and professionalism would cause them to avoid—may be merely misleading. *Deception*, however, is a legal term that involves a specific intent to mislead a buyer about a material (ie, decisional) fact. A comparative competitor claim ("Unlike our competitor's device, our device will reduce your patient's pain by 30%") may be an example of deception in advertising. An antagonistic competitor claim ("Unlike John Doe Physical Therapy Center, our clinic treats you like family") in some cases may be equivalent, in legal terms, to defamation of character. (For information on legal implications in advertising *physical therapy* services, see sidebar on page 55.)

To Ensure the Best Outcomes

It would be almost impossible for one therapist to seek out all the information about all the physical therapy products from all the companies that manufacture or sell them. If there were no advertisements, it would be very difficult for therapist-consumers to obtain the basic information they need to focus on the specific uses of specific products.

The reimbursement dollar is shrinking; physical therapy products and equipment are becoming more costly. To be cost-effective and quality-conscious in today's demanding health care environment, the therapist-consumer must view statements made in advertisements with the same spirit of professional inquiry used in clinical practice. Perhaps endorsements by therapists should be viewed as just another advertising format—one that, like any other format, requires the therapist-consumer to assess the value, quality, and appropriateness of the goods or services being advertised. From this perspective, then, the final judgment rests with the therapist-consumer.

The therapist's expectation ultimately is that certain results will occur with the use of a specific product. It therefore may be increasingly critical for therapists to communicate their needs for valid, reliable data to the companies that manufacture and advertise the products therapists want. *PT*

Carol Schunk, PsyD, PT, is Regional Director, Medicare and Rehab Specialists, Portland, Ore, and serves on the Board of Directors of APTA's Private Practice Section. Ron Hruska, MPA, PT, is Director of Physical Therapy and Rehab Services, St Elizabeth's Community Health Center, Lincoln, Neb. He serves on APTA's Judicial Committee and chairs the Nebraska Board of Examiners in Physical Therapy.

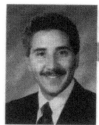

LIABILITY AWARENESS
Staying Informed in Risk Management
by Jonathan M Cooperman, MS, PT, JD,
and Ronald W Scott, PT, JD, OCS

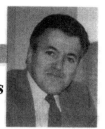

Disciplinary Action

When a member runs afoul of the APTA code of ethics,
there are consequences, both within
and external to the Association.

If asked, most physical therapists and physical therapist assistants probably would profess to practicing in a legal and ethical manner. However, it is an unfortunate reality for our profession that, occasionally, members are found to have violated APTA's *Code of Ethics*[1] or *Standards of Ethical Conduct for the Physical Therapist Assistant*.[2] Although all APTA members agree to abide by the Association's *Code of Ethics* as a condition of membership, few members may be familiar either with the sanctions that may be imposed if they do not abide by the *Code* or with the practical consequences of those sanctions.

A mark of our status as a profession is that we impose ethical standards upon our members and that we enforce them. APTA's Judicial Committee oversees both the interpretation of the *Code* and *Standards* (ie, by developing the *Guide for Professional Conduct*[3] and the *Guide for Conduct of the Affiliate Member*,[4] which are interpretations of the codes of ethics adopted by APTA's House of Delegates) and the disciplinary process.

Complaints of violations typically arise at the state level and initially are handled by the Chapter Ethics Committee (CEC). The *Procedural Document on Disciplinary Action*[5] ensures that all parties to the complaint receive due process. If a complaint arises, the CEC conducts an investigation, and the respondent (the person against whom the complaint is alleged) has a right to a hearing. Based on the information in the completed investigative file, the CEC will either dismiss the charges or recommend action to the Judicial Committee. If, after investigation, the CEC recommends that a specific sanction be levied, the Judicial Committee has several options: It may impose the disciplinary action recommended by the CEC, impose less severe disciplinary action, or dismiss the case. The Judicial Committee may *not* impose more severe sanctions than those recommended by the CEC.

Disciplinary Action

There are four specific disciplinary actions that the CEC may recommend to the Judicial Committee[5]:

Reprimand is a statement of recognition that the respondent's behavior was contrary to the *Code of Ethics* or the *Standards of Ethical Conduct for the Physical Therapist Assistant*. A reprimand is issued with the understanding that the respondent will correct the violation immediately (if he or she has not done so already). Ongoing conditions may not be attached to a reprimand, and this sanction is a private one; that is, it is not published.

Probation is a stronger sanction than a reprimand is, with conditions attached. The respondent must comply with the conditions within a specific time frame (which cannot be less than 6 months or more than 2 years). The CEC is charged with monitoring compliance with the conditions of probation. Failure to comply results in a review by the Judicial Committee, which may then impose more severe sanctions. For example, if a member is found to have violated the *Code* by failing to adequately document his or her involvement in patient care (Principles 2, 3.1), the CEC might require attendance at a continuing education course specifically related to documentation and/or might require the respondent to submit to random audits of his or her patient documentation. In cases in which the State Licensing Board has taken action, as in the case of substance abuse, the CEC will occasionally impose a probation that mirrors that required by the state. Probation, like a reprimand, is a private sanction and is not published.

Suspension is a temporary (not less than 1 year) removal of the rights and privileges of membership as outlined in the Association's Bylaws.[6] As a practical matter, the member must continue to pay dues and

~

Employers have a management prerogative to inquire of position applicants about relevant job-related matters, including any finding by APTA's Judicial Committee that an applicant violated the *Code of Ethics* or *Standards of Ethical Conduct for the Physical Therapist Assistant*.

~

will receive the Association's publications and nothing more. The suspended member loses all rights to vote, hold elected office, or serve on committees, at all levels of the Association. After the suspension has been served, and upon request, the respon-

Genome Research

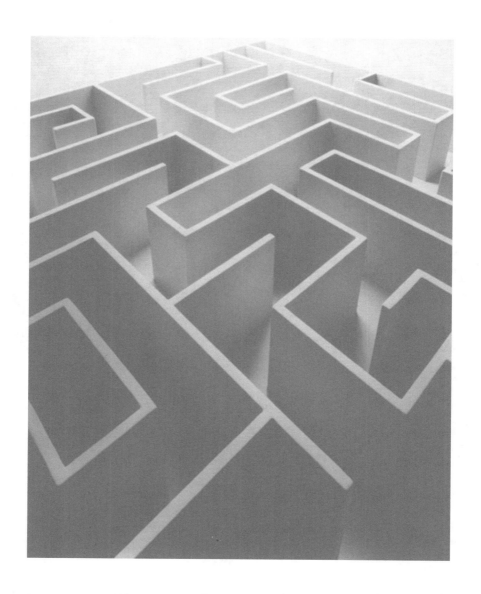

Physical therapists work with many patients with genetic-related conditions. Advances in human genome research will help prevent or treat many of these conditions but are raising other issues and concerns. Here is a look at how genetic testing and engineering will affect PTs and their patients.

By Lissa Poirot

Genetic Disorders and Engineering:
Implications *for* Physical Therapists

When my husband, Michael, began reporting lower back pain, it was his physical therapist (PT) who helped him receive a diagnosis for autosomal dominant kidney disorder. Michael saw a PT after reconstructive knee surgery, but when physical therapy didn't lessen his lower back pain, his PT asked a series of screening questions that included a detailed family history. The fact that Michael's mother, maternal grandfather, and uncle each had a kidney disorder raised a red flag with his PT, who suggested that Michael visit his physician. Sure enough, Michael had inherited the genetic disorder.

The Growth of Genetics

Genetic testing is a growing trend that allows more and more health care professionals to provide better screenings and interventions and to predict the future for their patients. With earlier diagnosis, patients—assisted by their health care providers—are able to take steps to stave off the negative conditions to which they are predisposed, while becoming better educated about the risks ahead.

The study of genetics has led to the discovery of links to a variety of conditions and diseases. For example, 5%-10% of hereditary breast cancers, 2%-5% of ovarian cancers, and 5%-10% of colorectal cancers can be linked to gene mutations. Recent genetic research has found links to rheumatoid and osteoarthritis, cerebral palsy, heart disease and stroke, Alzheimer's disease, and more than 1,200 other disorders.[1]

Genetics captured the headlines in 1990 with the Human Genome Project (HGP), a 15-year, government-funded initiative to identify all of the 100,000 genes existing in 23 chromosomes in the human body. Genes hold a sequence of an estimated 3 billion bits of information that can be categorized by one of four letters—A, C, T, and G. With these sequences and categories, researchers can map genes and store the information in a computer that will enable doctors to provide patients with information on their medical inheritance with just a drop of blood, saliva, or other DNA sample.

Allon Goldberg, PT, PhD, research fellow at the Institute of Gerontology at the University of Michigan, Ann Arbor says, "We know now that any two humans differ by approximately 0.1% in their genetic makeup. Ongoing research will let us know what these differences are and their importance."

Genetics and PTs

"Except for some cases of trauma, it is fair to say that virtually every human illness has a hereditary component," says Francis S Collins, director of the National Human Genome Research Institute (NHGRI) at the National Institutes of Health (NIH), Bethesda, Md.

Goldberg adds, "The most common problems seen in physical therapy practice, such as osteoarthritis in the knee joint, balance problems, and many other conditions, are now believed to have a genetic component, even though the specific gene may not yet be discovered. In some cases, the genes and specific mutations in the genes have been identified. As an example, in the early '90s, scientists discovered a gene on

Chromosome 4. When mutated, it produces a protein that ultimately leads to neurodegeneration and Huntington's disease."

"Even conditions related to lifestyle are now somehow connected to genetics," says Laura (Dolly) Swisher, PT, PhD, assistant professor of physical therapy at the University of South Florida, Tampa. "Think about all of the football players who end up with knee ligament problems. This condition is generally categorized as anterior cruciate ligament, or ACL. A small percentage of people who suffer with it enter therapy and go on to heal with no further problems. Others, however, may suffer for years, even throughout their lifetimes, with arthrofibrosis or fibrotic joint conditions. In this case the joint remains stiff, and it continues to cause the person problems. These people are more likely to have a gene that contributes to the ongoing condition."

Shreederi Pandya, PT, MS, clinical assistant professor of neurology and physical medicine and Rehabilitation at the University of Rochester, NY, offers another example. "Research today indicates that many conditions formerly attributed entirely to environment or lifestyle may be related to genetics, but an individual's lifestyle may cause the condition to manifest. In the case of carpal tunnel syndrome, it may explain why two people can sit at a computer keyboard typing every day, but the condition manifests in only one of them. It is these variations that make it imperative for PTs to understand the relationship between genetics and lifestyle conditions, and to be aware of the issues involved," Pandya explains.

Goldberg predicts that patient genotypes and other genetic information will become a part of each person's medical records. This will help practitioners assess

Genetic Disorders: An Overview

Genetic disorders can be divided into four categories: single gene disorders, chromosomal disorders, multifactional conditions, and mitochondrial disorders.

Single gene disorders also are known as Mendelian disorders. Occurring in approximately 1% of the population, single gene disorders are autosomal dominant, as is the case in Huntington's disease, breast and colon cancers, and achondroplasia. These conditions may be inherited or the result of a fresh mutation during egg fertilization.

Another single gene disorder is the autosomal recessive disorder, which is more rare and more frequent in ethnic or racial populations. Conditions include sickle cell anemia, most prevalent in black women; cystic fibrosis, most common in white children; and Tay-Sachs disease, most dominant in Ashkenazi Jewish families. Autosomal recessive disorders occur when both parents carry a gene mutation.

X-linked disorders, most prevalent in men because the disorder involves genes on the X chromosome, are another single gene disorder. Women are less affected because their second X gene compensates for the defective gene. X-linked disorders include Duchenne's muscular dystrophy and hemophilia.

Chromosomal disorders occur in only 0.7% of all newborns, but account for 50% of all first trimester spontaneous abortions and 10%-15% of people with severe mental disorders and/or congenital malformations. Disorders include Down syndrome and others characterized by mental retardation and unique physical features.

Multifactional disorders are the most common and account for the majority of birth defects, chronic conditions, and adult onset disorders. Instead of a single genetic mutation, multifactional disorders involve multiple variations that produce serious defects, including diabetes, arthritis, schizophrenia, coronary artery disease, cleft lips or palates, and spina bifida. Multifactional disorders also are affected by environmental factors, including toxins, allergens, and diet, as well as psychological and emotional stress.

Mitochondrial disorders are a special subcategory of single gene disorders involving genes structurally altered that result in defective energy production and severe adult onset disorders. Disorders include blindness, muscle disease, epilepsy, and aging dementia, as well as nerves, muscles, kidneys, livers, and other tissues.

Genetic Disorders

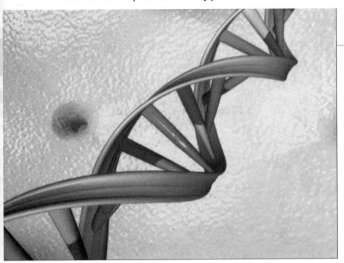

DNA double helix. The double helix is the structural arrangement of DNA. The sides of the "ladder" are formed by a backbone of sugar and phosphate molecules, and the "rungs" consist of nucleotide bases joined weakly in the middle by hydrogen bonds. Source: National Human Genome Research Institute, National Institutes of Health.

their patients' risk for conditions and provide individualize interventions, and may help PTs understand why some patients respond to the same or similar interventions faster or better than others who have the same or similar diagnosis.

By learning about genetic-related conditions, PTs can help patients become aware of their susceptibilities, Pandya says. He explains, "Most of my day-to-day work is with people who suffer from muscular dystrophy (MD), which we know is a genetic disease. Over 40 types of MD exist, however, and each one can manifest in a person at a different age. Even the manifestation age can vary, depending on the type of dystrophy and how many generations have carried the MD gene."

Following the physician's diagnosis of genetic-related movement disorders, the PT is often the first person the patient sees, and usually sees the most frequently and for longer periods of time. To provide

the best care, a PT needs to understand the origin of the diagnosis.

"How the condition or disease formulated is important. A diagnosis may reveal a missing chromosome that is the cause of the disorder, such as with Huntington's disease. Knowing the condition's origin will help the PT to determine if the patient will have nerve involvement or not, for example, or provide other valuable information related to the clinical picture," says Pandya.

Because the implications of genetic components are just now being understood, PTs have the opportunity to help define their role in this fast-

For More Information

Genetic Alliance: Advocacy, Education & Empowerment
4301 Connecticut Avenue, NW,
Suite 404
Washington, DC 2008-2369
Phone: 202/966-5557
www.geneticalliance.org

Georgetown University Center for Child and Human Development
3307 M Street NW, Suite 401
Washington, DC 20007
Phone: 202/687-8899
http://gucchd.georgetown.edu

National Coalition for Health Professional Education in Genetics
2360 W Joppa Road, Suite 320
Lutherville, MD 21093
Phone: 410/583-0600
www.nchpeg.org

National Human Genome Research Institute
National Institutes of Health
Building 31, Room 4B09
31 Center Drive, MSC 2152
9000 Rockville Pike
Bethesda, MD 20892-2152
Phone: 301/402-0911
www.genome.gov

growing field. If scientists or biologists provide PTs with information on their patient's genetic abnormalities, the PT then needs to determine how that abnormality will affect management of the patient, including prognosis and intervention.

Ethical, Legal, and Social Issues

Once patients receive genetic testing, PTs then can help them understand how their disorder may affect them, both in the present and in the future. Or, with simple interviews, PTs can pinpoint developmental or behavioral symptoms of patients that may suggest an underlying genetic disorder. PTs then can refer patients to their primary care physicians or a geneticist to receive a genetic diagnosis.

"When patients share information regarding their conditions with us, it is our responsibility to at least understand what they are talking about without assuming the role of their doctors," says Pandya. "I tell patients that I do understand their concern or question, but it is not in the realm of my practice to offer genetic advice. Our practice dictates that we guide our patients to their genetic counselors and physicians."

Nevertheless, PTs must deal with an increasing number of ethical, legal, and social issues when working with patients. In Michael's case, his mother had warned him that his kidney condition is incurable and would affect his life and heath insurance premiums. She suggested he avoid receiving an official diagnosis. [See "Genetic Discrimination and the Law."]

Michael, though, chose to be tested. His diagnosis was a troublesome blow. His grandfather had died of kidney failure, his uncle recently had undergone a kidney transplant, and his mother was just beginning dialysis. He wasn't ready to face his future of kidney problems. What would happen to his insurance? And the recent birth of our daughter raised additional questions. Did he pass along this genetic condition? Would she inevitably confront the same problem?

As the scientific and medical communities gain more information about genetics, patients and their health care providers increasingly will face dilemmas such as Michael's, while continuing to sort through who is privy to the information provided to them.

"We have to be advocates for our patients, but we also must remember that there may be controversy surrounding some of the questions they ask," says Michaele Smith, PT, education coordinator for the physical

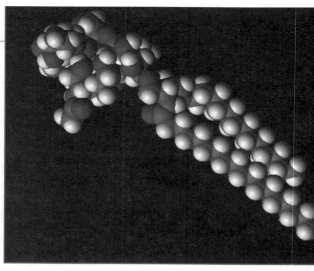

CPK diagram of the ganglioside GM2. The buildup of this molecule is the result of a genetic mutation in Tay-Sachs disease. Source: Accelrys, www.accelrys.com.

therapy division at the United States Public Health Service at the NIH. "A patient might ask if other family members should be tested for the condition because they wonder if it will affect their ability to secure health insurance in the future. Some may

Genetic Discrimination and the Law

The Health Insurance Portability and Accountability Act (HIPAA) provided the first federal protections against genetic discrimination in health insurance. The act prohibited health insurers from excluding individuals from group coverage due to past or present medical problems, including genetic predisposition to certain diseases. The law specifically states that genetic information in the absence of a current diagnosis of illness does not constitute a preexisting condition. On the other hand, HIPAA does not prohibit health insurers from charging a higher rate to individuals based on their genetic makeup, prevent insurers from collecting genetic information, or limit the disclosure of genetic information about individuals to insurers. Nor does it prevent insurers from requiring applicants to undergo genetic testing.[1]

Federal employees (and applicants) receive protection from Executive Order 13145, signed by President Bill Clinton in February 2000. It prohibits discrimination based on protected genetic information, a request for genetic services, or the receipt of genetic services. It says that federal departments and agencies may not discharge, fail or refuse to hire, or otherwise discriminate against any individual with respect to the compensation, terms, conditions, or privileges of employment because of protected genetic information or a request for, or receipt of, genetic services.[2]

A number of bills have been introduced into Congress to address genetic discrimination in health insurance and employment. Meanwhile, 41 states have enacted legislation related to genetic discrimination in health insurance and 31 states have adopted laws regarding genetic discrimination in the workplace. The state laws regarding health insurance conform to HIPAA.[1]

References

1 National Human Genome Research Institute. Genetic discrimination in health insurance. Available at www.genome.gov/10002328. Accessed December 2, 2004.
2 US Equal Employment Opportunity Commission. Questions and answers: executive order 13145. Available at www.eeoc.gov/federal/genetic/qanda.html. Accessed December 2, 2004.

not even know if testing is available for the condition. It's important that PTs know enough about genetics, including the ethical and moral issues involved, to be able to answer or direct their questions appropriately."

A University of Massachusetts study of more than 700 patients and 1,500 genetics services providers found that the majority of both agreed that no access to genetic information should be provided to insurers or employers without consent, and that patients should receive full disclosure of genetic findings.[2] Another study by the university surveyed geneticists and genetic counselors in 36 countries. More than 2,900 responded. Most United States' responses were more likely to respect patient autonomy; would not test children for adult onset disorders; would not report results to employers, insurers, and schools without consent; and would fully disclose genetic information to patients.[3]

A Georgetown University Medical Center study of 3,600 counseling and allied health professionals arrived at similar conclusions. Only 22 percent of those surveyed believe full disclosure should be made to insurers when health insurers pay for the genetic tests, even if it results in loss of insurance or higher premiums to the patient.[4]

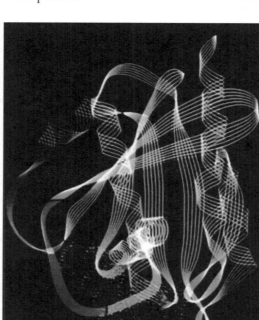

"Knowledge creates responsibility," says Swisher. "To know that people have predispositions to certain conditions and diseases, you have to know to what extent and to whom this knowledge can be shared. PTs are not always involved in the genetics' issues with their patients, but they are in a position to suspect genetic-related conditions. How you handle this is imperative to the patient's physical and mental health."

What PTs should do in these situations depends on the circumstance of the referral, or the routine screening. Swisher advises PTs to recommend patients seek additional medical testing from their private practitioners, and ultimately refer to their practitioner for further guidance on the condition.

If the patient has been referred to the PT by a practitioner, and the PT suspects a genetic condition that the practitioner did not detect, it is advisable that PTs consult with the practitioner directly to offer an opinion and suggest further medical examination and testing.

"If this is a direct access situation, the PT may be faced with the moral duty of suggesting the patient see a doctor," says Swisher. "Remember, there is a great deal more information available to the masses today, and many people are highly educated on their condition before they ever get to their health care providers. Others, however, do not use the Internet and so they know much less. You may frequently find yourself in a position to either confirm or dispute what a patient thinks is the cause of his or her condition. Given the demand on doctors today, you are likely spending

A 3-D protein structure. Source: US DOE Image Gallery, genome science gallery.

much more time with the patient than the physicians are and will be faced with addressing these issues."

Policy issues may be as difficult and sensitive to deal with as personal questions. Genetic information could easily stigmatize patients. "What happens in social and work relationships, for example?" asks Swisher. "We have seen the inhumanity of people being turned away from circles of their peers for physical and mental limitations or conditions. This is opening an entirely new realm that few of us have even considered. We don't know the questions that ultimately surface, let alone the answers to those questions."

With the increased responsibility placed on the health care community, and new research seemingly revealing new data every day, PTs must keep up with the rapid changes in genetic research and what those changes mean to their practices. The National Coalition for Health Professional Education in Genetics (NCHPEG), established in 1996 by the American Medical Association (AMA), the American Nursing Association (ANA), and the NHGRI, is committed to a national effort to promote health professional education and access to information about advances in human genetics. NCHPEG members are interdisciplinary groups from approximately 120 diverse health professional organizations, including APTA.

"Read literature and make gaining some level of knowledge regarding genetics an ongoing focus in your work and study," advises Goldberg. "The field is changing rapidly, and those professionals and practitioners who don't stay abreast of it may well be out in the cold one day soon."

The Future

Genetic research not only will affect patients and PTs vis-à-vis ethical responsibility and treatment options, but also may alter the very

services that PTs provide. Looking into the future, researchers may find ways to make genetic alterations that ultimately will eliminate certain diseases and conditions.

"The map of the genome looks at the genes that underlay common diseases such as diabetes, heart disease, cancer, and others. The next step will be to manipulate those genes to change them," says Marilyn Moffat, PT, PhD, FAPTA, director of the professional doctoral program and postprofessional master's program at New York University and former president of APTA.

Moffat says, "In the musculoskeletal arena, gene therapy and genetic

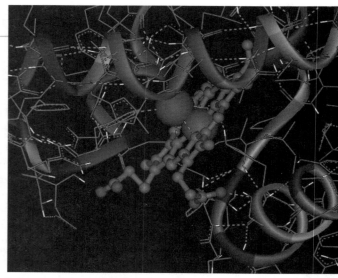
Ball-and-stick diagram of heme bound to a protein (colored by residue type). Source: Accelrys, www.accelrys.com.

engineering may eliminate the need for spinal surgery, may lead to new treatments of arthritis, and may open up new ways of dealing with osteoporosis. In the neuromuscular arena, genetic risk factors will be assessed in patients with multiple sclerosis, genetic deficiencies will be analyzed in patients with muscular dystrophy, and familial genetic mutations and dopamine-producing cell genetic codes will be determined in patients with Parkinson disease."

While PTs still will perform interventions, they may focus more on the health and fitness component. Genetics may be able to eliminate some conditions, but a full slate of work will remain as new diseases and conditions surface. PTs will be called on to address other categories as well—for example, childhood obesity and related diseases, such as diabetes.

"There always will be new diseases and new conditions, especially related to our increasingly aging population, trauma-related conditions, and the results of abusive behaviors that will lead to conditions requiring physical therapist interventions. One of our most important functions will be to help maintain a healthy population,"

says Moffat. "We must welcome the world of the genome that is to alter many facets of our practice and capitalize on all of the best that it will have to offer society. And we must always prepare for what future practice will be for us." **PT**

---

*Lissa Poirot is a freelance writer and editor. Primary research for this article was conducted by freelance writer **Christina DiMartino**.*

References

1 Smith M, Jain M, Long T, Danoff J. Genetic Disorders: Implications for Physical Therapists.

2 Wertz D. Patient and professional views on ethics: 12 clinic survey. Workshop abstract no. 104. In: Workshop abstracts of Human Genome Meeting; April 19-22, 2001; Edinburgh, Scotland. Available online at http://hgm2001.hgu.mrc.ac.uk/abstracts/publish/workshops/workshop15/hgm0104.htm. Accessed November 29, 2004.

3 Wertz D. Results of a 36-nation survey of geneticists' ethical views. Workshop abstract no. 105. In: Workshop abstracts of Human Genome Meeting; April 19-22, 2001; Edinburgh, Scotland. Available online at http://hgm2001.hgu.mrc.ac.uk/abstracts/publish/workshops/workshop15/hgm0105.htm. Accessed November 29, 2004.

4 Lapham EV. Genetics education of US health professional and public policy. Workshop abstract no. 106. In: Workshop abstracts of Human Genome Meeting; April 19-22, 2001; Edinburgh, Scotland. Available online at http://hgm2001.hgu.mrc.ac.uk/abstracts/publish/workshops/workshop15/hgm0106.htm. Accessed November 29, 2004.

New Genetics:
The Human Genome Project

by E Virginia Lapham, .PhD;
Toby Long, PhD, PT; and
Chahira Kozma, MD

Scientists are closer than ever to having access to complete genetic information that will help predict future health risks or determine the likelihood of passing on heritable diseases. As the number of patients with these "genetic diagnoses" increases, a basic knowledge of genetics and an understanding of related ethical, legal, and social implications becomes essential for PTs.

DNA Sequence
Photo Credit: FPG/VCG

The rapid advances now occurring in genetic research to identify and, in some cases, prevent or cure genetic diseases are among the most significant developments in health care in this decade. Although physical therapists typically are familiar with single-gene or rare hereditary diseases such as those described by Pandya (see page 86), the "new genetics" frontier includes identifying the genetic components of virtually all disease and disability, with the possible exception of trauma. (Even infectious disease, for example, has a hereditary component in that genetics can affect a host's susceptibility to the viral infection.[1]) From strokes and heart disease to cancers and behaviors leading to accidents, the role of genes is being uncovered in the laboratory and reported in the media almost daily. Incorporating this new genetic information and its implications into practice is a challenge for all health care professionals.

Genetic disorders and birth defects are among the leading causes of infant morbidity and mortality. Two to three percent of the newborn population is born with some type of birth defect, and one-third of infant mortality in the United States is due to birth defects with a genetic influence. Additionally, genetic disorders account for about 30% to 50% of all pediatric hospital admissions. Together, birth defects and genetic disorders are major contributors to developmental disabilities.[2]

Patients or consumers of genetic services (ie, individuals with identified or suspected genetic disorders and their families) are those most affected initially by genetic advances. They are often asked to participate in research designed to identify new genes, to try new treatments such as gene therapy, and, in some cases, to choose how much they want to know about their future health risks.

Predictive genetic testing now allows some diseases to be diagnosed years or even decades before the onset of symptoms. This diagnosis offers an advantage when there are preventive measures to be taken, but it can result in confusion and discouragement when it predicts a disease that is serious and for which few treatment options are avail-able. Consumers are faced with increasingly complex issues such as these yet, frequently, they have had little education on emerging issues in genetics other than what comes from the media.

Health care professionals who provide diagnostic and treatment services for patients with genetic disorders are already involved in genetics issues in several ways. For example, many PTs conduct intake interviews or take medical histories that suggest a genetic component to their patients' physical problems. Following examination, PTs frequently give a label to the developmental or behavioral symptoms of their patients, such as cerebral palsy or hyperactivity, that may be symptoms of a genetic disorder. PTs also may recommend that their patients seek additional medical evaluations, which can lead to a diagnosis of a genetic disorder. Providing guidance for patients is another role for PTs that requires them to keep updated on current developments, as PTs' responses to patients' questions might influence patient attitudes about whether or not to participate in genetic therapies or genetic research.

Much of the genetic research going on today is the result of a large, government-funded initiative, the Human Genome Project (HGP), which was started in 1990 with the goal of identifying all the genes in the human body in 15 years. It is one of the biggest scientific projects ever attempted, and its progress has been greatly assisted by continual advances in technology. In technical terms, the HGP aims to unravel the cells of our bodies and locate the estimated 100,000 genes (short segments of DNA) on our 23 pairs of chromosomes. These genes contain an estimated 3 billion bits of information represented by the four letters A, C, T, and G. Once the sequence of the 3 billion bits of information is known, the genes can be "read," and that information can be stored in a computer.[3] After the human genome mapping has been completed, it will be possible for scientists to take a blood, saliva, hair, or other DNA-containing sample from an individual and provide information about his or her medical inheritance, including risks of future diseases.

The ELSI Programs

The new genetics field raises a host of ethical, legal, and social implications. Table 1 summarizes some of the potential benefits and risks of information from the Human Genome Project.

As the table illustrates, concerns about

Table 1: Potential Benefits and Risks of the HGP

Potential Benefits	Potential Risks
Availability of new information about gene function and genetics of human development for medical research	Use of genetic information in ways that reduce issues of health and illness to genes, resulting in genetic discrimination in insurance and employment
Improved screening and diagnostic tools to allow early detection of genetic conditions	Overt or subtle coercion to use genetic technologies such as prenatal diagnosis or presymptomatic diagnosis
New treatments such as gene therapy	Unequal access to treatments based on location or ability to pay; possible side effects, lack of informed consent
New genetic products to increase commercial trade	Overcommercialization of genetic research without proper safeguards
New jobs, careers, and services in genetics	Less funding for programs other than genetic research

New Genetics:

patient privacy become paramount. For example, the results of some genetic tests can indicate an increased risk of future illness or reveal an increased risk of having a child with a genetic disorder or disease. In addition, PTs frequently write progress or summary reports of their work with patients to send to referral sources or other agencies or put notes in medical records. Often, this documentation includes information about or implies a genetic disorder. And, because related individuals may share genetic traits, information about one family member is also information about other family members, so privacy is more than an individual matter. When this information is passed on to health insurers, it could result in the insurer charging the patient higher premiums or even canceling his or her health care insurance. The potential for genetic discrimination in health insurance, disability insurance, and employ-

ment is among the many issues being raised by genetic research.[4]

The history of genetics in this century also raises concerns about eugenics, stigma, and discrimination that make it imperative to observe full protection of human rights with informed consent and other measures. A particular risk that must be avoided is the use of genetic information to rationalize the ethnic or racial prejudices that already fragment our society.[5]

Some of these concerns about the potential misuse of genetic information were anticipated by scientists and policy makers before the HGP was started. In the initial funding, Congress designated 3% to 5% percent of the HGP budget to be spent for studying the ethical, legal, and social implications (ELSI) of the genetic research and testing.[6] The funds were allocated to the National Institutes of Health (NIH) and the

Department of Energy (DOE) to set up ELSI programs, making the HGP the first major scientific program in history to have part of its funding designated for looking at the societal implications of what is being done as the project is developed.

The charge of the ELSI programs is to examine the ethical, legal, and social consequences of the new genetic information, stimulate public policy discussion, and facilitate the development of sound policy options. A particular emphasis is placed on

❖ privacy and fair use of genetic information,
❖ responsible clinical integration of new genetic technologies,
❖ ethical issues surrounding the conduct of genetics research, and
❖ professional and public education.

Each of these areas gives rise to issues that need to be considered by health care professionals, consumers, and the general public. The box on this page presents some important questions to consider regarding the issues emphasized by the ELSI programs.

The HuGEM Project

Of the four items above, the fourth issue, education of health professionals, has emerged as one of the highest priorities of the HGP. In 1994, a multidisciplinary committee formed by the Institute of Medicine (IOM) of the National Academy of Sciences noted that, as genetic testing and screening becomes more widespread, it is unlikely that there will be enough specialized genetics personnel to meet the need for counseling and education in the foreseeable future. The report recommends that all health care professionals be trained in basic genetics and in the ethical, legal, and social issues surrounding genetic testing. According to the report, health care professionals also need to be attuned to the broad spectrum of backgrounds that individuals and families with genetic disorders have and be sensitive to the implications of the disorders to those individuals.[7]

Among the education projects funded

(continued on page 82)

Questions to Consider

Privacy and fair use of genetic information

❖ Should genetic information be treated differently from other medical information in reports, charts, or other medical records?
❖ Should written informed consent be obtained from clients before their genetic information is shared with third parties?
❖ After taking a genetic test, should clients have the right not to be told the results?

Safe, effective explanation of genetic information

❖ Should health care professionals give developmental diagnoses that have genetic implications?
❖ Should parents be able to have their children tested for genetic conditions that do not show symptoms until adulthood if the conditions are neither treatable nor preventable?
❖ If a health care professional suspects that a patient has a genetic condition that is not diagnosed, does he or she have a professional obligation to share this information? If so, with whom?

Preventing stigmatization and discrimination based on genetic traits

❖ What role should society have to ensure fairness in the use of genetic information by health insurers and employers?
❖ What role should professionals have in helping to prevent stigmatization of people with genetic conditions?
❖ What are some of the racial/ethnic issues in genetics that professionals should consider?

Professional and public education

❖ What should professional associations do to help ensure their members' professional competence in the new genetics?
❖ What role should health care professionals have in educating their patients about the implications of the new genetics?

The Human Genome Project

Genetic Disorders

Genetic disorders encompass single-gene disorders, chromosome disorders, multifactorial conditions, and mitochondrial disorders.

Single-gene disorders are rare, with an estimated frequency of 1 in 500 in the general population, and are of three types:

❖ autosomal dominant conditions
❖ autosomal recessive conditions
❖ X-linked recessive conditions

Autosomal dominant conditions include Marfan syndrome, achondroplasia, neurofibromatosis, and certain forms of breast and colon cancers. The symptoms are variable and can range from mild to severe. In general, autosomal dominant conditions affect structures of the body such as bones, skin, and teeth. They need only one copy of a mutated gene to be expressed. They can be inherited or can occur as a result of a new mutation (a change that happens in the sperm or egg at the time of fertilization). An individual with an autosomal dominant condition has a 1 in 2 chance of passing the altered gene to his or her offspring during each pregnancy.

Autosomal recessive conditions include sickle cell anemia, Tay Sachs disease, and cystic fibrosis. In general, autosomal recessive conditions involve changes in the chemical substances (metabolic changes) in the blood or other tissues. Some autosomal recessive disorders have a higher incidence among certain ethnic or racial populations. Rare conditions tend to be more common among the offspring of couples who are blood related (consanguineous). It takes two copies of a mutated gene (one from each parent who is considered a carrier) for a recessive condition to be expressed in a genetic disorder. A carrier generally has no symptoms and is usually unaware of his or her status until he or she has a child who is affected. When both parents are carriers of a recessive gene, they have a 1 in 4 chance of having a child with the condition with each pregnancy. Testing for carrier and affected individuals is available for a large number of recessive conditions.

X-linked recessive conditions include Duchenne muscular dystrophy, hemophilia, and color blindness. The X and Y chromosomes are the sex-determining chromosomes. Females have two Xs, and males have one X and one Y. An X-linked genetic disorder occurs from an abnormal or mutated gene on the X chromosome. It affects males more frequently than females. A female who carries an abnormal gene on one of her X chromosomes is referred to as a carrier and, in general, has minimal or no symptoms. A female carrier has a 1 in 2 chance in every pregnancy with a male child of passing on the altered gene and thereby having a son with the condition. Genetic testing is available for many X-linked disorders.

Chromosome disorders include trisomy 21 or Down syndrome, trisomy 18, trisomy 13, Klinefelter syndrome, and Turner syndrome. In general, chromosome disorders are not inherited. Chromosome disorders may occur with any of the 23 pairs of chromosomes, and the risk increases with maternal age. Chromosome disorders are common, affecting about 7 of 1,000 live-born infants. An error may occur when either the egg or the sperm is forming and result in a fertilized egg having too many or too few chromosomes. This genetic imbalance is responsible for about half of all miscarriages or spontaneous abortions that occur in the first few weeks of pregnancy. When the pregnancy continues, chromosome disorders often result in the infant being born with multiple birth defects and mental retardation. An exception to this rule is the category of sex chromosome disorders, which tends to be associated with children with developmental problems and either tall or short stature.

Multifactorial disorders include many chronic conditions such as asthma, diabetes, coronary artery disease, hypertension, coronary diseases, schizophrenia, and certain forms of cancer. Multifactorial disorders result from the interaction of genes and environment. They often represent small variations in several genes plus one or more environmental factors. Multifactorial disorders are very common and account for the majority of birth defects and chronic diseases of childhood and adulthood.

Mitochondrial disorders come from genes that reside in cells but outside the cell nucleus, and mutations in them are passed only from the mother. They can be detected by molecular techniques and have been associated with certain kinds of blindness, muscle diseases, a type of epilepsy, and dementias associated with aging. Information about these disorders is a relatively recent development.

Adapted from: Lapham EV, Kozma C, Palinscar L, et al. Ethical, Legal, and Social Issues of the Human Genome Project: HuGEM Video Manual. Washington, DC: Georgetown University Child Development Center and the Alliance of Genetic Support Groups; 1996.

New Genetics: The Human Genome Project

by NIH through the National Human Genome Research Institute is the Human Genome Education Model (HuGEM) Project, a collaborative effort between Georgetown University Child Development Center and the Alliance of Genetic Support Groups, a national coalition of consumers, professionals, and support groups, to provide genetics education for health care professionals. HuGEM was started in 1993 with a focus on the education of two groups considered the most likely to be affected initially by the HGP: people with a genetic disorder in the family, and health care professionals who provide services to people with genetic conditions.

The health care professionals who participated in the first HuGEM project were primarily associated with medical centers. The consumers were recruited through genetic support groups across the country affiliated with the Alliance of Genetic Support Groups. The project started with surveys of the two groups to determine the experience, educational needs, and priority topics for genetics education. Telephone interviews were carried out with members of support groups across the country, representing 101 genetic disorders including single-gene, chromosome, multifactorial, and mitochondrial conditions. Mail questionnaires were sent to a variety of health care professionals, including PTs, psychologists, educators, physicians, social workers, physicians, nurses, nutritionists, occupational therapists, speech-language pathologists, and audiologists.

The large majority of health care professional respondents reported that they were working with individuals with genetic disorders in their practice, and many of the PTs in the study said they had discussed the genetic component of medical or developmental problems or were providing counseling about genetic concerns to at least a few of their patients. However, most of the health care professionals surveyed reported little education in genetics. For example, more than half the physical therapists in this survey population reported no formal training in genetics.

In the first project, the majority of health care professionals surveyed indicated a desire for continuing education in genetics. That finding led to the current HuGEM 3-year project, which started July 1, 1997, and is focused on educating six groups of health care professionals in collaboration with their national membership organizations. Collaborating organizations in the HuGEM II Project are

❖ the American Dietetic Association,
❖ the American Occupational Therapy Association,
❖ the American Physical Therapy Association,
❖ the American Psychological Association,
❖ the American Speech-Language-Hearing Association,
❖ the Council on Social Work Education, and
❖ the National Association of Social Workers.

In the summer of 1998, questionnaires were mailed to a random sample of the memberships of six of the collaborating organizations (the Council of Social Work Education and the National Association of Social Workers were combined). The purpose was to determine the needs, opinions, experiences, and knowledge of genetic testing and research related to the Human Genome Project and its ethical, legal, and psychosocial issues as well as to identify priority topics for education. The survey was carried out by the Survey Research Center, University of Maryland, and results will be used to develop educational programs for practitioners and educators.

During the first year, orientation to the HuGEM project was provided to the national staff and board members of the collaborating organizations. The presentation to APTA in June 1998 included content on the importance of genetics to PTs; an update on the Human Genome Project and its ethical, legal and social issues; a presentation from a consumer regarding her experience with physical therapy; and an overview of the HuGEM II Project. These four elements are part of each presentation and are the core of the education model.

In years 2 and 3, workshops for practitioners are being held at national and state conferences of the collaborating organizations (see page 64 for more information on the session to be held at PT '99). The purpose of these workshops is to provide information, training, and materials for participants to learn about genetics and genetic issues. Education kits including videos, manuals, curricula, and other resources will be provided for participants to use in their home communities to educate colleagues, students, and/or patients. The curricula will include an overview of basic human genetics, a look at the role of genetics in common disorders, identification of genetics resources for patients, information on racial/ethnic concerns related to genetics, and discussion of ethical, legal, and social issues.

Additionally, a 5-day course for educators, "Incorporating Genetics into Education and Practice of Health Professionals," will be held at Georgetown University, Washington, DC, in the spring and summer of 1999. APTA and the other collaborating professional organizations are selecting the participants; for more information and a copy of the selection criteria, contact APTA's Department of Information Resources.

Recent advances in identifying the genetic component of diseases and concerns about the ethical, legal, and social issues of genetic research have brought genetic issues to the forefront of health care. This has happened so rapidly that most health care professionals, including PTs, have had little time to understand and prepare for the implications of the new genetics to their practice. Modern health care practice includes recognition of the role of genetic factors in all health and disease. A basic knowledge of heredity and gene functioning, in addition to an understanding of interactions between genes and environments, is important in providing health care. Practitioners with these skills will better serve the increasing numbers of individuals and families diagnosed with genetic conditions. *PT*

E Virginia Lapham, PhD, is Principal Investigator, Human Genome Education Project II, Georgetown University Child Development Center, Washington, DC. Toby Long, PhD, PT, is Director, Division of Physical Therapy, Georgetown University Child Development Center. She is a consultant for the Human Genome Education Project II and is a member of PT's Editorial Advisory Group. Chahira Kozma, MD, is Medical Director, Human Genome Education Project II, Georgetown University Child Development Center.

References

1   Collins FS. Privacy, Confidentiality, and the HGP. In: Frankel MS, ed. *Exploring Public Policy Issues in Genetics*. Washington, DC: American Association for the Advancement of Science; 1996.

2   Jorde LB, Carey JC, Bamshad MJ, White RL. *Medical Genetics*. St Louis, Mo: Mosby Year-Book Inc; 1998:1-5.

3   *The Human Genome Project: From Maps to Medicine*. Washington, DC: US Department of Health and Human Services; 1996. DHHS/PHS Publication No. 96-3897.

4   Lapham EV, Kozma C, Weiss JO. Genetic discrimination: perspectives of consumers. *Science*. 1996;274:621-624.

5   Reilly PR. Rethinking risks to human subjects in genetic research. *Am J Hum Genet*. 1998;63:682-685.

6   Thomson E. The Ethical, Legal, and Social Implications Program at the National Human Genome Research Institute, NIH. In: Smith E, Sapp W, eds. *Plain Talk about the Human Genome Project: A Tuskegee University Conference on Its Promise and Perils.... and Matters of Race*. Tuskegee, Ala: Tuskegee University; 1997: 123-130.

7   Andrews LB, Fullarton JE, Holtzman NA, Mutulsky AG, eds. *Assessing Genetic Risks: Implications for Health and Social Policy*. Washington, DC: National Academy Press; 1994.

Resources

Human Genome Project Information
National Human Genome Research Institute, Bethesda, Md,
301/402-0911, www.nhgri.nih.gov.
HuGEM Project www.dml.georgetown.edu/hugem.

Genetic Support Groups
The following organizations provide information and referral for patients/clients to genetic support groups throughout the United States: Alliance of Genetic Support Groups, Washington, DC, 800/336-4363, www.geneticalliance.org.
National Organization for Rare Disorders (NORD), New Fairfield, Conn 800/999-6673, TDD 203/746-6927, www.rarediseases.org.

Ethical, Legal And Social Issues
National Resource Center for Bioethics Literature. Kennedy Institute of Ethics. Washington, DC, 202/687-3885, www.guweb.georgetown.edu/nrcbl.

Managed Care and Economics

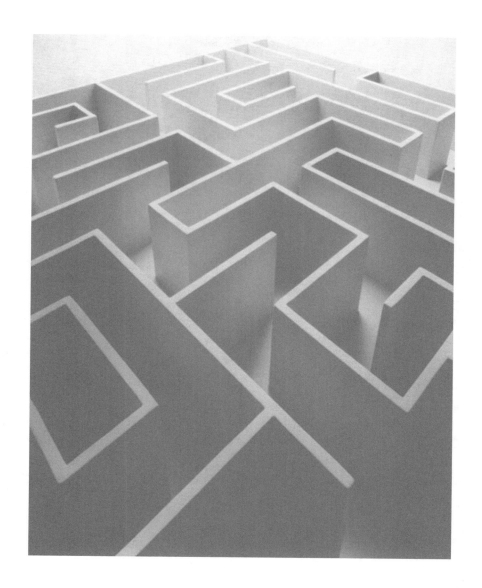

Principles and Objectives for the United States Health Care System and the Delivery of Physical Therapy Services

HOD P06-04-17-16

The American Physical Therapy Association (APTA) supports a health care system that provides all individuals within the United States with access to quality health care.

This system should provide comprehensive, cost-effective, and appropriate physical therapy services provided by a licensed physical therapist or by a qualified physical therapist assistant under the direction and supervision of a physical therapist. In primary care, physical therapists should be recognized as health care professionals who can and should play a major role in achieving clinically effective outcomes and cost efficiencies that are essential to comprehensive health care.

APTA endorses the following principles and objectives for a health care system in which physical therapy is acknowledged as an essential component of health care:

PRINCIPLE I: ACCESS TO CARE

The health care system should provide access for all individuals, and should:

- Enable patients/clients to select among providers, including physical therapists, who are qualified and authorized by state and other jurisdiction law to provide professional health care services.

- Permit patient/client direct access to physical therapists with no requirement of a referral from any other practitioner.

- Encourage employers to offer a choice of quality, affordable health care coverage to employees and their dependents.

- Enable patients/clients to select and participate in plans that allow the development of financial reserves to cover individual health care expenses, including those incurred for physical therapy and any catastrophic coverage.

- Include mechanisms to allow patients/clients to pay their provider of choice directly for health care services.

- Prohibit denials of coverage due to preexisting and/or congenital health conditions.

- Provide affordable fee-for-service options and other mechanisms to assure that patients/clients are able to choose their health care providers.

- Provide financial support for the education and training of sufficient numbers and types of health care professionals to assure appropriate access to care for all individuals.

- Include a requirement that all public and private health plans provide examination, evaluation, diagnostic, prognostic services provided by a physical therapist, and intervention services provided by a physical therapist or physical therapist assistant under the direction and supervision of a physical therapist in any setting.

- Provide coverage for programs and incentives that prevent injury, impairment, and illness, promote wellness and aid in maintenance of functional independence, and provide coverage for preventive and restorative care programs to reduce the incidence and long-term impact of disease, disability, and injury.

- Include a requirement that all public and private health plans provide adequate assistive technology, including but not limited to durable medical equipment.

PRINCIPLE II: QUALITY OF CARE

The plan of care for a patient/client should ensure that intervention is based on achieving appropriate outcomes specific to the patient's/client's needs. Although APTA endorses adherence to standards of practice and efficiency of care, the Association opposes any policy that places arbitrary limits on physical therapy services. To ensure quality of care and protection of the public's best interests:

- Professional practitioners should be involved in the development of practice parameters and guidelines specific to their scope of practice.

- Physical therapists should use clinical experience, literature-based evidence, and patient/client preferences and apply APTA's *Guide to Physical Therapist Practice* as the foundation of such parameters and guidelines.

- Decisions regarding the initiation, continuation, or discharge of a patient's/client's physical therapy should be determined by the physical therapist responsible for that patient's/client's management.

- Physical therapists should hold themselves accountable to the public and to third party payers through peer review, and should be recognized as the appropriate professionals to review the delivery and utilization of physical therapy services.

PRINCIPLE III: COST CONTAINMENT AND PAYMENT

Payment rates for health care services should be reasonable and equitable, and mechanisms to control costs in the health care system should not encourage providers to withhold, restrict, or deny essential patient/client services. Insurers should be required by law to disclose to patients/clients the services and types of care covered, including the extent of coverage of physical therapy services. To ensure appropriate payment and cost containment:

- Health care professionals should be involved in the development of standards, establishment of payment rates, and review of claims and utilization for their specific discipline.

- A referral from a physician or any other practitioner should not be required for payment for physical therapy services.

- No arbitrary criteria should be utilized to determine payment for physical therapy services.

- Practitioner self-referral arrangements, including physician ownership of physical therapy services, should be prohibited by law.

- The use of billing codes should be restricted to those professionals who are licensed to perform those services and payment for physical therapy services should be made only when the services have been provided by a physical therapist or by a physical therapist assistant under the direction and supervision of a physical therapist.

- Administration of health care benefits, coverage, and payment should be simplified, and patients/clients and providers should have access to a fair and expedited appeals process for denied claims.

- Payment for physical therapy services should occur only when adequate documentation exists, consistent with APTA guidelines, to support the need for physical therapy services.

- Payment for physical therapy services should be determined fairly in all settings, and guidelines should be consistent regardless of the setting in which the services are provided.

- Payment should cover all elements of the patient/client management model, including the education of the patient/client, family, and caregiver as a component of the physical therapist's plan of care.

- Health care professionals should seek optimal treatment effectiveness in consideration of cost efficiencies.

PRINCIPLE IV: STATE LICENSURE

The responsibility for licensure and regulation should remain exclusively within the purview of the state or other jurisdiction and should not be preempted by any federal or regional agency or process. There should be no credentialing of institutions that would override or eliminate the requirements of individual practitioner license laws.

Balancing Ethical Challenges

in a

Managed Care Environment

by Linda Resnik Mellion, PT, MS

An ethics instructor and utilization reviewer offers PTs guidance on weighing competing ethical demands and arriving at the "best" solutions.

Today's reimbursement environment has dramatically altered the delivery of health care, raising numerous new ethical challenges. Physical therapists (PTs) are struggling with the impact of managed care restrictions and care denials in many areas. Unfortunately, traditional health care ethics and professional codes have not offered much guidance on how to distribute health care resources fairly.

An ethical dilemma may arise early in intervention planning, at the initial visit when the PT is determining the nature and amount of physical therapy services to provide. The *Guide to Physical Therapist Practice*[1] states that the PT's responsibilities at the initial examination/evaluation include determining the prognosis and establishing the plan of care. This involves predicting the needed number of interventions based on the diagnosed practice pattern. But the PT, for example, might believe that the patient would benefit from 15 sessions, while the payer might have approved reimbursement for only eight.

150 ■ American Physical Therapy Association

This is particularly problematic when the number of visits is limited or the contract with the managed care provider is capitated—meaning the managed care provider is paid a specified amount per month, regardless of services provided.

Managed care can dictate what will be reimbursed, but it must not compromise the PT's judgment of what the patient truly needs. The ethical dilemma becomes balancing those two issues.

In the past, these types of conflicts were less prevalent. It was simpler for PTs to choose to offer more rather than less care to their patients, as reimbursement on a fee-for-service basis was the norm. In today's environment, however, reimbursement arrangements are having an impact on the amount and type of interventions delivered. A recent study of utilization of physical therapy services indicated differences depending on the payer source. Fee-for-service arrangements (as opposed to managed care payment arrangements) were associated with increased use of devices, therapeutic massage, strengthening, and endurance exercises.[2] The study did not identify the reason for this increased utilization.

There may be several reasons for these differences in utilization of services. It is possible that greater service utilization is the result of the PT's attempt to fulfill his or her duty of beneficence to the patient. That is, the therapist may believe that if some physical therapy is good, then more must be better.

A few recent studies seem to lend support to this premise. The amount of therapy has been linked to functional improvement in a variety of settings.[3-5] Roach et al conducted a retrospective study of inpatients with lower-extremity orthopedic problems. They reported that the duration of physical therapy was a predictor of functional status at discharge after controlling for baseline characteristics such as age, length of hospitalization, number of diagnoses, and initial functional status.[4] Kirk-Sanchez and Roach found that the amount of physical therapy and occupational therapy that patients with orthopedic diagnoses received during

Managed care can dictate what will be reimbursed, but it must not compromise the PT's judgment of what the patient truly needs.

inpatient comprehensive rehabilitation was related to their level of functional independence, as measured by the FIM (functional independence measure) at the time of discharge.[3] Guccione examined factors related to outcomes for hip fracture patients and reported that those who received physical therapy on average more than once a day had improved their odds of regaining independence in bed mobility, transfers, and ambulation.[5] These same patients had improved their odds of returning to their home environment.

Differences in utilization based on payer source might be a reflection of underutilization of services for patients who lack adequate health coverage. In contrast, some of the discrepancy in utilization of services may result from the delivery of unnecessary services. PTs may render more services to patients when reimbursement for those services is assured.

One preliminary study of rehabilitation treatment and outcome differences between fee-for-service and managed care patients in skilled nursing facilities confirmed that managed care patients did receive significantly fewer units of physical, occupational, and speech therapy and experienced significantly shorter lengths of stay.[6] However, the two patient groups did not appear to differ significantly in functional disability outcomes at admission or discharge.

Few studies have investigated the combined effect of reimbursement and utilization patterns on patient outcomes. Further research is needed.

Ethical Theory

According to ethicist Ruth Purtilo, PT, PhD, FAPTA, an ethical dilemma involves at least two morally correct courses of action that cannot each be followed; that is, taking one course precludes taking the other.[7] One way to resolve such dilemmas is to examine one's moral duties and determine which duty is the most binding and takes precedence over the others.

No one decision is right for everyone; however, there are specific ethical and legal obligations (or duties) that the PT should consider in resolving conflicts about managed care and the utilization review process.

In the preceding example, in which managed care limited the number of visits covered, the therapist believes that providing needed treatment to the patient is the right thing to do. To determine the appropriate amount of treatment, the therapist has to weigh the duty of beneficence to the patient (if he or she believes there is a chance of helping the patient) and the duty of justice (in helping to ensure the equitable distribution of health care services by helping to control costs). The PT also might have to factor in the duty of fidelity in complying with agreements made with managed care organizations and his or her beliefs about the patient's right to necessary physical therapy regardless of ability to pay.

In addition, a PT who participates in a capitated health plan may have an interest in delivering the most cost-effective care possible so that his or her institution can stay in the black or make a profit. The PT may feel torn between the duty to help the patient and responsibilities to the administration to avoid problems in obtaining payment for services rendered. In deciding the best course of action, the therapist must make a decision that he or she believes is more right than wrong.

Managed care may employ utilization reviewers to review the medical necessity, appropriateness, and reasonableness of services proposed or provided to a patient or group of patients. This review may be conducted on a prospective, concurrent, and/or retrospective basis.

Utilization reviewers and managed care

plans frequently refuse services that the clinician believes are essential. This is called an "adverse decision" or "adverse determination." Services may be denied because the reviewer does not consider them medically necessary, because the therapist's documentation does not support medical necessity, or because the services are not covered under the insurance policy.

An adverse decision can lead to other ethical dilemmas. If the payer refuses to cover a proposed intervention, the provider faces a difficult choice. If he or she refrains from offering care that will not be reimbursed, he or she risks harming the patient and incurring liability. If the therapist provides care regardless of cost, however, not only his or her own income but also the resources of hospitals and other institutions can be increasingly strained by the burden of uncompensated care.[8]

These situations certainly set up an adversarial relationship between the payer and the health care provider and between staff and administration when denials ensue. In addition, the payer's second-guessing of provider decisions can reduce the confidence that patients hold in the abilities of their providers.

A Fiduciary Duty

What is the provider's obligation when the third-party payer denies reimbursement for care? Must the provider deny giving care because reimbursement was denied?

Ethical standards such as the *APTA Guide for Professional Conduct* (intended to serve PTs in interpreting the *APTA Code of Ethics*; see box) point to the provider's fiduciary duty to ensure that the patient receives care of a certain standard. (The *Guide* is available on the Web at www.apta.org/PT_Practice/ ethics_pt/ pro_conduct.)

Principle 6 of the Code states, "A physical therapist shall maintain and promote high standards for physical therapy practice, education, and research." In the case of an adverse decision, the health care provider has a duty to continue to advocate for the patient's needs and best interests. This stems from the PT's basic duty of beneficence toward the patient—the duty to be guided by concern for the physical, psychological, and socioeconomic welfare of individuals entrusted to his or her care.

Section 7.1C of the *APTA Guide for Professional Conduct* specifies, additionally, "A physical therapist shall recognize that third-party payer contracts may limit, in one form or another, the provision of physical therapy services. Third-party limitations

APTA Code of Ethics

PREAMBLE
This *Code of Ethics* of the American Physical Therapy Association sets forth principles for the ethical practice of physical therapy. All physical therapists are responsible for maintaining and promoting ethical practice. To this end, the physical therapist shall act in the best interest of the patient/client. This *Code of Ethics* shall be binding on all physical therapists.

PRINCIPLE 1
A physical therapist shall respect the rights and dignity of all individuals and shall provide compassionate care.

PRINCIPLE 2
A physical therapist shall act in a trustworthy manner towards patients/clients, and in all other aspects of physical therapy practice.

PRINCIPLE 3
A physical therapist shall comply with laws and regulations governing physical therapy and shall strive to effect changes that benefit patients/clients.

PRINCIPLE 4
A physical therapist shall exercise sound professional judgment.

PRINCIPLE 5
A physical therapist shall achieve and maintain professional competence.

PRINCIPLE 6
A physical therapist shall maintain and promote high standards for physical therapy practice, education, and research.

PRINCIPLE 7
A physical therapist shall seek only such remuneration as is deserved and reasonable for physical therapy services.

PRINCIPLE 8
A physical therapist shall provide and make available accurate and relevant information to patients/clients about their care and to the public about physical therapy services.

PRINCIPLE 9
A physical therapist shall protect the public and the profession from unethical, incompetent, and illegal acts.

PRINCIPLE 10
A physical therapist shall endeavor to address the health needs of society.

PRINCIPLE 11
A physical therapist shall respect the rights, knowledge, and skills of colleagues and other health care professionals.

do not absolve the physical therapist from making sound professional judgments that are in the patient's best interest. A physical therapist shall avoid underutilization of physical therapy services."

Abandonment law prohibits the physician from discharging patients who are in need of continuing medical attention without first giving reasonable notice.[9] It appears that this body of law also would apply to PTs.[10] Therefore, therapists should provide ample notice to patients when limitations in their insurance coverage are anticipated. Additionally, if the patient needs more care, the therapist should discuss continuing treatment on a self-pay basis. If the patient is unable to pay privately, the therapist might arrange a payment plan or refer the patient to free or low-cost alternatives.

Section 7.1B of the *APTA Guide for Professional Conduct* states, "A physical therapist shall never place her/his own financial interest above the welfare of individuals under his/her care." If the patient will be harmed by discontinuing treatment, the provider has an ethical obligation to continue treatment until other arrangements can be made for care. Experts argue that, although payers make important economic decisions, physicians remain responsible for the medical decisions, and a payer's denial of reimbursement should not dictate the patient's care.[8] In fact, providers may have a professional obligation to help the patient appeal the adverse decision.

Court decisions seem to support this idea. For example, in the case of *Wickline v State of California* the court absolved the health plan of liability because the physicians did not protest utilization review decisions that they felt were not in the best interest of the patient.[11] This responsibility extends to PTs and is supported by sections 7.1C and 7.1D of the *APTA Guide for Professional Conduct*, which state in part, respectively, that, "A physical therapist shall avoid underutilization of physical therapy services" and "A physical therapist shall avoid overutilization of physical therapy services."

> *If the patient is unable to pay privately, the therapist might arrange a payment plan or refer the patient to free or low-cost alternatives.*

Who Determines Medical Necessity?

The burden of proof ultimately rests with the health care professional to provide evidence to support the need for or the intensity of an intervention. There is a general understanding that it is not the utilization reviewer's responsibility to prove or disprove the efficacy of care; the provider is responsible for demonstrating that the care he or she provides is necessary and reasonable.[12] The PT has a duty of fidelity to the patient to ensure professional standards of practice and to prevent adverse decisions based on substandard care.

The issue of reimbursement frequently rests on the strength of the clinical documentation, and review criteria typically incorporate documentation guidelines and standards. Poor documentation of care, or provision of care that violates state practice standards, may harm the patient by leading to a denial of care. The PT has a duty of non-maleficence (meaning the duty to do no harm) to prevent this situation. Clear guidelines for documentation are provided within the *Guide to Physical Therapist Practice*, the *APTA Guidelines for Physical Therapy Documentation*,[13] and the *APTA Standards of Practice*.[14] The PT also has a responsibility to accommodate reasonable payer requirements and requests.

The provider has a duty, too, to be honest with the patient regarding adverse managed care determinations. Disguising a denial of treatment by the insurer as a recommendation based on the provider's professional judgment and ordinary practice violates the basic principle of truth-telling in health care.

Certainly, there are reasons why a provider might be uncomfortable sharing this type of information with patients. First, the PT may be concerned that the patient will discontinue needed treatment if he or she cannot afford to pay for it out of pocket. Second, the PT may not want to undermine the patient-therapist relationship and the patient's confidence in his or her professional judgment. Many patients feel torn between their provider's judgment that an intervention is medically necessary and the payer's claim that it is not.[15]

In addition, the PT may be uncomfortable sharing the reasons for a denial if his or her own behavior has resulted in the decision. The provider may find it easier to tell a patient that the insurance company will not allow a specific intervention rather than admit that poor documentation or substandard care delivery led to a denial. Scapegoating, or blaming managed care for adverse decisions caused by the provider's actions, is considered unethical. If the patient does not know that a choice is to be made and does not know who controls or participates in that choice, that patient's ability to appeal decisions and to pursue claims for treatment against the insurer is diminished.[8]

The insurer and the provider have very different moral and legal obligations to the patient. The insurer's obligations are dictated by the terms of an insurance policy and compliance with state and federal regulations.[16] Insurers and subscribers for the most part can decide for themselves what sorts of coverage and limits they want to insure. Once these are contractually agreed upon, insurers are legally entitled to enforce those limits.[8]

continued on page 68 ▶▶▶

Balancing Ethical Challenges
continued from page 51

For example, a health care plan might agree to pay for medically necessary care but offer only limited days of coverage for rehabilitative services, restrict the number of physical therapy visits allowed per diagnosis or per year, or specifically exclude maintenance care. An insurance policy that limits physical therapy treatment to 60 calendar days per diagnosis, for instance, would legally be allowed to deny care beyond the 60-day period even if that care were considered medically necessary.

Hope for the Future

Managed care evolved as a strategy to provide necessary health care services within budget constraints. The continuing challenge for our health care delivery system is to balance costs and benefits in a truly just fashion. Future enactment of patients' rights legislation may offer some degree of consumer protection, but it will not offer a method for controlling health care costs, and it will not assist the provider in making ethical decisions regarding utilization of services.

Development of clinical research knowledge, however, may ultimately help to resolve some of these ethical problems. One of the most promising initiatives in health care is the growing focus on evidence-based practice. A rapidly expanding body of scientific knowledge regarding intervention efficacy is beginning to be used to identify not only effective interventions but also ineffective and costly procedures that offer limited results. As data are accumulated and patterns are identified, the hope is that best practices will be identified and integrated into care delivery, resulting in improved patient care.

Application of ethical theory supports the move toward an evidence-based approach to health care management. The health care provider has a duty to perform a service that is beneficial for the patient; in other words, in order for health care to be ethical care, it must demonstrate patient benefit.[17] Providing interventions that do

In order for health care to be ethical care, it must demonstrate patient benefit ... Proving our intervention efficacy is in the best interests of our patients.

not clearly lead to a better outcome is self-serving and costly to the patient. Providing ineffective interventions potentially violates the ethical basis of the clinical relationship. Proving our intervention efficacy is in the best interests of our patients.

Ultimately, evidence regarding intervention efficacy will guide third-party payers in the determination of medical necessity. Evidence about intervention efficacy also might justify decisions about the need for physical therapy services. Research that identifies the most effective kinds of interventions, as well as their optimal intensity and duration, will be invaluable in influencing public opinion, guiding reimbursement policy, and prompting regulatory action to ensure coverage of necessary services. **PT**

Linda Resnik Mellion, PT, MS, is Instructor of Ethical/Legal Issues in Health Care in the University of Rhode Island's physical therapy program. She also is a doctoral candidate at Nova Southeastern University in Fort Lauderdale, Florida. She serves as a utilization reviewer for a major third-party payer and is former chair of the Rhode Island Board of Physical Therapy Examiners in the Rhode Island Department of Health.

References

1. *Guide to Physical Therapist Practice, Second Edition.* Alexandria, Va: American Physical Therapy Association; 2001.
2. Jette DU, Jette AM. Physical therapy treatment choic- es for musculoskeletal impairments. *Phys Ther.* 1997;77:145-154.
3. Kirk-Sanchez NJ, Roach KE. Relationship between duration of therapy services in a comprehensive rehabilitation program and mobility at discharge in patients with orthopedic problems. *Phys Ther.* 2001;81:888-895.
4. Roach KE, Ally D, Finnerty B, et al. The relationship between duration of physical therapy services in the acute care setting and change in functional status in patients with lower-extremity orthopedic problems. *Phys Ther.* 1998;78:19-24.
5. Guccione AA, Fagerson TL, Anderson JJ. Regaining functional independence in the acute care setting following hip fracture. *Phys Ther.* 1996;76:818-826.
6. Wilbur K. *An Analysis of Post-Acute Treatment and Outcome Differences Between Medicare Fee-For-Service and Managed Care* [dissertation]. Los Angeles, Calif: University of Southern California; 1999.
7. Purtilo R. *Ethical Dimensions in the Health Professions, 3rd Ed.* Philadelphia, Pa: WB Saunders; 1998.
8. Haavi Morreim E. Whodunit? Causal responsibility of utilization review for physicians' decisions, patients' outcomes. *Law, Medicine & Health Care.* 1992;20:1-2.
9. Bennett JJ. APTA examines patient abandonment. *PT— Magazine of Physical Therapy.* 1999 1999;7(7):24-28.
10. Scott R. *Health Care Malpractice: A Primer on Legal Issues for Professionals.* New York, NY: McGraw Hill; 1999.
11. Wickline v State of California, 228 192 Cal App 3d 1630,1645-1646, 239 *Cal Rptr* 661 810,819 (Cal App 2 1986).
12. Clifton DW Jr. Review criteria: cookbook medicine or professional tool? *PT—Magazine of Physical Therapy.* 1995;3(9):37-40.
13. *APTA Guidelines for Physical Therapist Documentation.* Alexandria, Va: American Physical Therapy Association; 2001. Available at www.apta.org/PT_Practice/Patient Client_Management/doc.../guidelinesforptdocumenta.
14. *APTA Standards of Practice and the Criteria.* Alexandria, Va: American Physical Therapy Association; 2001. Available at www.apta.org/PT_Practice/PatientClient_Management/Standards/Standards.
15. Rimler G, Morrison R. The ethical impacts of managed care. *Journal of Business Ethics.* 1993;12:493-501.
16. Banja J, Johnston ME. Part III: ethical perspectives and social policy, outcomes evaluation in TBI rehabilitation. *Arch Phys Med Rehabil.* 1994;75:19-26.
17. Olsen, D. Ethical cautions in the use of outcomes for resource allocation in the managed care environment of mental health. *Arch Psych Nurs.* 1995; IX(4):173-178.

Saying "No" to Patients for Cost-Related Reasons

Alternatives for the Physical Therapist

RUTH B. PURTILO

Physical therapists express their respect for patients by providing competent, compassionate care. Constraints may be imposed on realizing this ideal when treatment must be refused or discontinued because patients lack the financial resources to pay for physical therapy services. The purposes of this article are 1) to review key features that have contributed to the current high cost of health care, 2) to describe approaches being proposed to curb costs, and 3) to suggest ways physical therapists can have a constructive role in creating rational cost-containment policies that are consistent with professional ideals. Seven activities by which physical therapists can become involved at the health care policy level are discussed.

Key Words: *Cost control; Costs and cost analysis; Ethics; Physical therapy profession, patient services.*

Ethical codes of the health care professions are predicated on a moral ideal that human beings should be treated with respect.[1] The *Code of Ethics* of the American Physical Therapy Association includes an explicit commitment to this ideal, stating that Association members must strive to protect the patient's rights and dignity.[2] The most direct way this ideal is realized is for physical therapists to apply their professional skills competently and compassionately in response to the legitimate health care needs of patients whose condition warrants physical therapy intervention. For the most part, physical therapists can—and do—respond according to this ideal. Moreover, many physical therapists are looking ahead to identify future trends in patient needs and ways that those needs can best be met. Illustrative of this trend is a recent *Physical Therapy* article entitled "The Graying of America: Opportunities for Physical Therapy" that begins

> The specter of an excess population of sick, poor, disabled, aged Americans who are retiring earlier, living longer, and costing more per case to care for has riveted the attention of public policy on the "graying" of America. The projection of a major increase in our elderly population and changes in longevity patterns present tremendous opportunities and responsibilities for physical therapists. . . .As our patient population becomes increasingly older, the application of our clinical expertise must change to provide the necessary physical therapy services.[3]

At the same time that physical therapists are eagerly responding to immediate and future health care needs, some characteristics of the current health care system make it difficult for therapists to accept or to continue treating certain qualified patients. The constraints are imposed by these patients' lack of resources to provide payment for physical therapy services. Daniels points out that health care professionals are understandably distressed when their commitment to competent, compassionate care for all patients is thwarted

by financial considerations, especially because in the United States the dollars saved on one patient are not necessarily channeled to other more pressing health care priorities (or to health care at all).[4] In addition, for many health care professionals, the idea of refusing care on the basis of financial criteria seems morally repugnant.[5]

The purposes of this article are 1) to review some key features of the current situation wherein physical therapists at times forego or discontinue treatment of a patient because of cost constraints; 2) to describe current approaches to curbing costs; and 3) to explore constructive alternatives to accepting cost-driven policies that compromise the physical therapy profession's commitment to the ideal of providing competent, compassionate professional services.

CONTRIBUTING FACTORS TO THE HIGH COST OF HEALTH CARE

Costs have become a major focus of concern in health care, and there is good reason for concern. The United States has the costliest health care system per capita in the world.[6] Actual dollar costs have risen steadily since the 1960s. Between 1975 and 1985, the United States almost doubled its health care expenditures, from $247 billion in 1975 to $425 billion in 1985.[7] A 1987 Institute of Medicine study predicts that this upward trend will continue.[8] According to the US Department of Commerce and the Congressional Budget Office, in 1987 the United States spent about 11.5% of the gross national product (GNP), over half of $1 trillion, on health care. In other words, about $1 billion is being spent every day, about $600,000 during the reading of this article.

Although many reasons are advanced, a consensus does not exist regarding the primary cause of the recent steady increase in costs. There is more agreement, however, about the range of probable interdependent factors that combine to create the persistent increase.

Most often earmarked as a key contributing factor is the modern dependence on and success of lifesaving technology. Reiser, a medical historian, concludes that the use of technology was firmly linked to diagnosis and was increasingly being linked to therapeutics by the end of the nineteenth

R. Purtilo, PhD, is Henry Knox Sherrill Professor of Medical Ethics, MGH Institute of Health Professions, and Ethicist-in-Residence, Massachusetts General Hospital, 15 River St #410, Boston, MA 02108-3402 (USA). She was Professor and Chairman, Department of Medical Jurisprudence and Humanities, University of Nebraska Medical Center, 42nd St and Dewey Ave, Omaha, NE 68105, when this article was written.

This article was submitted July 14, 1987; was with the author for revision 17 weeks; and was accepted March 3, 1988. Potential Conflict of Interest: 4.

century, a process that had begun as early as the scientific revolution in the seventeenth century.[9] By the first half of the twentieth century, such cost-efficient biotechnological breakthroughs as vaccines, antibiotics, and the iron lung had gained widespread acceptance, demonstrating beyond doubt the crucial role of technology in the delivery of high-quality health care.[9] In the mid-1950s onward, the development of improved ventilation and resuscitation technologies to maintain the severely compromised organs of patients with poliomyelitis helped to further wed technology and medicine.[10] At the same time, intensive care units, renal dialysis, and early attempts at transplantation of vital organs were developing. As the potential for lifesaving intervention has continued to increase, so has the cost of equipment to effect it.[11] Currently, even the traditionally more "hands on" professions (eg, medical rehabilitation professions) increasingly depend on expensive technology.[12]

A second major component adding to the increase in overall costs of health care has been brought about by the numbers of persons requiring these expensive technologies. More persons, including newborns, are living longer because of the use of expensive technology, although many individuals continue to require expensive, long-term care throughout their life span.[13] Attempts to suggest limits on expensive interventions are often viewed as prejudicial.[14] Furthermore, expensive technological care is increasingly expected by patients. In a study of problems confronting small community hospitals, for example, a common theme was that patients demand to be transferred to tertiary care centers, where the latest diagnostic and treatment equipment is available, even when health care professionals disagree that a good clinical reason exists for the transfer.[15] Health care professionals do often comply with transfer requests for various other reasons, including the fear of litigation and the desire to honor the patient's wishes.[16]

A third component purported to foster increased costs of health care is the third-party payment systems of remuneration for services. Open-ended government reimbursement programs (eg, Medicare) are believed to have greatly increased the amount of services rendered, thereby increasing overall costs. One reason offered is the belief that both private and governmental third-party reimbursement arrangements effectively relieve the health care professional and the patient from having to be accountable regarding expenditures.[17] Controversy continues regarding the relationship between third-party reimbursement plans, spending, and costs.[18] The Rand Corporation, for example, conducted a large health insurance experiment and concluded that persons receiving free care used significantly more than those who paid at least 25% of the costs incurred. Among the Rand Corporation's conclusions was that cost consciousness could ensue through the use of co-payments and deductibles.[19] Fuchs, a leading economist, is among those who disagree with the Rand Corporation's conclusions. He contends that a more governing reason is that patients and their families often lack the relevant information to make informed decisions and may be too emotionally overwrought to make on-the-spot choices to limit treatment; therefore, costs are not an important consideration to most people regarding treatment decisions.[20]

These proposed reasons for the high costs of health care in the United States are not exhaustive. They do point, however, to three pervasive themes in analyses of the current cost predicament in health care. Physical therapists find themselves drawn into the web of issues generated by the focus on high costs.

RESPONSES TO THE HIGH COST OF HEALTH CARE

The current high cost of health care is frequently referred to as a crisis. Responses to this crisis entail two main lines of thinking and action, with many proposals attempting to embrace aspects of the two extreme positions. At one extreme are those who maintain that the continuing escalation in costs threatens to "break the back" of the US economy and that the best solution is to reduce costs by means of market forces. Some services will necessarily be eliminated. At the other extreme are those who insist that in a society as affluent as that of the United States, the challenge is to find ways to pay for services. Attempts to eliminate services as a means of containing costs is a value-laden political statement and nothing more. Economists, politicians, ethicists, and health care providers are found in both camps.

Havighurst and Hackbarth are representatives of the first position.[21] They place the blame for runaway costs on the communal organization of health care and the collective responsibility assumed by society for reimbursing health care costs. They propose that the ultimate effective check on further increased expenditures for health care is to "remove government encroachment" and "support a competitive market in which total health care spending and the level of doctors' incomes are determined by smoothly working market forces."[21] In this way, they argue, US society will eventually realize that health care is a product, no different than other consumable products such as a summer vacation package or a new hat or trash masher. With time, the cost that US citizens are willing to pay for this valuable commodity will become clear, and only then will we know how much of the GNP health care is really worth.

Daniels[4] and Thurow[6] are representatives of the second position. According to them, health care costs are a problem but do not threaten to devastate the US economy. Emphasis on the elimination of services, therefore, is neither necessary nor morally correct. Instead, emphasis on more cost-efficient methods of providing services is needed. Daniels, a philosopher, argues that health care traditionally has been viewed in western societies as a special type of good offered in response to a basic human need, that need being the form of human suffering created by illness or injury.[4] His interpretation has been the approach that has guided treatment decisions focused on the benefit to individual patients and has been the philosophical underpinning for arrangements that enable the provision of basic services to those unable to pay for them. Indeed, they believe that the presence of human need in the form of illness places a moral claim on citizens in society. Consequently, there is a collective responsibility to provide services to the extent possible, taking into account actual limits of available resources.[22]

Economist Thurow[6] worries that the ideas contained in recent cost-containment proposals that rely on market forces threaten the traditional values and approaches delineated by Daniels.[4] Thurow explains:

The federal government used to view health care as a social problem. Today it views it almost solely as a budget-deficit problem. The shift in perspectives is important. . . .Since governments provide health care primarily to the elderly and the poor, government deficit-reduction measures systematically dismantle the existing system of paying for health care for these groups. . . .[He adds, however, that this is a transformation that will not affect only the poor and the elderly.] Cutting health care costs is going to be a central business objective in the next five years too. Whereas government cost-containment measures focus attention on the elderly and the poor, corporate cost-containment focuses attention on the health care systems for the middle class. . . . Business magazines have started to publish articles on how corporations can and must shake costs out of their health care systems.[6]

Arnold Relman, editor of the *New England Journal of Medicine*, agrees with Daniels's[4] and Thurow's[6] approach, finding it consistent with a medical ethics point of view. Nonetheless, he is pessimistic because he believes US society is experiencing a social climate that supports the privatization of most social services, including medical care, and accepts a competitive market as the appropriate means of containing societal expenditures.[23]

Many physical therapists probably are not in a position to have thought through these issues, especially the various political, economic, and ethical implications of these two extreme approaches. It is reasonable, however, to assume that, because parts of both approaches are currently being tested in the United States, some therapists are anxiously contemplating what might happen if rehabilitation services are further reduced for various groups of patients. Others are already expressing anger about having had to refuse or discontinue therapeutic services. Refusing treatment to patients for cost-related reasons is the worst possible alternative. Constructive approaches are needed to contain mounting and unnecessary health care costs.

ALTERNATIVES TO SAYING "NO" FOR COST-RELATED REASONS

Assuming that physical therapists want to avoid working under policies and practices that are harmful to some patients, the challenge is to seek alternatives to unnecessary refusals. What does this task involve in a period during which lively discussion still exists regarding the appropriateness of current approaches to cost containment? Ultimately, the cost-related issues are a society-wide problem, requiring the cooperation and diligence of many groups. In working toward a consensus, however, health care professionals should be active participants from the start. In contrast to the majority of activities physical therapists have engaged in during their maturation as a professional group, however, the current health care costs challenge requires that large numbers of physical therapists become involved in the formation, review, and refinement of health policy at the institutional, local, regional, and national levels. Only by informed, substantive, and widespread involvement in cost-related policy issues can the profession gain insight into and develop strategies to affirm acceptable approaches to cost containment while rejecting those that unnecessarily compromise the quality of health care. The following seven alternatives are among those available to members of the profession.

Increased Awareness of Concepts and Terminology

First and foremost, physical therapists must become well aware of the concepts and vocabulary being used to discuss the problem. An excellent starting place is a special section in *Clinical Management in Physical Therapy* entitled "Insurance Reimbursement and the Physical Therapist."[24] Educational programs introducing students and practitioners to basic economics concepts will help. Because the language of health care policy currently is so governed by economics, business,

and the related notions of profits, management, and products, the formal and continuing education of physical therapists must be structured to encourage understanding of these concepts. Subscription to basic health care economics journals, business ethics newsletters, or a lay newspaper such as the *Wall Street Journal* can help ensure that physical therapists do not become "conversation dropouts" at this critical period in their professional practice.

Documentation and Development of Cost-Effective Methods of Providing Services

Physical therapists have a responsibility to document instances in which saying "no" on the basis of costs compromises good clinical judgment. For example, Medicaid or Medicare reimbursement policies that control the number of days of treatment for patients sometimes place therapists in such a position. Record keeping specifically designed to highlight the negative effects of having to alter treatment regimens because of cost constraints can ensure useful and welcome data for policy makers. Additionally, physical therapists must continue to engage in studies of cost-efficient means of providing services to show why certain expenditures are merited. One useful approach for designing a data-gathering system for such purposes is presented by Ginzberg in the April 17, 1987, issue of the *New England Journal of Medicine* in an article entitled "A Hard Look at Cost Containment."[25]

Improved Availability of Data

Physical therapists can be agents of change by publishing their data and clinical impressions in professional journals and by presenting the material at professional meetings. These professional activities not only make the data available to readers who want to become informed but also encourage others to do likewise.

Mechanisms for Recommending Change

Physical therapists can work directly with institutional administrators. Almost every institution has mechanisms in place for making recommendations regarding reasonable alterations to present practices and policies. Therapists should offer to serve on committees that are designed to review potential problem areas related to patient care, and supervisors should accommodate requests by their staff therapists who wish to serve on such committees by relieving them of some other tasks.

Legislative Involvement

There has never been a more compelling time than now to link arms with legislators. Health care professionals are in a prime position to have their voices heard if they share their expert opinions with state and federal congressional representatives and testify at hearings. To be sure, physical therapists rally en force when the legislature is voting on issues such as physical therapy licensure or physical therapy without referral. Where are physical therapists when Medicaid changes are being debated? Being willing to provide data and offer a considered opinion, and also sending a thank-you note to legislators for their support, is not only appreciated but helps to ensure that tasks are accomplished that therapists perceive as important. Furthermore, only by such engagement can therapists learn firsthand what legislators' worries and constraints are.

Innovations at the Departmental Level

In addition to these suggestions for "going to the top," innovations at the departmental level may be useful for assessing the strengths and weaknesses of cost-related policies. One approach would be to establish a regularly scheduled morbidity and mortality conference similar to those held in clinical departments. At these conferences, the participants retrospectively examine their mistakes and prospectively plan approaches to prevent repeating them. There is no reason why this "M and M" conference could not be structured to examine cost-related departmental policies. What could be a bigger "mistake" than a policy that leaves physical therapists in the situation of saying "no" to patients for the wrong reasons? The examination might reveal that poor policies are partly a result of physical therapists' mistakes and thus provide a forum for forging new approaches to serious problems related to the high cost of health care interventions.

If such a format were implemented, five questions could be used as a framework for guiding therapists' thinking about whether a policy that seems poor is indeed the best possible option available under the circumstances:

1. What important ends are being served by the chosen policy?
2. Is an unacceptable portion of the policy (eg, the action to exclude whole groups from treatment) a "last resort" move?
3. Are the limits of due proportion being honored? That is, are the least hurtful policies possible being adopted in instances in which harm necessarily will ensue to some groups?
4. Is the action being carried out with just intentions?
5. How does this policy help to save the high ideals that have characterized health care and does it convey respect for the dignity of persons, regard for the individual, and compassion?

When the strengths as well as the problems inherent in a policy are identified, therapists will be better equipped to engage in useful negotiations with policy makers regarding needed reforms.

Participation in Charitable Activities

Finally, physical therapists do have the option of treating patients who cannot pay for services, simply accepting that in some instances remuneration for services will be in the form of a patient's gratitude. In the December 1987 issues of *JAMA* and the *ABA Journal*, an identical editorial, coauthored by the editors of these two important journals, prods physicians and lawyers to share in the task of caring for indigent patients:

How many members of the legal and medical professions now deliberately care for the poor in a voluntary and uncompensated way? Many, but not enough. What percentage of their time is spent doing so? Much, but not enough. Accompanying articles in this issue of both the ABA Journal and JAMA explore these questions in some detail. . . .Doctors and lawyers in our society have benefited greatly from the abundant opportunities made available to them from the fruits of our plenty. We believe that all doctors and all lawyers, as a matter of ethics and good faith, should contribute a significant percentage of their total professional efforts without expectation of financial remuneration. This percentage will vary depending on time, setting, opportunity, and need, but all should give something. This is the proper behavior of a learned professional. We believe that 50 hours a year—or roughly one week of time—is an appropriate minimum amount. . . .There is a

great tradition behind the giving of this gift. In the church, it is called stewardship. In law, it is called *pro bono publico*. In medicine, it is called charity. In everyday society, it is called fairness.[26]

Although a whole health care system cannot be built on unremunerated services, the professional ethic long has held that one characteristic of a true profession remains its special relationship with the poor. As physical therapists move steadily toward a status of professionalism equal to those traditional professions of medicine, law, and clergy, the onus of responsibility rests fully on their shoulders to participate in charitable activities as the occasion requires it.

Presumably, these seven suggestions for how physical therapists can contribute to discussions of how best to effect reasonable constraints on health care costs will be an incentive to think of other suggestions as well. The suggestions presented in this article are but representative of the many constructive alternatives available.

CONCLUSION

Physical therapists can be proud to be part of a profession that responds constructively to challenge. Physical therapists who served in wartime rehabilitation settings, those who persevered during the poliomyelitis epidemics, and those who have served in underserved areas of the United States and the world stand as models against which all can strive when the occasion calls for it. In each of these situations, physical therapists have demonstrated courage, compassion, and competent attention to the challenge they faced. Today, the occasion again calls for a constructive response to a serious health care problem, that of health care costs. The challenge is to again respond with courage, compassion, and competent attention as various approaches are taken to help curb high health care costs. Each approach has ramifications for the professional practice of physical therapy, although not all of the ramifications are fully known yet. As new policy approaches are discussed and tested, physical therapists as individuals and as a profession must assume an active role in shaping the health care system by exercising the seven avenues of involvement suggested in this article. The resulting health care system should be built on realistic constraint, but also on unremitting commitment to the ideals of high-quality health care.

REFERENCES

1. Jameton A: Nursing Practice: The Ethical Issues. Englewood Cliffs, NJ, Prentice Hall, 1984, pp 126–129
2. Code of Ethics and Guide for Professional Conduct. Alexandria, VA, American Physical Therapy Association, 1987
3. Jette AM, Bottomley JM: The graying of America: Opportunities for physical therapy. Phys Ther 67:1537–1542, 1987
4. Daniels N: Why saying no to patients in the United States is so hard. N Engl J Med 314:1380–1383, 1986
5. Brock DW, Buchanan AE: The profit motive in medicine. J Med Philos 23:1–35, 1987
6. Thurow L: Medicine versus economics. N Engl J Med 313:611–614, 1985
7. Office of the Actuary, Health Care Financing Administration: Health care spending hike. AMA News, August 15, 1986, p 4
8. Gray BH (ed): For-Profit Enterprise in Health Care. Washington, DC, National Academy Press, 1986
9. Reiser SJ: The machine at the bedside: Technological transformations of practices and values. In Reiser SJ, Anbar M (eds): The Machine at the Bedside: Strategies for Using Technology in Patient Care. New York, NY, Cambridge University Press, 1984, pp 8–9
10. Pontoppidan H, Wilson R, Rie MA: Respiratory intensive care. Anesthesiology 47:96–116, 1977
11. Pichler JA: Capitalism in America: Moral issues and public policy. In DeGeorge RT, Pichler JA (eds): Ethics, Free Enterprise, and Public Policy:

Original Essays on Moral Issues in Business. New York, NY, Oxford University Press Inc, 1978, pp 19–40

12. Caplan AL, Callahan D, Haas J: Ethical and policy issues in rehabilitation medicine. Hastings Cent Rep 17(Suppl):1–20, 1987

13. Frohock FM: Special Care: Medical Decisions at the Beginning of Life. Chicago, IL, University of Chicago Press, 1986, pp 138–158

14. Callahan D: Setting Limits: Medical Goals in an Aging Society. New York, NY, Simon & Schuster Inc, 1987

15. Purtilo RB: Rural health care: The forgotten quarter of medical ethics. Second Opinion 6(3):10–33, 1987

16. Flannery M: Simple living and hard choices. Hastings Cent Rep 12(4):9–12, 1982

17. Health and Public Policy Committee, American College of Physicians: Medicare payment for physicians' services. Ann Intern Med 106:151–153, 1987

18. Somers AR: Containment of health care costs: A diagnostic approach. Forum Medicine 2:106–112, 1979

19. Newhouse JP, Manning WG, Morris CN, et al: Some interim results from a controlled trial of cost sharing in health insurance. N Engl J Med 305:1501–1507, 1981

20. Fuchs VR: A Time to Reap—Adults 45–64: How We Live—An Economic Perspective on Americans from Birth to Death. Cambridge, MA, Harvard University Press, 1983, pp 159–184

21. Havighurst CC, Hackbarth GM: Private cost containment. N Engl J Med 300:1298–1305, 1979

22. Hannan EL, Rouse RL, Barnett B, et al: Methods for developing relative need criteria to accompany a health care capital expenditure limit. J Health Polit Policy Law 23:113–136, 1987

23. Relman AS, Reinhardt U: An exchange on for-profit health care. In Gray BH (ed): For-Profit Enterprise in Health Care. Washington, DC, National Academy Press, 1986, pp 209–223

24. Horting M: Insurance reimbursement and the physical therapist. Clinical Management in Physical Therapy 7(2):21–40, 1987

25. Ginzberg E: A hard look at cost containment. N Engl J Med 317:1151–1154, 1987

26. Lundberg GD, Laurence B: Fifty hours for the poor. JAMA 258:3157, 1987

HABITS OF THOUGHT

By Charles J Dougherty, PhD

Ethical Principles in Health Care Reform

Health care reform isn't just a political debate—it's an ethical dilemma as well.

President Clinton opened the health care reform debate in earnest 2 months ago with a major address before a joint session of the US Congress. In that address, the President articulated six principles to guide health care reform: *security, simplicity, savings, choice, quality, and responsibility*. As is called for on such an occasion, the President developed the *political* meaning of each of these principles. But they also have important *ethical* content, a dimension that should play a role in the public policy debate.

Security

Politics: The politics behind the principle of security are captured by the Clinton Administration's slogan for its plan: "Health care that is always there." A primary goal of health care reform is to provide comprehensive coverage for all Americans and to end the exclusion of preexisting conditions that is so common in contemporary insurance plans.

Ethics: The ethical issue behind the politics of security is the *right* to health care. The status of personhood confers a dignity that must be respected by a framework of rights—rights that provide 1) protection from interference and 2) access to basic goods and services. In modern developed societies, health care has been counted among these basic goods and services. This international consensus—which holds regardless of whether a society embraces an explicit concept of health care as a right—has led all of our peer nations to guarantee a basic package of health care to all of their citizens. The ethical challenge at hand for America, then, is the recognition of health care as a basic human right.

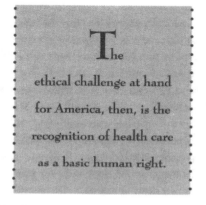

The ethical challenge at hand for America, then, is the recognition of health care as a basic human right.

Simplicity

Politics: To illustrate the principle of simplicity, Clinton displayed a health care credit card during his address to symbolize a way to reduce paperwork and bureaucracy both for patients and for providers. He emphasized that the United States spends more money on the *administration* of health care than does any other nation and that administration remains the fastest growing component of the health care economy.

Ethics: Simplicity itself is an aesthetic ideal or an organizational virtue more than it is an ethical value. But two very important ethical values are closely *associated* with simplicity: consumer access and professional satisfaction. A difficult, frustrating, highly bureaucratic system of health care can keep people *away* from needed care even when there is universal insurance, thus undermining the intention to respond to the citizen's right to health care. A system in which physicians and other providers spend inordinate time on paperwork and are constantly called upon to justify treatment decisions can sap practitioners' motivation—and could drive them out of the health care arena altogether. Simplicity therefore is a means to realize the ethical value of

1) access to health care that 2) is provided by highly motivated and caring professionals.

Savings

Politics: Despite large numbers of uninsured and underinsured persons, the United States spends more money—and more funds as a percentage of gross national product—on health care than does any other nation. Moreover, the rate of increase in health care spending continues to outstrip general inflation. Clinton made the point that financial restraint in the health care sector is necessary for the health of the American economy.

Ethics: Three important ethical issues are raised by the principle of savings. First, there is a general ethical obligation not to waste natural and human resources: If needs can be met with less spending, they should be. Second, in addition to the direct financial costs of health care, there are "indirect-opportunity costs"—services that cannot be funded adequately because limited resources have been allocated to health care. Ironically, some of these services, such as education and economic development, can have just as large an impact on a population's health status as health care delivery itself has. Finally, the need to save money raises the thorny ethical issue of health care rationing. No health care system can provide everything to everybody. Priorities must be set, and difficult choices must be made.

Choice

Politics: One of the central political realities of the health care reform debate is the importance that Americans attach to the freedom to choose their own physicians and that American physicians attach to the freedom to choose their own style of practice. Any reform measure perceived to deny or limit these choices would not be politically viable—in spite of the fact that the current system *already* denies or limits these choices for many patients and physicians.

Ethics: The ethical issue behind this political attachment to choice has two dimensions. The most obvious dimension is the value that Americans traditionally place on individual freedom. Our concept of the *person* entails a right of self-determination, a right to choose that encompasses the way we seek and provide health care.

The second dimension is less obvious but potentially more important in the context of health care: trust in the patient-provider relationship. The patient's ability to choose a physician, and the physician's ability to choose an organizational style of relating to patients (eg, fee for service, health maintenance organization, participating provider organization), allows the maximum opportunity for building trust in individual therapeutic relationships. Patients generally want a physician who is "*their* physician," who puts *their* interests first, and who advocates on *their* behalf. Physicians also generally want this type of relationship. And care generally is enhanced by the trust created in these types of relationships.

Quality

Politics: The political *sine qua non* of health care reform is quality. In spite of the many problems in the health care delivery system, most Americans believe that the current US health care system provides the highest-quality health care in the world. Reform that is perceived as a threat to that standard of quality would be rejected by consumers and providers.

Ethics: The surface issue here is plain: Everyone deserves health care of the highest possible quality. But below the surface is a difficult question: *What is high quality?* High quality in health care has several alternate meanings. It may mean the best medical outcomes: The highest-quality system obtains the best outcomes for patients. It may mean the "right" processes: The highest-quality system uses the most appropriate pathways to care and the most appropriate procedures at the most appropriate time. It may mean consumer satisfaction: The highest-quality system is the system that is most satisfying to patients.

Each of these variables is problematic, both in itself and in relation to the others.

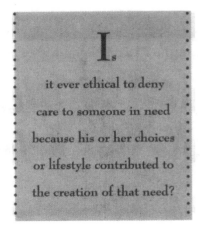

Is it ever ethical to deny care to someone in need because his or her choices or lifestyle contributed to the creation of that need?

Medical outcomes, for example, are affected by a patient's state of health at the outset of treatment and may be negative even when all the right procedures have been followed. And patient satisfaction can be affected by a myriad of factors, some of which—such as "amenities" or "pleasantness"—do not have a *direct* connection with health care. Moreover, providing the highest possible quality for all persons inevitably requires that some choices be made among these various meanings. Achieving better outcomes overall may require less spending on appropriate but high-cost procedures. Better monitoring of procedures may leave fewer dollars for amenities. Spending on amenities may raise consumer satisfaction even if it results in worse medical outcomes.

The ethical commitment to high quality is far easier to *state* than it is to *realize and enforce*.

Responsibility

Politics: Clinton called for a new emphasis on three areas of responsibility: political, social, and personal. In the political realm, he asserted that all citizens have a responsibility to contribute to financing the health care system. He held *society* responsible for efforts to improve health status, especially through lessening the violence that plagues our cities. Finally, he urged individuals to take greater responsibility for their own health.

Ethics: The ethical dimensions of each of these kinds of responsibility are critical to health care reform. The health care system could be financed progressively; as with income tax, progressive funding would ask the wealthy and the well to pay more to support the poor and the sick. On the other hand, funding could come primarily from cost-sharing and other forms of "user fees." This

approach may help restrain utilization, but it also may discourage some people from seeking out needed care. Social and environmental factors—especially poverty, joblessness, and violence—create substantial inequities both in health status and in access to health care. Efforts to minimize these factors could yield significant health dividends, increasing the number of productive years and improving the quality of Americans' lives.

Encouraging greater *personal* responsibility for health runs immediately into two thorny ethical problems. Given what we know about genetics and the impact of early childhood development, how responsible *is* an individual for the state of his or her health? And if individuals are called to greater responsibility for their own health, what is to be done with those who are *irresponsible*? Is it ever ethical to deny care to someone in need because his or her choices or lifestyle contributed to the creation of that need?

Clinton's speech officially opened the health care reform debate. The principles he offered provide an important political framework. But if health care reform is to create a genuinely better health care system for all Americans, the ethical challenges raised by these principles cannot be overlooked. *PT*

Charles Dougherty, PhD, *is Director, Center for Health Policy and Ethics, Creighton University, Omaha, Neb. Dougherty has served as an advisor on health care reform to Senator Bob Kerry (D-Neb), to the Catholic Health Association, to the National Health Policy Council, and to President Clinton's health care transition team. Dougherty currently chairs the Hospital Ethics Committee, St Joseph's Hospital, Omaha, and serves on the Ethics and Grievance Committee, Metro Omaha Medical Society. He is the author of* Ethics at Work *(Belmont, Calif; Wadsworth Inc, 1990) and* American Health Care: Realities, Rights, and Reforms *(New York, NY: Oxford University Press Inc; 1988).*

HABITS OF THOUGHT

By Nancy T Watts, PhD

Physical Therapy as a Career

Our "habits of thought" need to take us in new directions—not to disregard quality, but to add equal concern for cost; not to abandon logic, but to test it with research.

Few habits of thought affect our lives as profoundly as the way we visualize our own careers. This image shapes our personal expectations, the design of our education programs, and the goals of our professional association. It is a complex vision. Although having a job means simply doing work for pay, having a career means that an occupation is lifetime work and that we progress within it as we gain experience. Both the diversity and duration of careers in physical therapy have changed greatly over the past few decades, and those changes now create appealing opportunities and strong challenges to our traditional ways of thinking about physical therapy education and practice.

Because objective data on work patterns in physical therapy are scarce, I must rely on personal impressions to describe these changes. When I entered the field in the late 1940s, I began work—as did most of my classmates—as a staff therapist in a general hospital, spending much of my time treating patients who were recovering from poliomyelitis. Most of my colleagues were women, and, as was the case in most other occupations, the majority of them stopped working after only a few years to marry and raise children. Part-time jobs were rare, and so was private practice. Graduate programs in physical therapy did not exist. Those of us who continued to work found that progress often meant moving away from provision of direct patient care. If we became teachers or administrators, the required qualifications emphasized job performance rather than advanced academic credentials. This pattern is summarized in Figure 1.

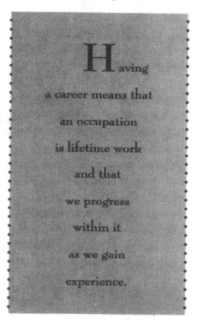

Having a career means that an occupation is lifetime work and that we progress within it as we gain experience.

In contrast, in today's pattern (Fig 2), many graduates remain active in physical therapy for more than 40 years. Their career options are varied and include rewarding opportunities to remain active as clinicians and to combine clinical work with teaching, consulting, administration, or research. Whatever path they choose, today's graduates will find that continued study and advanced credentials are needed to compete for most choice positions.

Where, then, are the challenges? Consider the following questions.

What role should professional ("entry-level") education play in lifetime career development?

In the past, most thinking about physical therapy education focused on initial preparation for practice. During the past several decades, these professional education programs have been hard-pressed to keep pace with changes in responsibility and with the rapid growth of knowledge in the field. Longer programs, higher degrees, and ever more tightly packed curricula have helped, but it is futile to expect initial professional education to fully prepare graduates for a 40-year career.

The problem of preparing practitioners for long careers was clearly analyzed by West[1] when he wrote of medical education:

1. Only a small portion of the current body of medical knowledge can be taught in four years.
2. Much of the knowledge that will be employed in the student's future career is not known today and, therefore, cannot be taught.
3. Not all that is taught is learned.
4. A small part of what is taught is erroneous.
5. A small portion of what is taught will soon be obsolete.
6. The physicians of the future (including family physicians) will be specialists. Thus, some of what they learn will have limited relevance to their careers.
7. Of that which is taught, and learned, and relevant, much is quickly forgotten.

If all this is equally true of physical therapy, a realistic plan for career development must then involve education as a lifelong process in which preparation for many specialized roles is deferred until the graduate has had enough experience to make initial career choices. In this design, both independent study and periodic return to the classroom play an important part.

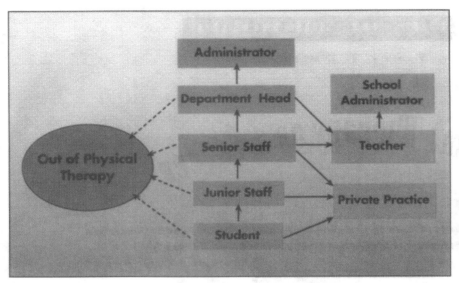

take us in new directions—not to disregard quality, but to add an equal concern for cost, access, and safety, and not to abandon logic, but to test it with research on the outcomes and efficiency of our services. As we plan new strategies for career education and design new ways to test our professional beliefs, the habits of thought we employ should help us both to respond to change and to create new opportunities for the future. *PT*

Nancy T Watts, PhD, FAPTA, is Professor Emerita, Massachusetts General Hospital Institute of Health Professions, Boston, Mass.

Figure 1. *Typical physical therapy career progressions—then. (Adapted from Watts NT. Considerations for the future.* **Proceedings from the Symposium for Physiotherapy Educators, London, England, August 5-7, 1991.** *Winnetka, Ill: Health Professionals International; 1991.)*

REFERENCES

1   West K. The case against teaching. *Journal of Medical Education.* 1966;41:766-771.

Is a clinical ladder justified in terms of the public interest?

These pathways offer experienced clinicians 1) progressive increases both in material rewards and in autonomy, 2) responsibility, and 3) a sense of accomplishment. However, the value of advanced clinical expertise is now being questioned by planners, administrators, and reimbursement managers, who ask

- Is the "master clinician" really cost-effective?

- Is direct access to physical therapy really safe?
- Will the profession's efforts to raise the qualifications of its practitioners jeopardize public access to needed services?
- Where are the objective data to support the contention that advanced skills are needed and useful?

In the past, our thinking emphasized logical explanation of the contributions that clinical experts could make to the quality of care. Our habits of thought now need to

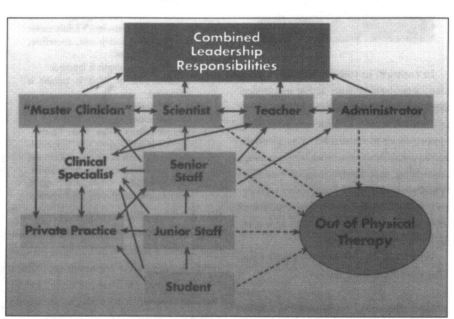

Figure 2. *Typical physical therapy career progressions—now. (Adapted from Watts NT. Considerations for the future.* **Proceedings from the Symposium for Physiotherapy Educators, London, England, August 5-7, 1991.** *Winnetka, Ill: Health Professionals International; 1991.)*

HABITS OF THOUGHT

By Janet A Coy, MA, PT

The Community Perspective

How can we balance the interests of patient, profession, and society?

*a*llocation of health care resources is an issue that illustrates the tension among the sometimes competing interests of the individual patient, the physical therapy profession, and the larger community of which we physical therapy practitioners are a part. Resource allocation requires careful reflection—both at the level of practice and at the level of policy.

A Keen Focus on the Individual
When I interview students for admission into the physical therapy program at the State University of New York Health Science Center at Syracuse, most of them comment that one of the features that attracts them to the profession is the emphasis on *individual patient care*. Rarely does anyone mention policy issues or concerns about resource allocation.

Physical therapists generally have more opportunity than most other health professionals to work with individual patients for extended periods of time. We typically gain intimate knowledge of a patient's goals, fears, limitations, hopes, and life circumstances. We also become acutely aware of the difficulties faced by individuals who do not have adequate insurance or other resources to pay for all the treatment or equipment that would maximize their ability to function at home, school, or work or in the community.

In addition, the American Physical Therapy Association's (APTA) *Code of Ethics* (1992) and *Guide for Professional Conduct* (1992) place a high priority on concern for the individual patient. As stated in the *Guide,* "Physical therapists shall recognize

> Protecting the interests of our profession or individual patients or both, then, may come into conflict with allocations that better provide for members of society as a whole.

that each individual is different from all other individuals and shall respect and be responsive to these differences" (Principle 1.1A) and "Physical therapists are to be guided *at all times* [italics added] by concern for the physical, psychological, and socioeconomic welfare of those individuals entrusted to their care" (Principle 1.1B). Purtilo[1] also correctly points out that, as we move toward becoming independent practitioners, we morally are obligated to be "intensively responsive to patients' needs and intensively focused on pa-tients' satisfaction." We can no longer so easily blame the physician or "the system" when patient needs go unmet. With increasing professional autonomy comes increasing moral responsibility for treatment outcomes.

Several disparate forces—the nature of how we deliver care, our own *Code of Ethics,* our push toward autonomy—converge, then, to keenly focus our attention on the needs of individual patients.

"But Have We Done *Enough?*"
The drive toward professional autonomy also alerts us to the need to protect and enhance our interests as a profession. As we struggle to alter reimbursement regulations, change practice acts to allow independent practice of physical therapy, and prevent "encroachment" on our work by other groups, we more clearly articulate our unique contribution and become aware of our interests.

Having discerned and protected the interests both of our patients and our profession, however, we must ask, "Have we done *enough?*" I believe that, as a "habit of thought," we need to adopt another, broader perspective: the perspective of "the community"—in particular, we need to focus on resource allocation.

An Issue of Justice
As a nation we have become concerned about the inexorable growth of health care costs. Many people have argued that improving efficiency and eliminating waste and unnecessary or unwanted procedures alone would solve the problem. There is compelling evidence, however, that these measures would have only a relatively small impact—and, even then, only in the short run. (For an in-depth discussion of these issues, see Daniel Callahan's *What Kind of Life: The Limits of Medical*

Progress.[2]) In the final analysis, it is—and will continue to be—financially impossible to do *everything* that might benefit *every* individual patient. Thus we must consider not only *how* health care dollars should be spent, but also what *portion* of taxpayer monies should be spent on health care versus other public goods such as education, the environment, and defense. We face an issue of justice: How should social benefits and burdens be allocated to members of society?

Principle 8 of our *Code of Ethics* enjoins physical therapists to "participate in efforts to address the health needs of the public." But what does this mean? If we protect the individual rights and interests of our patients, as well as the interests of our profession, have we fulfilled this duty? No. We also must develop our sense of responsibility to society as a whole; that is, we must develop a sense of community. As Callahan has stated, "Without a powerful sense of community, there will be only the transitory alliances of those who find it convenient to serve their autonomy by banding together," but community "requires constraints, limits, and taboos, just as it requires shared ideals, common dreams, and a vision of the self"—or the profession—"that is part of a wider collectivity."[3]

There invariably will be conflicts: what is best for a particular patient versus what is best for our profession versus what is best for the community. Acknowledging and accepting the inevitability of these types of conflicts will help us—as individuals and as a profession—to avoid knee-jerk reactions to various health care reform proposals and to encourage reflection and participation in meaningful dialogue. Consider the following example.

Under the state of Oregon's plan for health care reform, more than 700 health services were "prioritized." Those services rated as having the highest priority qualified for full coverage by public dollars. Because of the state's financial situation, only the top 587 services were covered. Treatment for tendinitis was not of a sufficiently high priority to receive coverage. If I am a physical therapist in Oregon who works frequently with pa-

tients who have tendinitis, I may become indignant, pointing out how this type of injury interferes with my patients' abilities to perform their jobs and carry out primary life activities. For the sake of my patients, I may lobby for a change for the proposed policy. Because I realize that tendinitis is a condition for which physical therapy typically is indicated, I also may lobby to protect the well-being of my profession.

However, in making the case that physical therapy for tendinitis should be financed—for the sake of patients as well as for the sake of the physical therapy profession—I also need to consider who would not get treatment. The fact is that some individuals will receive government-financed care and some individuals will not. Unless the selection is to be totally arbitrary—as many would argue is the case today[2]—there is a need to establish a principled way of determining precisely who will receive those benefits. Protecting the interests of our profession or individual patients or both, then, may come into conflict with allocations that better provide for members of society as a whole.

One partial remedy to these tough decisions is pro bono work. Scott[4] argued well for the need for our profession to engage in pro bono service. Nevertheless, pro bono health care will never be able to address all the unmet needs. As Scott notes, the underprivileged continue to be poorly served even by the profession of law, which has "the most extensively documented history of pro bono expectations and requirements." And even if the physical therapy profession *could* meet all the unmet direct physical therapy needs of the uninsured and underinsured, *indirect* needs such as equipment would remain problematic.

Other measures can contribute to the simultaneous protection of patient, professional, and societal interests. Ensuring the efficacy and cost-effectiveness of our services through valid research and proper utilization of support personnel, especially physical therapist assistants, would have a positive impact on cost-related policy issues. We must realize, however, that even with full implementation of

such measures, conflicts will persist. Justice may require some patient or professional interests to be less well-served to secure larger societal interests. It would be morally irresponsible to lobby for narrow patient or professional interests that are contrary to the interests of the commonwealth.

Finding a Balance

Although I have argued for the importance of the community perspective, I also must reinforce the importance of the individual perspective. Rather than devaluing the individual autonomy of our patients or of our profession, we must find a *balance* between the ideal of autonomy and the responsibility to community. We must continue to focus on our ethical duties to the individual: informed consent, the patient's right to know, and confidentiality, to name a few. Furthermore, we must continue to develop high standards as a profession. Ensuring the stability and growth of our profession will itself serve to meet many important patient and societal needs. Thus, let us not abandon the perspectives of patient and profession, but rather expand our perspectives to include the community. 𝖯𝖳

Janet Coy, MA, PT, is Assistant Professor of Physical Therapy, College of Health Related Professions, State University of New York Health Science Center at Syracuse.

References
1 Purtilo RB. To move beyond private opinion. *PT—Magazine of Physical Therapy.* 1993;1(1):94-95.
2 Callahan D. *What Kind of Life: The Limits of Medical Progress.* New York, NY: Simon & Schuster; 1990.
3 Callahan D. Autonomy: a moral good, not a moral obsession. *The Hastings Center Report.* 1984; 14(5):42.
4 Scott RW. For the public good. *PT—Magazine of Physical Therapy.* 1993;1(1):82-85.

HABITS OF THOUGHT

by Ruth B Purtilo, PhD, PT, FAPTA

Protecting the "Care" in Managed Care

Several trends in emerging managed care plans may challenge the PT's commitment to keeping the "care" in health care policies and practices.

Care has long been associated with what health professionals do. At times, we've even been characterized as the "caring professions."[1] It therefore comes as no surprise that the term "managed care" has been chosen to describe the current movement to integrate the delivery and financing of health care in the United States.

In the literature on the managed care approach, however, discussions of care are few and far between. Some of you might say that this also comes as no surprise, because you believe that managed care deals more with *structures* than with the caring dimensions expressed in the professional/patient relationship. Others, however, might take the view that I promote, which is that we must move away from old habits of thought that characterize caring as a function of individuals only. We must create new habits of thought that include the idea of *caring environments* and *caring structures*, not just caring individuals. I further suggest that the ability to carry out our best intentions to be caring as individuals has always been determined in large part by the types of structures in which we work and by the types of policies that guide our practice.

The Caring Environment

If you were a patient, what would *you* consider to be a caring health care environment? Your answer might include procedures that

> We must create new habits of thought that include the idea of caring environments and caring structures, not just caring individuals.

make you feel as though you are being treated with dignity, policies that reassure you that you are not being discriminated against, physical surroundings that create a sense of security and allow you to stay in touch with family members and other sources of emotional support, tolerance and forbearance toward your idiosyncracies, and freedom from undue worry about how you will pay for your treatments. Each of these aspects of a caring environment would take a specific form in a physical therapy clinic, health promotion center, or nursing home.

What type of environment is a caring environment for you as a health professional? It probably is one in which you are allowed to realize some of the same goals, securities, and comforts that your patients want to realize. Such an environment would allow you to carry out your best intentions to be caring within the professional/patient relationship.

Does managed care meet the basic criteria of caring? In a recent *New England Journal of Medicine* article, Emanuel and Dubler[2] assessed the extent to which managed care fosters individual dimensions of caring. They proposed six criteria for evaluating whether the policies of managed care plans preserve the ideals of the professional/patient relationship:

- Patient choice of health care providers and sites.
- Assurance of competence of health professionals.
- Effectiveness and continuity of communication.
- Compassion shown by professionals.
- Continuity of services.
- Absence of conflict of interest within the system.

The authors concluded—correctly, I believe—that managed care plans are too new and too diverse for their effects to be fully known; however, they also urged health professionals to thoughtfully observe and discuss the potential threats to the age-old idea of care.

Seeds of Compromise

Thoughtful discussion about managed care is taking place in the physical therapy profession. The programs and presentations at the 1995 APTA Combined Sections Meeting were one example of the breadth and depth of analysis being undertaken as our profession deals with the impact of managed care on our values and practices.

Several trends in emerging managed care plans pose special challenges to our commitment to keeping the "care" in health care policies and practices. Although each trend has some positive value, each trend also carries seeds of compromise. As you thoughtfully observe the managed care environment, pay close attention to these three important trends:

Reliance on outcomes data to measure quality of care. This trend may lead to the laudable result of more cost-efficient physical therapy interventions. Outcomes research can measure only the "technical" interventions, however; it has difficulty detecting communications activities, coordination of the patient's overall treatment plan, and those interventions that help a patient maintain function. Serious questions must be raised about how outcomes approaches can be refined to more fully include our contributions

to the patient's other needs and life situation. If we become solely technically oriented, we will fail to meet the criterion of treating persons with dignity.

Plans that offer coordinated care—but only within the plan. Managed care plans coordinate delivery and financing of interventions among health professions that previously may have worked in more isolation from each other. This certainly can be of benefit to the patient. In closed-panel managed care plans, however, therapists, physicians, and other professionals are not able to refer patients to qualified professionals who are not in the plan, even when such referrals are in the patient's best interest (see "Managed Care, ERISA, and PT," page 62). This policy cannot be judged as caring—regardless of how cost-efficient it may be.

Patient focused care (PFC). Designed to provide continuity of interventions throughout the patient's course of diagnosis and treatment, the PFC concept deserves

support. But some practices inherent in some PFC approaches—such as cross-training of health professionals and downsizing—may lead to less-than-competent interventions. Trading continuity for competence meets neither the health professional's ideal of treating patients with respect nor the reasonable expectations that patients bring to the health care setting.

Your Influence

No doubt you have identified aspects of managed care that either support or challenge a caring environment. As you think about this, consider the two very different views of managed care that follow.

In June's Letters to the Editor (page 15), Donna Zorn, MPH, PT, wrote:

> Managed care will enhance professional autonomy... The [physical therapy] profession previously worked under the old idea that the more that is done for the patient, the better. Today, with limited resources, professionals will have to

look at what is reasonable for the patient, what is efficacious, and what will help him or her achieve the treatment goals.

If nothing else, managed care is making us look at how we have been practicing and how we can streamline and still maintain quality.... It is good for us every once in a while to take stock of what we do.

In this month's Letters (page 13), however, Lynn Hutchinson, PT, has this to say:

I remember being schooled in the ability to treat—efficiently—two to four patients at a time. After a few years of doing just that, I discovered burnout and dissatisfaction. Therapists need time to listen and touch with beneficence or they lose the reason for being in a medical service profession. I enjoy educating patients in the prevention of future injury and refuse to give up the quality of care that years of experience allow me to give to my patients.

Now I must call and write letters to patient care coordinators and referral coordinators to plead for authorization to treat beyond evaluation. We have lost our autonomy to insurance companies and paper-pushers who are not educated in our profession or even in the medical care aspects of medicine. Sometimes they listen, but more often they read from a well-rehearsed script of denial. This isn't what I've been called to as a therapist...

Whose vision of managed care is "right"?

Clearly, the basic idea of managed care will continue to evolve. Yours can be among the influential voices that will help ensure that practices and policies governing managed care approaches are responsive to the cherished values of the health care professions.

....

 Ruth Purtilo, PhD, PT, FAPTA, is Professor of Clinical Ethics, Creighton University Center for Health Policy and Ethics, Omaha, Neb, and is Past President, American Society of Law, Medicine and Ethics. She is coordinator of Habits of Thought.

References

1 Reich W. Historical dimensions of an ethic of care in the health professions. In: Reich W. *Encyclopedia of Bioethics, vol 1, 2nd ed*. New York, NY: Macmillan & Co Inc; 1995:331-336.

2 Emanuel E, Dubler NN. Preserving the physician-patient relationship in the era of managed care. *N Engl J Med*. 1995;273:323-329.

Suggested Readings

Purtilo R. Interdisciplinary health care teams and health care reform. *American Journal of Law, Medicine, and Ethics*. 1994;22:212-126.

Purtilo R. Managed care: ethical issues for the rehabilitation professions. *Trends in Health Care Law and Ethics*. In press.

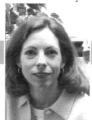

government affairs
by Karen Stavenjord

The Keys to Compliance

Systematic self-monitoring is central to meeting regulatory requirements—and averting risk.

With recent implementation of the Health Insurance Portability and Accountability Act (HIPAA) and the Centers for Medicare and Medicaid Services' (CMS) Comprehensive Error Rate Testing program (CERT), the regulatory landscape is more complex than ever for physical therapists (PTs). Much of what you need to do to comply with these and other federal requirements, however, involves self-monitoring and is grounded in common sense. Let's look at some potential trouble areas for PTs—and the keys to achieving and maintaining compliance.

False Claims

Fraud occurs when an individual practitioner or entity *intentionally* deceives or misrepresents, with the knowledge that the deception or misrepresentation could result in the practitioner or entity gaining an unauthorized benefit. We've all seen news reports about health care practitioners accused of over-billing Medicare or charging for services that never were rendered. When substantiated, such instances are clear examples of fraud.

A number of federal statutes related to fraud prohibit providers from intentionally submitting erroneous claims to and receiving payment from federal health care programs. The civil False Claims Act (31 USC §3729-33), for example, can be invoked when a health care practitioner *knowingly* submits, causes to be submitted, or conspires to submit a fraudulent claim, or a claim for which there is a false record (such as a certification for physical therapy on which the physician's signature has been forged). "Knowingly" has been interpreted by the courts and federal enforcement agencies to mean that the practitioner had actual knowledge that the information on which the claim was based was false, that there was deliberate ignorance of the truth or falsity of a claim (such as intentionally ignoring provider guidance issued by a Medicare carrier), or reckless disregard (such as hiring an inexperienced person to do the practice's billing).

Depending on the applicable statute, penalties for violation can include civil monetary penalties, imprisonment, or exclusion from the Medicare program. Monetary penalties for violating the False Claims Act, for instance, are three times the amount of the fraudulently submitted claims, plus $5,500 to $11,000 per claim.

When a practitioner receives payment to which he or she is not legally entitled for items or services, but *without knowingly and/or intentionally* having misrepresenting facts in order to obtain payment, abuse—not fraud—is taking place. Abuse can occur without the practitioner having actual knowledge of any wrongdoing. The False Claims Act relates to instances of fraud, not abuse.

A Compliance Plan

Types of false claims that may be filed by PTs include:

- ❖ Billing for services furnished by aides or technicians,
- ❖ Providing inadequate supervision,
- ❖ Billing one-on-one codes for a group therapy session,
- ❖ Failure to comply with the 8-minute rule for billable treatment under Medicare,
- ❖ Failure to comply with Medicare Correct Coding Initiative (CCI) edits,
- ❖ Up-coding or unbundling of services,
- ❖ Failure to obtain necessary physician visits for the patient,
- ❖ Failure to obtain certifications or re-certifications from referring providers,
- ❖ Acceptance of cash payment from a patient without having first provided him or her with advanced beneficiary notice (ABN) that the services for which he or she has paid might not be covered by Medicare,
- ❖ Billing for services not furnished,
- ❖ Billing for services performed by a student,
- ❖ Improper documentation or fraudulent modifications to the medical record, and
- ❖ Fraudulent use of a provider number, such as use of an enrolled provider's number for services provided by a non-enrolled physical therapist.

Mary Daulong, PT, CHC, of Business and Clinical Management Services Inc, a health care compliance consulting company, says that while coding and reimbursement issues are key focuses in investigation of fraud and abuse, there are plenty of other risk areas for PTs, as well.

"Per the conditions of participation and coverage, CMS states that an organization, its staff, and/or individual providers must be in compliance with all applicable federal, state, and local laws and regulations," Daulong notes. "So, failing to comply with regulations promulgated by the Occupational Health and Safety Administration, or under the Americans with Disabilities Act, could result in a fraud or abuse claim. Comprehensive compliance, therefore, is what should be strived for at all times."

In October 2000, the Department of Health and Human Services' Office of Inspector General (OIG) issued a document, *Compliance Program Guidance for Individual and Small Group Physician Practices*, that addresses many of these issues. (See box on page 29 for link.) It was written with physician practices in mind, but its elements are relevant to all health care providers.

continued on page 29 ▶▶

government affairs

continued from page 26

Web Resources

APTA:

❖ Fraud and Abuse: www.apta.org/Govt_Affairs/regulatory/fraud_abuse

❖ Assistants, Aides, and Students: www.apta.org/Govt_Affairs/regulatory/Medicare/assistants_aides_students

❖ Coding: www.apta.org/Govt_Affairs/regulatory/Medicare/coding

❖ Documentation: www.apta.org/Govt_Affairs/regulatory/regulatory_documentation

US Department of Health and Human Services, Office of the Inspector General:

❖ Compliance Program Guidance for Individual and Small Group Physician Practices: www.oig.hhs.gov/authorities/docs/physician.pdf

Centers for Medicare and Medicaid Services:

❖ Therapy Resources: www.cms.hhs.gov/medlearn/therapy

❖ Program Memorandums, Transmittals and Manuals: www.cms.hhs.gov/manuals

❖ National Correct Coding Edits: www.cms.hhs.gov/providers/hopps/cciedits/default.asp

❖ HIPAA Information: www.cms.hhs.gov/hipaa/hipaa2

❖ HIPAA Privacy Rule Guidance: www.cms.hhs.gov/ocr/hipaa/privacy.html

certainly contributes to minimizing the chances for fraud and abuse."

A well-crafted set of compliance standards and procedures is an excellent way to protect your practice or place of employment from liability, and to reduce risk in the event of a complaint or audit. PTs should view compliance efforts as wellness and prevention programs for the long-term health of their practice. APTA strongly recommends that PTs—especially those in private practice—strengthen their compliance programs.

HIPAA

APTA encourages PTs to view meeting HIPAA requirements as another facet of their overall regulatory compliance efforts. (See box at left.)

Under its privacy provisions, HIPAA establishes standards for the treatment of

The document lists seven components of an effective compliance program:

❖ Conducting internal monitoring and auditing,

❖ Implementing compliance and practice standards,

❖ Designating a compliance officer or contact,

❖ Conducting appropriate training and education,

❖ Responding appropriately to any detected offenses and developing corrective action,

❖ Developing open lines of communication, and

❖ Enforcing disciplinary standards through well-publicized guidelines.

The OIG maintains that these voluntary steps can be taken by a practice of any size without incurring significant expense. Daulong agrees.

"Most physical therapy practices could develop a compliance plan with some enhancements to their existing policies and procedures," she says. Daulong adds that, while "establishing a compliance plan is not a regulation or even a requirement, I think it is a great insurance policy, and it

government affairs

protected health information. The regulations also outline a complaint procedure for patients who feel that their protected health information has been improperly disclosed, and every physical therapy practice must have an updated manual of policies and procedures to address these standards. Ed Shay, a partner with the Philadelphia, Pennsylvania, law firm of Post and Schell, PC, notes that HIPAA "for the first time, and in a comprehensive manner, forced an industry-wide evaluation of how health information is used and disclosed. The privacy rule," he notes, "also imposed a uniform set of minimum standards for privacy in every state—subject, of course, to the applicability of more stringent state laws."

Shay believes "the existence of the privacy rule has been instrumental to coming developments in electronic prescribing and electronic health records that have been foreshadowed in the recent Medicare pre-

scription drug legislation." HIPAA, he points out, mandated the changes that were needed to enable the health care delivery system to benefit from available technological advancements.

PTs haven't seen the end of new HIPAA provisions, either. Most recently, regulations were released to establish the National Provider Identifier (NPI). When these regulations are implemented, PTs and other health care providers will have a single unique provider number assigned to them that will be used with all payers, further streamlining the electronic claims process. The process of applying for an NPI won't begin until May 2005, so watch for more information on the application process as that date approaches.

"CERTain" Impact

In 2003, CMS implemented CERT, a new system for monitoring the accuracy of

payments. CERT asks practitioners to provide CMS with claims from randomly selected beneficiaries; every carrier and fiscal intermediary is involved. AdvanceMed, the current contractor for this program, uses existing Medicare guidelines, processing guidelines, and local medical review policies (LMRPs) to determine error rates and their causes.

The first report using data generated by the CERT process was released last November. While it found that the overall error rate has been fairly stable in the past few years, it also showed that PTs had one of the highest error rates—18.2%, excluding non-responses. There are still many unanswered questions about the calculation of those error rates, but, regardless, the result is that physical therapy is under increased scrutiny. In this environment, the importance of self-monitoring cannot be overstated.

The good news is that CMS has expressed its intent to provide outreach and education on Medicare guidelines and to work with member groups such as APTA on solving the error rate problem.

A Culture of Compliance

The process of identifying potential weaknesses, training employees in what they need to know, and appointing a person or people to be responsible for compliance is the backbone of establishing an effective compliance program. Compliance is not a matter of discussing written standards once and then filing them away. It is an ongoing process, involving living documents that are used every day and updated frequently to address trouble areas and changing regulations. The benefits of fostering a culture of compliance are numerous—and well worth the expenditure of time and resources. **PT**

Karen Stavenjord is assistant director of the Government Affairs Department at APTA. She can be reached at karenstavenjord@apta.org.

HABITS OF THOUGHT

By John D Banja, PhD

On Fraud and the Rehabilitation Profession

Suspicions about integrity and fiscal responsibility in health care.
Fraud and allegations of fraud in rehabilitation. How can the physical therapy community respond?

*A*llegations of health care fraud are disconcerting to all health professions, and the physical therapy profession is no exception.

Rehabilitation professionals—especially those providing services to people with traumatic brain injury—recently may have felt some shock waves when charges of fraud targeted certain postacute brain injury treatment facilities. Rather than basing patient discharge on functional or clinical criteria, it is alleged, these facilities retained patients until third-party reimbursement was exhausted. Patients and their families further complained that the facilities under investigation not only failed to provide contracted services, but virtually imprisoned patients by staunchly refusing discharge requests made both by the patients themselves and by their families.[1]

Health professionals naturally have been shocked by these charges. The coercion and illicit financial gain implied by the charges are thoroughly at odds with professional values. Society insists not only that health care providers exert a considerable effort to protect and assist persons who seek their services, but that providers also practice a professional morality *explicitly prohibiting* the subordination of health care consumers' interests to professionals' interests. The ease with which health professionals could potentially take illicit advantage of health care consumers has long been noted; values associated with trustworthiness and integrity thus are communicated by educators early in academic training programs.

The *hope*, of course, is that fraudulent practices such as those cited above occur only in the rarest of instances—if they occur at all. Even if this is true, however, rehabilitation professionals should be morally anxious

> *M*any treatments are routinely used in rehabilitation despite the fact that their efficacy is in doubt... But is this really fraud?

about another phenomenon that is not altogether unrelated to fraud: the everyday provision of rehabilitation services *in the absence of an adequate clinical assurance of efficacy.* How often, for example, does a physical therapist discuss a patient's poor prospects for functional improvement with the managing physician, only to be told, "Keep trying for a while longer. You never know. Just see what you can do." And how many treatments are routinely used in rehabilitation despite the fact that their efficacy *in general* is in doubt (eg, coma stimulation, cognitive retraining, and certain psychotropic medications)? [2,3]

But is this really fraud? Decisions to allocate rehabilitation interventions of uncertain value, after all, are not made furtively behind closed doors. Indeed, the provision of rehabilitation to patients for whom the benefits may be questionable typically is *justified* through the language of ethical propriety in statements such as, "Everyone deserves a chance at rehabilitation." Rehabilitation pro-

fessionals therefore may believe that the uncertainty inherent in rehabilitation treatment outcomes is light years removed from the fraudulent practices of the rehabilitation professionals currently under investigation. It is important to realize, however, that the absence of empirically grounded expectations for the efficacy of a particular treatment may help "justify," for example, an extended hospital stay. Appeals to ignorance (eg, "We just don't know whether this treatment will work" and "We won't know for a while")—appeals that ordinarily discourage potential purchasers of services or products in other sectors of the economy—ironically pass as excuses in health care environments for the continuation of treatments and, consequently, of third-party billings.

The rehabilitation professional's adherence to society's standards of professional accountability falls short, then, to the extent that he or she does not or is reluctant to:

1. *Discuss the meaning and probability of an intervention's "success"* with patients and third-party payers.
2. *Allocate services according to scientifically demonstrable indexes* of clinical success or warrant (instead of according to the availability of third-party reimbursement).
3. *Disseminate outcomes research results* that provide empirical grounds for prognoses and an objective gauge to use in determining criteria for rehabilitation candidacy.

This discussion is not intended to impugn the accomplishments of the rehabilitation profession or the extraordinary successes that are an everyday occurrence in rehabilitation settings. The objective of this discussion simply is to acknowledge the relative frequency of admission for certain types of patients for whom the potential for functional improvement is debatable—either because of the severity of their impairments or because of the limitations of available treatment modalities. The fact that "rehabilitation potential" remains largely uninvestigated terrain is an invitation for the rehabilitation community to sustain a serious effort in outcomes research during the next decade. In the years before 2000 and beyond, the cost-conscious environment of health care will *insist* that rehabilitation consumers be identified on clinically—rather than financially—meritorious grounds.

If we as rehabilitation professionals voluntarily take up the challenge of determining "rehabilitation potential" on scientific grounds and allocate rehabilitation treatments according to the findings, our professional integrity will be preserved and our presence in society will be magnified. Indeed, the current suspicions about the integrity of health professionals in general, the demands for cost containment, the predictable penalties for greed or fiscal irresponsibility, and the increasing need for rehabilitation services mean that rehabilitation professionals can no longer afford—literally or figuratively—to avoid this challenge. *PT*

John D Banja, PhD, is Associate Professor of Rehabilitation Medicine and Assistant Professor of Community and Preventive Medicine, Emory University School of Medicine, Atlanta, Ga.

References

1. Centers for head injury accused of neglect. *New York Times.* March 16, 1992:A1.
2. Cope N. Legal and ethical issues in the psychopharmacologic treatment of traumatic brain injury. *Journal of Head Trauma Rehabilitation.* 1989;4:13-22.
3. Brooks N. The effectiveness of post-acute rehabilitation. *Brain Inj.* 1991;5(2):103-109.

JUDGMENT CALL

Allocation of Care: Readers Respond

In October 1996, Jim Dunleavy, PT, presented a dilemma in which a PT was faced with the possibility of being forced to offer different plans of care to patients with similar conditions, based on the patients' health care coverage. Following is a reprint of that scenario, with excerpts of reader responses and commentary by Ruth Purtilo, PhD, PT, FAPTA.

brenda is a staff physical therapist in a medical center outpatient department. She has been assigned to treat two patients with the same diagnosis: anterior cruciate ligament (ACL) tear. Brenda knows from experience that she can most likely get these patients back to their previous level of function using the treatment program she has developed for ACL repairs, which involves 2 months of two or three visits per week.

After Brenda has been assigned to treat both patients, she finds that the two patients' health care plans are very different. Patient X has traditional insurance coverage that will pay 80% of reasonable charges for as long as Brenda provides documentation that shows that treatment is warranted. Patient Y is covered by a managed care plan that allows a maximum of 12 visits for this diagnosis.

Brenda has many concerns related to this situation, including the outcome of treatment for Patient Y.

QUESTIONS FOR THE READER:

1. Does Brenda face a dilemma (ethical, professional, practical, or otherwise)?
If you answered "yes," describe the dilemma.

2. What strategies would you suggest to help Brenda deal with this situation?

3. Should Brenda alter her treatment plan for Patient Y to fit the managed care organization's guidelines?

4. Should Brenda tell Patient Y about the difference between her ideal care plan
and the one she is being asked to offer?

5. Upon what professional standards, ethical principles, ideals, character traits,
and other guidelines do you base your conclusions?

Guidelines Must Not Be Set in Stone

Does Brenda face a dilemma? Yes, ethically, because she may seem to be providing or favoring more care for patients with traditional insurance coverage. Professionally, because Brenda knows that she must provide the same quality of care in a limited time and must tactfully explain this to Patient Y without belittling his or her managed care plan. Also, Patient Y's doctor may have recommended more than 12 visits to completely rehabilitate an ACL tear.

Brenda should provide as much patient education, instruction in self-care, and home exercise programs as possible. She can utilize a PTA and help the PTA devise a detailed outline of an exercise protocol, including precau-

tions and expectations for outcome. Brenda can also try cutting back Patient Y's treatment sessions to 1 or 2 visits per week, with an emphasis on patient education, and she can monitor Patient Y by phone, thereby actually overseeing Patient Y over a 2-month time period.

When 12 visits have been completed and Brenda still feels the patient may benefit from

(continued on next page)

further sessions, she can contact Patient Y's primary care physician and make the recommendation, explaining why. Patient Y's managed care plan may allow for further care if the physician deems it medically necessary.

Brenda can also discuss her strategy with Patient Y to determine what each is trying to accomplish. Patient Y may want to consider paying out-of-pocket, or the facility may agree on some services to be performed free of charge.

Should Brenda alter her treatment plan? I don't think Brenda or we as health care professionals have much of a choice. We would definitely have to alter Patient Y's treatment plan to fit the new guidelines. If all parties involved remain open-minded and flexible, the degree to which the treatment plan is altered may not have to be so serious.

Brenda can tell Patient Y what the insurance company is willing to cover and ask how they can work within these guidelines. I wouldn't offer any further information unless the patient asks. There is no ideal care plan for all patients with any given diagnosis. Progression is dependent on many factors, including patient motivation, continuity, and consistency of care.

Professionally and ethically, the bottom line is to provide high-quality care to our patients. The human aspects must be taken into consideration in all our decision making. Our patient discharge summaries don't always paint a rosy picture, whether a patient is covered by traditional insurance or by managed care.

Certainly, guidelines, rules, and regulations may make our jobs more difficult or challenging, but they are a part of life. As professionals, we want to maintain honest and trusting relationship with our patients, as this will help in instructing them in self care. Setting guidelines may be cost-effective, but they must not be set in stone.

Katie Isgate, PTA
American Rehab Center
Pottsville, Pa

Conclusions Based on Survival
Yes, Brenda faces a dilemma, because Patient Y may not be ready for discharge after 12 visits. Patient X will be able to be seen until he is close to 100% of his previous function. In all practicality, Patient X will make more revenue for the clinic.

Twelve visits should enable Brenda to see

the patient for his medical necessity. Brenda should teach the patient a good home program and have the patient join the gym at the clinic, where he or she can obtain some supervision.

Should Brenda tell Patient Y about the difference in care plans? No. Here in California, we are under a "gag order" that stipulates that we cannot explain details of a patient's plan or we are dropped from the plan. We also cannot explain how little we are reimbursed.

We have been on a capitated managed plan for 4 years. Our clinic has written critical pathways for trying to provide the best care under our restraints. Our conclusions are based on survival.

A private practice outpatient facility
(name withheld by request)
San Francisco Bay area

Be Flexible and Creative
I don't see this situation as a dilemma. I see it as a challenge. Have a positive attitude—see it as an opportunity to grow through the challenge. Be objective—look at the situation for what it is: Two individuals with similar problems. Look at individual differences in the two cases. The therapist should be both flexible and creative enough to arrange her care plans to fit within the parameters of the patient's medical benefit plans.

The therapist should absolutely not reveal differences between a perceived "ideal" plan and the plan she is using. What would it accomplish? The therapist should be mature and professional enough to resist that notion. The patient deserves to have his or her own unique, "ideal" care plan.

Guidelines for conclusions: I referred to my copy of the Illinois practice act. I interpret it as requiring therapists to have high morals, ethics, *always*. My personal values system: 1) respect others, 2) " the golden rule": Do unto others as you'd want them to do to you, 3) empathy. My personality/character traits? I am persistent, I try to be realistically flexible and adaptable, and I like to be creative.

Mary C Wilson, PTA
Coal Valley, Ill

Every Case Must Be Considered on an Individual Basis
Brenda does not face a dilemma. A competent therapist knows that every case must be considered on an individual basis. Only in com-

The scenario I proposed here emphasizes the responsibilities of a professional caregiver to take many factors into account in the professional decision-making process. A caregiver cannot be lulled into the habit of making health care decisions based only upon what is best for the financial survival of the practice. A physical therapist must recognize his or her responsibility to consider the interests of the patient, profession, and society and to devlop a solution to meet their needs. In a managed care environment, the attempt to achieve a balance among all of these partiescan be difficult at best. Managed care requires us to try to *do more with less*. Our responsibility to the patient, the profession, and society is not to allow this to have an adverse impact on the outcome of our care.

This dilemma is another example illustrating the importance of measuring outcomes. Measurement of outcomes will provide us with an opportunity to make better ethical decisions about our care, and it will give us a clear position from which we can argue for the best interests of the patient, profession, and society, including a quantity of service provision that is required to meet the outcome, or quality of care, that they demand.

Jim Dunleavy, PT
Department of Rehabilitation Medicine
St Luke's—Roosevelt Hospital Center,
New York, NY
President, Acute Care Section

placent—and incompetent—physical therapy is the treatment the same for every patient with a particular injury. Brenda has been given the parameters for treatment: One patient has health care coverage that allows Brenda an unlimited amount of time in which to treat. The other patient must be treated within 12 visits. The goal for each is the same: For the physical therapist to devise innovative and successful therapy treatments.

Brenda should gather as much information as she can about the patient, both from the medical record and patient interview. For example, is this person motivated enough to work independently at home? Does he or she this medical center, and as long as the medical center accepts the two "very different" health care plans, she has an ethical obligation to provide the services as dictated by both payer and employer.

A much larger issue is that Brenda has the perception (most likely, from my clinical experience, an incorrect perception) that ACL repairs somehow require 16 to 24 postoperative visits. This view is contrary to that of myself and others. Brenda needs to rethink what is truly clinically necessary.

Brenda needs to determine whether she is willing to adapt to the system mandated by her employer, and, if not, resign her position. If she is willing to adapt to the needs of the employer and the employer's payers, then she needs to review the literature, which is certainly contrary to her perception regarding number of physical therapy visits. Once her literature review is complete, she needs to adopt a new value-efficient care path for treating ACL problems.

Should she tell Patient Y about the difference in care? Only if Patient Y questions the care that he or she is receiving.

The literature concerning postop ACL rehabilitation is nebulous and sketchy as to the need for large number of visits. A major goal of physical therapy is to empower patients toward self-care and responsibility. When looking at ethical principles, it is important to understand the needs of all parties concerned, in this case the patient, the payer, the employer, and, finally, the physical therapists. It is the task and professional responsibility of the professional caregivers in the United States to adapt to the needs of all parties concerned in such a dilemma as the one above.

Until outcomes data and peer-reviewed research support the need for extensive postoperative physical therapy visits (which is not the case in most orthopedic problems), we need to look to ourselves as caregivers to develop goal-oriented phase programs, with an emphasis on home programs when the patient has reached certain goals and a certain phase and when progressing to another phase requires only time, based on healing constraints (perceived or real).

More importantly in this hypothetical situation, we are viewing a health care plan that is basically traditional and based on therapists' documentation for more visits, and a managed care plan that allows a maximum of only 12 visits for this diagnosis. Physical therapists should consider the relevance and greater value of accepting a capitation plan rather than either of these two plans mentioned above. In a capitated setting, particularly if there could be some financial risks on Brenda's part, she might be motivated to look toward improved clinical efficiencies.

James E Glinn, Sr, PT, President
Glinn & Giordano Physical Therapy Inc
Bakersfield, Calif

Individualizing Programs
Each patient should receive the same treatment program. Frequency of visits will be different because of the insurance guidelines, but a few therapy visits are better than none, and it's unlikely either payer will change its policies (although a maximum of 12 for an ACL repair is ridiculous—I hope the patient isn't an athlete).

No change is necessary for Patient X, except maybe twice a week versus three have the proper equipment at home? What kind of lifestyle does he or she have? Brenda then should look at her treatment program and identify the elements that require a therapy visit, and the elements that can be performed by the patient. Finally, she should set treatment goals, and determine the strategy and tactics that will accomplish them, prior to beginning therapy. It would be impossible for Brenda to plan a successful treatment without keeping the imposed time limit in mind.

Brenda should inform the patient about the difference between her ideal care plan and the one she is being asked to offer. There have been occasions in the history of physical therapy when a patient was willing to pay for extra visits that the insurance company didn't cover. The patient should be consulted during development of the treatment plan, and ultimately, should make the decision of whether to receive the gourmet 2-month treatment plan or the abbreviated version.

I base my conclusions on the *Code of Ethics* of the American Physical Therapy Association, particularly those principles that state that 1) physical therapists accept responsibility for the exercise of sound judgment; 2) physical therapists maintain and promote high standards for physical therapy practice; 3) physical therapists provide accurate information to the consumer about the profession and about those services they provide; and 4) physical therapists accept the responsibility to protect the public and the profession from unethical, incompetent, or illegal acts.

Also contributing to my conclusions is my belief that the patient's needs are the highest priority in physical therapy decision making. Therapists, of course, can't give away their services for free; in today's health care systems, I guess the best we can do is make the best decisions in consultation with the patient, within the framework of existing finances.

Kathleen Doehla, SPT
Virginia Commonwealth University/
Medical College of Virginia
Richmond, Va

A Hierarchy of Needs

Yes, Brenda has a dilemma. Brenda's expectation is that 16 to 24 treatments are necessary to reach an optimal therapeutic outcome for Patient Y. Reducing the treatments by 50% should certainly make her feel uneasy; other-

wise, the implication is that she was not providing "medically necessary" treatments to patients with ACL injuries like Patient X in the past.

Besides the professional dilemma, Brenda does have an ethical problem. She fears an unfortunate rehabilitation outcome for Patient Y after an already messy situation of an ACL injury and reconstructive surgery, unless Patient Y is given 8 to 12 additional treatments. She might believe that Patient Y has a "right" to these additional visits, based on how medical coverage has worked in the past. In those former days, she just followed the frequency orders that were handed to her and only asked questions when something was really askew, but rarely made her own judgments and decisions.

Brenda's strategies should begin by recog-

∾

"Does patient Y have a 'right' to the Gold plan? Since there is certainly a need for health care cost containment, could there not be an acceptable Silver or Bronze plan?"

∾

nizing her own assumptions in this situation. Questions she might ask herself: Is Patient Y capable of an independent home program under specific instruction? Would this be an adequate alternative? Are there other known cases involving ACL rehab with fewer treatments? What were the outcomes? How were those cases like or unlike Patient Y's? Could there be optimal outcomes apart from the 24-treatment (Gold) plan? Do all patients with ACL injuries need 16 to 24 treatments? Could some patients do well with fewer treatments, or would others do better with more than 24 treatments?

Does Patient Y have a "right" to the Gold plan? Since there is certainly a need for health care cost containment, could there not be an acceptable Silver or Bronze plan? If yes, then why not just try to work with the 12 visits?

If Brenda believes that Patient Y clearly needs the 24-treatment Gold Plan and that nothing less will do, are alternative financing, reduced rates, or even brief, no-fee treatments

(partly on Brenda's time) an option? Brenda would then have to force one of these options to get out of her dilemma.

Brenda should alter the treatment program by staggering the treatments earlier in the program and placing more responsibility on the patient.

If Patient Y's health plan is clearly restrictive compared with other health plan options, *and* this difference would clearly have a detrimental effect on the patient's long-term outcome, then, yes, Brenda should bring this to Patient Y's attention. Brenda should be aware, however, that the choice of health plans may be based on factors that serve the patient's needs other than just physical therapy coverage, such as hospitalization, affordability, etc. In many cases, there are better choices, but if the current choice is adequate, it's probably better to leave well enough alone.

I believe that in the real world there is a hierarchy of needs. Life-threatening needs in an intensive care unit take precedence over gait difficulties from bed to bathroom and running 5 miles without pain.

I believe our relatively affluent society has a responsibility to address those most urgent needs by dispensing its resources. However, for the lesser needs (eg, jogging 5 miles without pain), the individual ought to be willing to carry a heavier financial burden for treatment beyond a minimal starting point begun by an insurance plan.

Patients and their therapists should be free to accept the limits of insurance coverage or to explore payment options for further treatment. The government's role should be to ensure that prospective subscribers are provided clear information by health plans when making insurance choices.

Vincent Gatto, PT
Reading Physical Therapy
Reading, Mass

Adapt to the Needs of All Parties

Brenda's dilemma is simple. a) She is a staff physical therapist employed by b) a medical center outpatient department. In accepting that employment, she has tacitly approved agreements that her employer may make with third-party payers. In short, as long as she is a staff physical therapist employed by
(continued on next page)

times a week, to keep the patient's 20% payment down. Twice a week falls within the therapist's guidelines. Patient Y can receive the same 2-month program with properly managed frequency and a very detailed home program. The patient can be scheduled for twice a week for 4 weeks, then once a week for 4 weeks. Patient Y can borrow weights, tubing, whatever, from the therapy department, trading out as progression is made, then purchasing at discharge what is needed. Even home electrical muscle stimulation can be made available, if necessary, and usually just in the first 2 or 3 weeks. Walking can be utilized as the aerobic activity versus the stationary bike in the department. The patient can be instructed in self-mobilizing and self passive-range-of-motion techniques if range of motion is a problem.

A patient shouldn't be "punished" with a skimpier care plan because of the insurance plan's guidelines. With clever designing from the therapist, patients can receive the same program. (Exercise programs are easier to manipulate than a modality program.)

Should she tell the patient about the difference in plans? NO. She can still offer her ideal care plan, but home management will be a larger factor. Care needs to be taken that the insurance isn't "bad mouthed" and the patient ends up distrusting the payer. The program can be made to work in 12 visits over 8 weeks without causing bad relations between patient and insurance/therapist and insurance/patient and therapist.

I've been in this situation (Medicare edits). Individualizing programs to patients is something I feel strongly about. What if Patient Y had a fine insurance plan, but because of transportation problems could only come 1 or 2 days per week? The patient shouldn't be made to feel something is wrong with the insurance plan or that his or her therapy will be any different from anyone else's.

Proper and thorough documentation will keep the therapist on the insurance's "good" side. In the long run, this could lead to insurance guideline changes.

S Monique Brownlee, PT,
Certified Personal Trainer
Rehabworks/ARA
Jonesboro, Ark

An Advocate for Her Patient

The following conclusions represent a compilation of ideas from 34 about-to-graduate physical therapy students with a variety of backgrounds and clinical rotation experience.

We disagreed about whether Brenda faces an ethical dilemma. Some believed that Brenda is not facing an ethical dilemma, that Brenda should be flexible with her rehab protocol and realize that with recent changes in health care, there will be more cases limited to a certain number of visits. Others believed that Brenda faces both ethical and professional dilemmas. Ethically, she has a responsibility to her

~

Care needs to be taken that the insurance isn't "bad mouthed" and the patient ends up distrusting the payer.... The patient shouldn't be made to feel something is wrong with the insurance plan or that his or her therapy will be any different from anyone else's.

~

patient to provide the most appropriate care within her abilities. Professionally, she has a responsibility to her employer to provide reimbursable care.

Brenda should educate Patient Y about the severity of her injury, surgery, and the extensive rehabilitations that follow ACL reconstruction. This could motivate the patient and make the patient responsible for her rehabilitation through home exercise programs. If Brenda does not see appropriate range of motion and strength gains in her patient with home programs, then she should be an advocate for her patient by calling the insurance company. Brenda could provide the insurance company with documentation and research showing that her patient is not making significant

progress, and request more visits.

We believe Brenda should alter her treatment plan to fit into the managed care guidelines. Brenda should be flexible to meet the needs of both her patient and her employer.

We disagreed about whether Brenda should tell Patient Y about the difference between the two care plans. Some of us believed Brenda should not tell her about the differences, because this might have a negative psychosocial impact on the patient that would eventually affect the patient's status. Also, the patient might think that because Brenda was limited to 12 visits, those 12 visits are enough, and Brenda should be able to work with them. Furthermore, it is possible that the patient knew what type of insurance plan he or she had and was aware that there would be limited access to physical therapy services. Finally, this group thought Patient Y should not be informed until it was evident that under this plan, he or she was receiving inadequate care.

Other members of the class felt that Brenda should inform her patient of the differences between the care plans and that the patient could be a spokesperson for him- or herself and call the insurance company to request more visits. Also, they felt this would further motivate the patient.

We based our decisions on professional standards and ethical principles stated in the APTA *Code of Ethics*. Furthermore, our decisions are based on information received through the University of Indianapolis academic program, which has increased our awareness, not only of health care changes, but also of how managed care will influence our practice.

Physical Therapy Class of '96
University of Indianapolis

(continued on next page)

Published responses to Judgment Call are the opinions of their authors. They should not be construed as the opinions or positions of *PT* or of the American Physical Therapy Association.

Commentary

These thoughtful responses create a context for several comments I will add.

The good news is that the challenge Brenda faces is not new. In our professional lifetimes, the extent and type of treatment offered to patients have in large part been governed by third-party reimbursers (eg, Medicaid, Medicare, private insurers), and these reimbursement sources frequently have supported different types of interventions, lengths of stay, and other variables for a given condition. Brenda's worry that Patient Y may not receive optimal or even adequate treatment because of the constraints imposed by the third-party payment source is familiar to every reader who has spent any time in practice. Therefore, Brenda—and we as a profession—have a long and rich experience to draw from in trying to respond ethically to this type of situation.

In a nutshell: *The patient's best interests always have been, and must continue to be, the guiding beacon in deciding when the therapist has fulfilled her or his professional duty.*

Brenda's act of voluntarily accepting employment helps to set her future decisions. Several respondents suggest what she may or may not be able to do based on what they are able to do in the different settings where they work. Like all of us, she has agreed to conduct herself according to the plan's rules and expectations. Philosophers call this type of agreement a "social contract," meaning that what is right and wrong, or good and bad, is determined by the parties involved. Because almost all employment agreements are social contracts, therapists should examine diligently the conditions to which they are agreeing when signing an employment contract. Brenda's contract with her employer is the appropriate ethical standard for her behavior if, and only if, its stipulations enable her to fulfill her duty of due care for patients. The "duty of due care" is the way society (eg, the law) describes professionals' duty to protect patient interests by providing *at least* the minimal type and amount of intervention that a patient's condition calls for. Most therapists would like to go beyond that minimal standard (described today as doing what is "medically necessary") to do what's optimal for each patient, but no one has the ethical or legal prerogative to offer less than the minimum.

Most of the respondents are creative in helping Brenda find a just and humane approach to her situation. They note that if Brenda is correct (ie, if adequate coverage is not provided through Patient Y's plan), she must seek alternatives that will approximate the preferred course without falling below a minimally acceptable regime.

Several respondents urge Brenda to evaluate whether she really needs to offer as many treatments as Patient X's plan allows. Others suggest home care or other alternatives. Their comments highlight the need for vigilant resistance to accepting norms of treatment based simply on "the way things are done" as well as for continued research into what is indeed medically necessary.

Suppose that Brenda cannot discern even a minimally acceptable alternative because of the constraints built into Patient Y's plan. Gatto is correct in suggesting that in this case Brenda should inform her patient. At least 16 states have already passed "anti-gag rule" legislation regarding managed care organizations, recognizing that the integrity of the professional-patient relationship is seriously compromised if professionals are prevented ("gagged") from disclosing relevant information; in this case, the professional cannot offer what she believes is the preferred course of treatment because it is not available through the patient's health plan. For some patients, disclosure of this information would enhance their freedom of choice, since they could decide to go elsewhere. Unfortunately, not every patient has that option. And, as for Brenda, if time after time she is faced with this course of action, she may be better off to seek employment elsewhere (again, unfortunately a choice not every professional has the freedom to make).

Glinn's consistent attention to society's needs and interests reminds readers that physical therapists sometimes have taken solely self-interested positions that have not served society well. Assuredly everyone's interests must be taken into account in policy decisions. However, I join respondent Doehla in placing the role of the physical therapist more squarely as patient advocate than Glinn's comments seem to recommend. Members of society still depend on professionals to be advocates for them in matters that the public cannot always best gauge. We cannot be all things to all people, and in our role as professional we are given license (literally) with all of its privileges, to speak on behalf of protecting patients' interests (their healthfulness itself being a social good) above the interests of taxpayers, above happiness, or above any other social good.

Current managed care arrangements, which integrate delivery and financing of health care services, are but a beginning attempt to address the serious problems our society has created in the way that health care services currently are provided. Many refinements will be attempted, and it will take the involvement of everyone, especially health care professionals, to create a morally justifiable balance of interests. The loyalties and thoughtfulness that Brenda brings to this moment of decision making will go beyond what patient Y receives. Through such decisions, patients will come to know what to expect, practitioners will decide what their future role will be, and policymakers will learn what they can and cannot tinker with when it comes to the traditional professional duty of placing the patient's interests first.

Ruth B Purtilo, PhD, PT, FAPTA, is Professor of Clinical Ethics and Director, Creighton University Center for Health Care Policy and Ethics, Omaha, Neb, and Past President, American Society of Law, Medicine, and Ethics.

JUDGMENT CALL

by Ruth Purtilo, PhD, PT, FAPTA

Modality Utilization: Readers Respond

In March's Judgment Call, Ron Hruska, MPH, PT, presented a dilemma in which the director of a physical therapy department was instructed by an administrator to increase provision of "billable" services. Following is a reprint of that scenario and excerpts of reader responses, with commentary by Hruska and Ruth Purtilo, PhD, PT, FAPTA.

*m*ark is the director of a suburban, hospital-affiliated, outpatient physical therapy clinic. He supervises five other PTs on site.

Mark is a relatively new supervisor. Shortly after assuming supervisory duties, he had instructed his staff to consider whether, in some cases, modalities were being used unnecessarily when patient education might be just as beneficial to the patient.

Bill is the administrator of the hospital affiliated with the clinic. Bill receives a monthly report from Mark summarizing activity and revenue related to procedures, modalities, and other services provided. Approximately 70% of the revenue generated by the clinic reflects contractual discounted fee-for-service activity.

Over a period of several months, Bill notes that although there is a consistent pattern of referrals, there is a slow but steady decrease in revenue as a result of the decreased use of modalities and the increased time spent on patient education. Bill calls Mark and expresses his concern about the budget projections and current revenue patterns. He tells Mark, "I suggest you look closely at improving the number of procedures per patient visit, or you may be asked to decrease staffing."

Mark is concerned about his staff's job security. He also feels the pressure to account for the decline in revenue that resulted from the drop in modality and procedure utilization. He cannot increase the current fees being charged for services without risking the loss of his current fixed-fee contracts.

Mark reluctantly considers encouraging the staff to increase modality or procedure utilization per visit whenever possible.

QUESTIONS FOR THE READER:

1. How will Mark's decision affect his staff's ability to serve as advocates for their patients?

2. What ethical and/or professional responsibilities lie ahead for Mark and his staff?

3. What alternatives exist for Mark and the other PTs on staff?

4. Upon what professional principles, ethical principles, ideals, character traits, and other guidelines do you base your conclusions?

Author's Comments

The ethical dilemma I presented for this installment of Judgment Call illustrates the impact that cost-containment can have on the quality of service provided.

Managed care implies a demand for higher efficiency in briefer time periods. It also frequently means lower rates of reimbursement for procedures. Discounted fee-for-service arrangements, reduction or waiver of coinsurance arrangements, acceptance of Medicare assignment only, and other fixed-price-per-service arrangements can force the provider to look at other cost-shifting measures to meet revenue targets or demands. With these increasing restrictions in third-party reimbursement, physical therapists are finding themselves faced with ethical dilemmas resulting from conflicts between financial obligations and moral obligations. For example, maintaining balances between utilization of modalities and patient advocacy can be difficult; for some, it may not be possible. This real-life dilemma reflects that reality.

Ron Hruska, MPA, PT
Saint Elizabeth
Community Health Center
Lincoln, Neb

Emphasizing Skilled Treatment

We see Mark in a position in which many hospital department directors, physical therapist administrators, and private practitioners have found themselves over the years, particularly as the profession of physical therapy has become identified—both within and outside of our immediate professional circles—chiefly with the provision of and reimbursement for modalities.

Certainly, ethical, professional, and other issues will need to be addressed by Mark and Bob, as well as by the staff they employ, as they attempt to resolve real or perceived conflicts. Clearly, we as PTs are bound by our *Standards of Practice, Code of Ethics, Guide for Professional Conduct*, and our own consciences in providing physical ther-apy-related services. The answer to Mark's conflict is not necessarily in opposition to what our code or our consciences should direct us to do.

There has been a long history of overutilization and abuse of modalities. Despite the diversity of both licensed and nonlicensed professionals responsible for this trend, physical therapists have been the primary professionals blamed for these excesses, which have cost insurers billions of dollars and have been a chief reason for the aggressive focus on cost-containment in physical therapy by outside agencies. The incentives for the ongoing use and billing of primarily modality-oriented treatments have often been identified as 1) modalities' ease of application relative to more intensive therapeutic procedures, 2) the limited human resources required in providing modality services, and 3) a relative value scale that provided the same financial reward for a hot pack as it allowed for 30 minutes of a more resource-intensive therapeutic procedure. It did not take long for providers of all types to recognize that greater modality use meant greater profitability and less work. Historically, payment methodologies throughout the country have inadvertently encouraged modality billing through financial incentives.

Today, however, there have been significant modifications in the Resource-Based Relative Value Scale (RBRVS) of the Physical Medicine and Rehabilitation CPT codes. Relative value methodology is the cornerstone of the Medicare payment system, which the payer community is quickly adopting as the universal methodology for payment for all medical services, including physical therapy.

The relative values for supervised modalities have been decreased, while the relative values for therapeutic procedures have increased. There has also been a reduction in the time increments for therapeutic procedures, from 30 to 15 minutes, which more closely resemble the times associated with "unit" structures used by clinics and hospitals. This means that if facilities are utilizing an RBRVS fee schedule to bill for services and payers are utilizing an RBRVS-based fee schedule to reimburse for those services, facilities will see a decrease in the reimbursement allowances for modalities and an increase in the reimbursement allowances for skilled therapeutic procedures, including patient education.

Why is this important to Mark and Bob? Quite simply, if Mark has a good understanding of RBRVS, he can very effectively demonstrate to Bob that a treatment paradigm of modality-focused care not only may be based on poor clinical judgment, be in conflict with our ethical code, and not be in the best interest of the patient, but that utilization of multiple modalities in place of more skilled, functionally based restorative treatment interventions might have a negative impact on the department's bottom-line profitability. Mark should be able to demonstrate that the more emphasis that is placed on skilled or educational treatment approaches, the greater the reimbursement per visit, and, therefore, the greater the department's profit margin. Now *that* is something that will attract Bob's attention!

Mark also should be able to accurately code the patient education services he is performing in his clinic so that appropriate reimbursement is obtained. He should encourage Bob to assess how a shift from modality-based treatment to more therapeutic and educational interventions will affect patient outcomes and length of stays in his clinic. Mark should be confident that his instructions and advice to his staff regarding the focus on patient education and other skilled therapeutic procedures is sound and consistent with ethical and professional standards. Through the incorporation of this advice, his physical therapy clinic should see an increase in revenue as a result of performance of skilled therapeutic and educational procedures and an improvement in patient outcomes as a result of this more skilled intervention, not to mention an increase in the level of professional respect from the payer community, the public, and other medical professionals.

Stephen M Levine, PT
Spine and Sports Rehab
Timonium, Md
APTA Representative to the
AMA Relative Value Update Committee
of the Health Care Provider Advisory
Committee Review Board

(continued on next page)

"Re-engineering" to Fit

An important starting point of this discussion is that Mark has identified a specific treatment philosophy for his staff and department. Bill gives Mark the autonomy to decide how to handle the situation. However, carrying out the treatment philosophy creates a quandary for Mark as a neophyte director.

Although the system envisions and encourages his current behavior, it has not fully embraced it by modifying reimbursement mechanisms to make it feasible, and although Mark and his staff's decisions regarding the clinical needs of their patients are appropriate, he must adjust the practice environment to achieve implementation.

Initially, Mark has a responsibility to understand and verify the "budget projections and current revenue patterns" of which Bill is speaking if he is to effectively manage change.

Let's assume that Mark and his staff continue to support a clinical decision-making model in which patient education is more appropriate than modalities in some situations. Mark then needs to work with Bill to re-engineer his department and the hospital to achieve this model. Through interaction with major payers in the market, the case for appropriate use and reimbursement of selected services can be made. Future hospital contracts can be modified to reflect the nature of the physical therapy services they offer. Mark and his staff can show the payers that patient education converts to dollars saved in terms of patient outcomes and satisfaction.

To achieve improved client outcomes through education, the department needs to select or develop effective patient educational materials, including brochures, videos, lectures, and World Wide Web sites. Standardization of education approaches will be important to document outcomes showing that education as a treatment choice is comparable to use of modalities in terms of positive patient outcomes and thus is equally reimbursable.

From a practice standpoint, Mark must recognize that the financial resources of the disappearing fee-for-service environment are no longer the norm. The new model of efficiency and effective visits is characterized by per-visit and case-based caps, DRGs, and capitation. Gone is the assumption that increased costs of labor or materials can easily be passed on to the patient and the payers.

Mark must diversify his staff, staffing, and practice activities. For example, Mark and his staff need to explore other areas of practice, both by specialty and practice site, that might bring additional revenue to the hospital. By aggressively seeking to diversify services, Mark and his staff show a commitment to maintaining control over their clinical decision-making while recognizing the realities of the current health care environment. This proactive stance is a somewhat new behavior now required of the PT who cannot hope for his or her director's protection in a system where the rules change daily. This is not "someone else's problem."

I base these conclusions on the professional standards of maintaining control over what type of physical therapy treatment is or is not needed and on the ethical principles of assuring the patient that a decision is patient-centered and is not driven by financial incentives.

Francis J Welk, MEd, PT
Susquehanna Physical Therapy Associates
Bloomsburg, Pa
(Member, APTA Board of Directors,
APTA Risk Management and Member
Benefits Committee, and
Private Practice Section Board of Directors)

Presenting Alternatives

Managed care has forced us as PTs to examine practices such as the use of modalities. We had become complacent practitioners, continuing to use physical agents, sometimes without good research to support their usage.

To respond to the decrease in revenue by restoring increased modality use would be a temporary and irresponsible solution. This type of response has led us to the situation where we are today, when professional decisions made by licensed PTs are questioned by third-party payers.

To respond to the ever-present and real bottom line of lost revenue, Mark needs to present alternatives. He has already taken a step in the right direction by moving toward patient education as a treatment focus, but this does not need to take more of the PT's time than use of modalities! Use group treatment sessions for patients with similar diagnoses. These group sessions can be alternated with individual treatment sessions or modified as needed for the patient's and the practice's needs. Another revenue-generating alternative along this same line of practice philosophy may be "back school," group educational sessions, or wellness programs for patients to continue exercising after skilled physical therapy is no longer indicated. Depending on the state practice act, qualified support personnel may be able to run these alternatives, with the supervision and guidance of a PT.

Mark can make some very positive changes for his practice, as long as he doesn't back down. He can respond to the concerns of the hospital administrator while serving as a patient advocate and providing the best possible care.

Patricia M Adams, MPT
Clinical Instructor of Physical Therapy
Rutgers University/University of
Medicine and Dentistry
Camden, NJ

Taking the Middle Ground

I believe the dilemma presented was very real, and does occur often in the workplace, not only on the corporate level but in independent practice settings. Insurance intermediaries have customarily reimbursed for the technical parts of medical and physical therapy practices instead of professional components of the practice. CPT codes are the most often-utilized descriptive entity in reimbursement for practice, but most active practitioners don't feel the codes adequately reflect the practice of physical therapy. The dilemma has softened with the new CPT codes reflecting direct, one-on-one time with the patient by the therapist (97530, 97535, and others), which can be offered to third-party payers in place of the traditional modality codes.

Mark cannot offer free services to the patients seen in the hospital outpatient clinic without the direct acceptance of this practice by the hospital administration. He also cannot force his physical therapy staff to perform services that are not necessary for the recovery of function of the patients of the clinic. Mark must take the middle ground, practicing reimbursable physical therapy, utilizing the existing CPT codes to define the services rendered, and reducing staff if these codes do not render enough reimbursement to meet the financial goals of the hospital and outpatient clinic.

I do not believe that modality usage and patient education are diametrically opposed to one another. Modalities would be used as a component of preparation of tissues, comfort to the patient, or alleviation of inflammation and its symptoms. Application of modalities can also be delegated to acceptable support personnel when possible to free the PT for other activities. Patient education is a necessary component of almost any treatment plan of care, and it can and should be billed separately from other care components. Both can easily coexist in most treatment protocols and regimes. Mark was right to ask his therapists to utilize more patient education, but he did not have to do this at the exclusion of other intervention.

Bill is acting within his job requirements in asking the physical therapy staff to show appropriate billings for the time utilized in the treatment of patients in the clinic. If he is asking for procedures to be done just to increase revenue, he needs to be reprimanded by Mark. However, I took Bill's message to Mark as saying that he wanted to see billed time equal to time spent with the patient in the clinic by the therapists. Shouldn't an administrator *expect* billed time to equal time spent on work activities by his employees?

I see minimal conflict in the *Standards of Practice for Physical Therapy*, the *Code of Ethics*, or the needs related to patient/therapist advocacy if all parties perform in the following manner: Treat the patient in the most appropriate manner, use the appropriate billing terminology to receive adequate reimbursement for services rendered, utilize appropriate support personnel to help in the administration of services at the most cost-efficient level, and reduce staff if necessary to maintain cost-efficient care of the patients, keeping the other criteria in mind.

Steven W Forbush, MS, PT
Millhopper Physical Therapy
Gainesville, Fla

Commentary by Ruth Purtilo, PhD, PT, FAPTA

Welk summarizes one part of the ethical dilemma posed by this situation in his statement, "Mark has identified a specific treatment philosophy for his department. Bill gives Mark the autonomy to decide how to handle the situation." He identifies the other part of the dilemma in his observation that Mark faces serious constraints when he attempts to carry out that philosophy.

An ethical dilemma is a situation in which the person responsible for the outcome (the "agent") is presented with two or more right courses of action but finds that to act on one will necessarily compromise the other. Ancient Greek tragedies portray moral agents in these types of situations. The moral agent in our story is Mark.

Almost all of the respondents correctly identified the two right courses of action: One is to provide high-quality physical therapy interventions on the basis of good clinical judgment. That is the mark of a true professional, and the foundation on which society "licenses" PTs to practice. As Levine and Forbush note, this mark of professionalism is the governing theme in our ethical codes and professional documents (eg, *Standards of Practice for Physical Therapy, Code of Ethics*, and *Guide for Professional Conduct*). Mark judges that modality use as a means of increasing revenues is inconsistent with his best clinical judgment. Adams concludes that if Mark does not act on his best clinical judgment, "increased modality use would be a temporary and *irresponsible* solution" (italics mine).

The other right course of action that Mark recognizes is to devise and honor measures designed to ensure that the department will remain financially responsible. The mechanisms currently designed to achieve those ends are addressed by several of our respondents. The basic conceptual orientation of managed care, which will affect many—some predict all—physical therapy practices, is to provide high-quality services at the lowest cost possible. The strength of this orientation is that pro-

fessionals have an ethical duty not only to individual patients, but also to society's larger needs. Levine suggests that physical therapy has sometimes neglected this aspect of its professionalism through a "history of overutilization and abuse of modalities."

How irresolvable is Mark's dilemma? Does it have the characteristics of a true Greek tragedy, in which fate has placed Mark in the hapless position of necessarily compromising one cherished value for the other? Is high-quality physical therapy treatment at an irresolvable moral standoff with financially viable approaches?

All of the respondents believe that Mark still has "elbow room" to at least partially diminish the harm that would be done if the conflict were irresolvable. In the fashion so reflective of PTs, the respondents identified alternatives that would help Mark resolve the dilemma.

Some of the suggestions focus on changing times and PTs' willingness to accommodate in areas that *do not compromise quality*. Old habits and entrenched practices sometimes become mistaken for high-quality care; another major theme in the responses is the ethical responsibility to evaluate and revise such habits and practices. For example, outcomes approaches should not be dismissed out-of-hand based on our lack of familiarity with this way of determining quality. Among the suggestions offered by respondents: paying attention to practices that incur high overhead, diversifying areas of practice, and understanding how the RBRVS works.

The suggestions made by respondents show an optimistic view that although the challenges facing PTs' deepest values are real, now is by no means the moment to claim that moral tragedy is the only possible result. The diligent search for alternatives and our participation in refining our mechanisms are tools for preserving our ethical standing as professionals.

Ruth Purtilo, PhD, PT, FAPTA, is Professor of Clinical Ethics, Creighton University Center for Health Care Policy and Ethics, Omaha, Neb, and Past President, American Society of Law, Medicine, and Ethics.

JUDGMENT CALL

by Christopher J Hughes, PhD, PT

A Move to the Competition: Readers Respond

In December 1996, Ron Hruska, MPA, PT, presented a dilemma related to philosophy of care and job security in today's managed care environment. Below are some responses from readers, with commentary by Hruska and by ethicist Ruth Purtilo, PhD, PT, FAPTA.

Kim works in an independent practice, Northside Physical Therapy, with five other physical therapists. The practice has grown successfully, with an average annual increase of 12% to 15% in caseload volume—until this year. The group is finding managed care organization (MCO) contracts more difficult to accept because of low payment rates and increasingly higher discount demands. Last year's business reflected an increase of MCO activity by 50%; this year, MCO activity has been reduced by 20%.

Kim has always respected this independent therapists' group for its philosophy of high-quality care, reasonable caseloads, and realistic functional outcome expectations. Now, she worries about the pressure being exerted by managed care (eg, increased discount demands, orientation toward a higher volume of patients, and contracts establishing insufficient capitated reimbursement rates). In addition to agreeing to discount some services and increase the caseload volume, the group has increased utilization of support personnel, extended its hours of operation, and shortened the time slots for new evaluations. However, group members are holding fast in their opposition to new contracts that offer what they feel are unreasonably low reimbursement rates, citing concerns about the potential negative impact on the level of care they will be able to provide.

Practices with longer MCO contracting histories are able to command higher reimbursement rates, which is frustrating for Kim and her associates. Kim has been approached by one of these longer-established practices, Southside Physical Therapy, to work with them. Based on visits to the facility and conversations with PTs who have worked there, Kim believes that the practice philosophy at Southside Physical Therapy is oriented more toward the business aspects of practice and less toward the high-quality care on which her group prides itself. However, after considering her associates' lack of success in establishing competitive rates of reimbursement with local MCOs, Kim is seriously contemplating a move to the competition, for her own job security.

QUESTIONS FOR THE READER:

1. Describe the dilemma Kim is facing. What is the nature of the dilemma—ethical, professional, legal, practical, or other?

~

2. Would Kim's dilemma be different if her current group had agreed to contract at the lower rate?

~

3 What are Kim's options in this situation? What are her associates' options?

~

4. Upon what professional standards, ethical principles, ideals, character traits, and other guidelines do you base your conclusions?

Hierarchy of Needs

The psychologist Maslow proposed that human needs are arranged into a hierarchy, with basic needs such as food and warmth at the bottom and higher needs, including safety, love, and self-esteem, in ascending order above the basic needs. At the top of the hierarchy, Maslow placed "self-actualization," the need to be and do what one is born to do (ie, a person's "calling").

As managed care has an impact on practice procedures, business practices, and possibly quality of care, physical therapists will be challenged to re-address their own hierarchy of needs in order to advocate effectively for their patients. The ethical and all-too-real professional dilemma I proposed addresses job security and the impact that managed care can have on care-givers' hierarchy of needs.

As reimbursement practices change, so does the need for PTs to identify the shifting values that moti-vate these changes, so that self-actual-ization can occur.

Because the paradigms of managed care influence physical therapy service, we will be challenged to define, defend, and clarify our personal and professional ethics and hierarchical needs sooner, pos-sibly through the use of negotiation skills to prevent moral and legal dilemmas.

Ron Hruska, PT
Saint Elisabeth Community Health Center
Lincoln, Neb

A Bit Rash?

The dilemma Kim is facing appears to be both practical and professional. We are not told specifically about Southside Physical Therapy and their practice pat-terns, but from what is said, it appears that they remain legal and ethical, though not optimal in Kim's view. It is likely that Kim would not have this dilemma if her current group had agreed to contract at lower rates, since this would have likely necessitated practice patterns similar to those of the competition, Southside Physical Therapy.

From a practical standpoint, Kim must now decide if she is willing to move to Southside Physical Therapy, where she knows the practice patterns are at a stan-dard that she feels is less optimal, or remain at Northside Physical Therapy, where she is more comfortable with the practice patterns but unsure of the long-term viability of her job. Is Kim certain that the move to Southside Physical Therapy will truly offer greater long-term job security, or might Southside Physical Therapy's willingness to compromise qual-ity suggest that her professional position may be replaced by less expensive "care extenders" in the future, as MCO pressure increases?

Kim's lowering of her standards for greater job security might not be as much of a sure thing as she thinks. If Kim truly is more comfortable practicing at Northside Physical Therapy, her first step should be to sit down with the own-ers/managers to dis-cuss her concerns. It may be that her per-ceptions of the future are different from those of the managers, and management may have information that will alleviate her fears. The acuity of her sit-uation might also depend on her position with Northside Physical Therapy, based on seniority, experience, or whatever other criteria Northside Physical Therapy man-agement will use to decide which PTs will be relieved of their jobs—if and when that situation occurs. After talking with man-agement, Kim may find that Northside Physical Therapy's position has stabilized within the managed care environment, and, if Northside management believes efficiency has been improved to a level that they find satisfactory, a move by Kim to Southside could be unnecessary.

I believe Kim must be willing to exam-ine her professional standards and ideals and decide if her resistance to some changes at Northside Physical Therapy is founded on habit rather than on the best ways to practice. She must also examine completely whether her fears are reality based, and the only way to do that will be to completely examine the situation and gather all information before making a decision. From reading the scenario, it sounds like she is being a bit rash and may be about to put herself in a more uncom-fortable position based on what may or may not be unfounded fears.

Gordon Eiland, PT, SCS, ATC
Tyler, Tex

"Resistance is Futile"

In the latest installment of the *Star Trek* movie series, the crew of the Starship Enterprise is engaged in a battle with the Borg, a collective of cybernetic beings of one mind, bent on the domination of all other cultures in the universe. The Borg always warn others to lower their defenses, submit to the process of becoming one of them, to simply com-ply and begin to work as they are ordered for the good of the collective. The Borg call this "assimila-tion," and their battle cry, "Resistance is futile," is essentially true.

The nature of Kim's dilemma is not legal, but ethically and professionally she might face conflicts if her personal stan-dards are breached. These standards are often a function of our education. If, for example, you are confident that adequate care can be provided by support personnel, you will have no problem turning it over to them. But, if through additional train-ing and experience, you find that your per-sonal skills far exceed those of others, and that these skills are necessary for your patients to progress, you cannot easily relinquish direct care without at least some pangs of guilt.

The Borg often succeed by sheer force

> "If Kim truly is more comfortable practicing at Northside Physical Therapy, her first step should be to sit down with the owners/managers to discuss her concerns."

(continued on next page)

(continued from previous page)

of numbers. Similarly, some practices succeed by providing large numbers of low-paid staff to manage patients. If the physical therapist is satisfied that this will replace the care he or she might personally provide, there's no ethical dilemma. The Borg Queen doesn't seem to worry about it.

Then again, she's not actually trying to make anyone better.

I can't see how deciding to take less money earlier would help in any way. Timing makes no real difference to the outcome of assimilation. And in today's health care environment, there are no options. That being the case, our personal standards,

our profession's standards are not relevant. The Borg—er, I mean the MCOs—don't care. They don't want to destroy us, and they don't want our jobs. They simply insist that we become one of them.

And, truly, resistance is futile.

Barrett L Dorko, PT
Cuyahoga Falls, Ohio

Commentary

The author of the case and the respondents to Kim's dilemma raised some common themes. In reading these responses, I was reminded that there is a systematic method[1] of assessing situations that can help us to know both the type of ethical problem we are facing (if any) and how we can move toward its resolution in the less-than-ideal circumstances of everyday life. In the process of adding commentary, I will review the five steps of this method.

1. *Gather the relevant facts.* What does Kim know about this situation? In high-stress situations, "fight-or-flight" solutions are common, and Kim is considering abandoning ship to begin employment with a different physical therapy practice. Having more information would be beneficial—even wise—before Kim decides to leave Northside. For example, the commentators point out correctly that Kim should want to know more about the specific differences in practice patterns between the two sites, Southside's position regarding the use of care extenders to keep costs down, and the criteria that will be used by Northside to downsize if and when it does. Dorko makes an assumption that the process of assimilation already is upon the health care world. Does Kim know if the inevitability Dorko proposes about managed care is going to express itself in her life? These data are important because accurate, relevant information is one tool to use in conscientiously assessing a situation.

2. *Determine the type of ethical problem present.* Once all the relevant data are in, Kim will be better able to determine the type of ethical problem

she has. Kim's case is presented as a dilemma. In more technical terms of ethics, a dilemma is one important type of technical problem. A dilemma has two ethically correct courses of action, but to act on one of them necessarily causes the person to break faith with the other one. Conversely, in a situation of ethical distress, a person such as Kim may know what is right but be frustrated by the belief that she will not be able to reach her goal.

Eiland points out the two horns of her possible dilemma: It is right to maintain high standards of practice, but it is also right to seek job security. Dorko suggests that institutional arrangements occasioned by managed care organizations may create a situation of ethical distress for Kim, but no dilemma necessarily exists. What do you think? Given the information we have about this case, I judge this to be more of an ethical distress situation. She does not know her job is threatened. If she receives this information, however, then she will have a true dilemma.

3. *Decide which ethical theory to use.* In a full ethical analysis of this case, we would give thought to whether Kim's ethically justifiable course of action could be realized by looking at the duties and rights of Kim and other relevant players in this drama (the deontological approach). We could also decide whether the right answer to this ethical problem could be ascertained by weighing the consequences of the various courses of action Kim might take (the utilitarian theory method). We'd also want to think about the kind of person Kim should be in this role, and which character traits would support it (the

virtue theory approach). Dorko seems to argue using the utilitarian approach of weighing the consequences to resolve the problem (ie, less money won't help, so she might as well stay put), while Eiland appeals to the deontological approach, arguing that Kim's decision should be governed by a desire to fulfill the profession's duty to give the best care. These two commentators highlight that both consideration of duties and rights and a weighing of consequences may help Kim know how to proceed.

4. *Look for alternatives.* Even when Kim has thought through what she ought to do, ethically speaking, our commentators correctly emphasize that in the less-than-perfect world of everyday practice, the actual solution must be sought within the range of realistic options open to Kim. Each commentator was thoughtful in trying to help Kim sort through her options.

5. *Take action.* Finally, the end point of the ethical reflection is action. The commentary in these pages provided several decisive checkpoints on the way to Kim's next career move. Whatever Kim does, the breadth and depth of the ideas presented here gives her the opportunity to make an ethically right decision.

Ruth Purtilo, PhD, PT, FAPTA, is Director, Center for Health Care Policy and Ethics, and CC and Mabel L Criss Professor, Creighton University, Omaha, Neb, and Past President, American Society of Law, Medicine, and Ethics.

Reference

1 Purtilo R. *Ethical Dimensions in the Health Professions.* 2nd ed. Philadelphia, Pa: WB Saunders Co; 1993:49-58.

Selected Readings

Banja JD. Rehabilitation and empowerment. *Arch Phys Med.* 1988;71:614-615.

Barnitt R. Ethical dilemmas in occupational therapy and physical therapy: a survey of practitioners in the UK National Health Service. *J Med Ethics.* 1998;24:193-199.

Homenko DF. Overview of ethical issues perceived by allied health professionals in the workplace. *J Allied Health.* 1997;26:97-103.

Ethical Considerations in the Business Aspects of Health Care. Woodstock Seminar in Business Ethics, Georgetown University. 1995. Available at: http://www.georgetown.edu/centers/woodstock/business_ethics/health.htm. Accessed on September 20, 2005.

Purtilo R. *Ethical Dimensions in the Health Professions.* 2nd ed. Philadelphia, Pa: WB Saunders; 1993.

Purtilo R. Interdisciplinary health care teams and health care reform. *J Law Med Ethics.* 1994;22(2):121-126.

Purtilo R. Managed care and the rehabilitation professions. *Trends Health Care Law Ethics.* 1994;10:1105-1110.

Purtilo R. Teams: health care. *Encyclopedia of Bioethics*, Vol 3. 2nd ed. 1995:2469-2472.

Scott R. *Professional Ethics: A Guide for Rehabilitation Professionals.* St Louis, Mo: Mosby; 1998.

Swisher LL, Krueger-Brophy C. *Legal and Ethical Issues in Physical Therapy.* Boston, Mass: Butterworth-Heinemann; 1998.

Thomasma DC. The ethics of managed care: challenges to the principles of relationship-centered care. *J Allied Health.* 1996;25:233-246.

Veatch RM, Flack H. *Case Studies in Allied Health Ethics.* Upper Saddle River, NJ: Prentice Hall; 1996.